Amplification for
the Hearing-Impaired

6. Amplification for Young Hearing-Impaired Children   213

Richard C. Seewald and Mark Ross

Contents

Those of us who learned from him, were intellectually stimulated by him, and saw many advances in Audiology arise as a result of his research and teaching are indebted to Dr. Raymond Carhart. To his memory this book is dedicated.

Michael C. Pollack

Library of Congress Cataloging-in-Publication Data

Amplification for the hearing-impaired.

    Includes bibliographies and index.
    1. Hearing aids.   2. Audiology.   I. Pollack,
Michael C. [DNLM: 1. Hearing Aids—instrumentation.
WV 274 A526]
RF300.A46   1988   617.8'9   87-21227
ISBN 0-8089-1886-9

Grune & Stratton, Inc.
Orlando, Florida 32887

Distributed in the United Kingdom by
Grune & Stratton, Ltd.
24/28 Oval Road
London NW 1 70X

Library of Congress Catalog Number
International Standard Book Number 0-8089-1886-9
Printed in the United States of America
87 88 89 90   10 9 8 7 6 5 4 3 2 1

Amplification
for the
Hearing-Impaired
Third Edition

Edited by Michael C. Pollack, Ph.D.

with an Introduction by Raymond Carhart, Ph.D.

Grune & Stratton, Inc.
Harcourt Brace Jovanovich, Publishers
Orlando   New York   San Diego   London
San Francisco   Tokyo   Sydney   Toronto

Contents

Contributors

Kenneth W. Berger, Ph.D.
Professor Emeritus
School of Speech Pathology and Audiology
Kent State University
Kent, Ohio

Daniel L. Bode, Ph.D.
Psychologist
Psychiatric Services, Ltd.
Belleville, Illinois

Robert G. Glaser, Ph.D.
President
Audiology Associates of Dayton, Inc.
Dayton, Ohio

Earl R. Harford, Ph.D.
Hearing Care Specialists, Ltd.
St. Louis Park, Minnesota

Eugene R. McHugh, Ed.D.
McHugh Center for Hearing
Colorado Springs, Colorado

Joseph P. Millin, Ph.D.
Professor of Audiology
School of Speech Pathology and Audiology
Kent State University
Kent, Ohio

Randy Morgan
President
Westone Laboratories, Inc.
Colorado Springs, Colorado

Michael C. Pollack, Ph.D.
President
Professional Hearing Services, Inc.
Akron, Ohio

Mark Ross, Ph.D.
Professor
Department of Communication Sciences
University of Connecticut
Storrs, Connecticut

Derek A. Sanders, Ph.D.
Professor of Audiology
Department of Communication Disorders and
Sciences
State University of New York at Buffalo
Amherst, New York

Richard C. Seewald, Ph.D.
Assistant Professor
Department of Communicative Disorders
Elborn College, University of Western Ontario
London, Ontario, Canada

Kenneth E. Smith, Ph.D.
President
Hearing Associates, Inc.
Shawnee Mission, Kansas

Preface

In the twelve years since the publication of the first edition of this text, a number of major changes have taken place in our profession. Many, if not most, clinical audiologists are now involved in the direct dispensing of hearing aids; so many, in fact, that the Academy of Dispensing Audiologists was formed to meet and represent their needs and interests.

New experimental and clinical methods are now available to provide us with better indications of real-ear responses of hearing aids. KEMAR data have greatly altered many traditional views of earmold acoustics and hearing aid responses. Improved earmold and hearing aid technologies have led to new developments in both areas, allowing us to do a better job for our patients.

Perhaps most importantly, easily usable probe microphone systems are now available that allow us to directly measure the acoustic signal reaching the tympanic membrane of the hearing aid user.

All of these changes led me to realize the need for an updated edition of this book. It is quite different from the first two editions, and also quite similar. New chapters on formula fitting techniques (Chapter 7) and the business of hearing aid dispensing (Chapter 11) have been added. New contributors such as Robert Glaser, Earl Harford, Eugene McHugh, Randy Morgan, and Richard Seewald bring fresh perspectives to subjects from the prior editions. Ken Berger, Dan Bode, Joe Millin, Mark Ross, Derek Sanders, and Ken Smith have updated and expanded their already outstanding contributions.

The orientation in this edition is toward the dispensing audiologist, the future of our profession.

Acknowledgments

Without the support of many of the contributors to this book, as well as my staff and friends, during a recent time of great emotional upheaval in my life, this text would never have been completed. As a result of their support, I believe that this edition is better than it would otherwise have been. Much of what I have learned during the past year has resulted in my having a greater empathy and openness, both of which make me a better person, clinician, and author. My heartfelt thanks go to all those who offered the much-needed support during that time.

Michael C. Pollack

Raymond Carhart

Introduction

Dr. Carhart completed the introduction to our first edition shortly before his death. As far as I know, it was his last completed work. It is reprinted here essentially intact as a memorial to him. The only changes I have made are deletions of references to material in the first two editions that are not included in this edition. The fact that so many of his comments, written in 1974, are still pertinent today is a tribute to his insights and suggests that our profession has not truly grown as much as we would like to think it has. There are still many unresolved issues, as Dr. Carhart pointed out.

MCP

Let us start with some obvious but necessary remarks. First, a hearing loss becomes a handicap only when it keeps listeners from perceiving sounds of importance to them. Second, modern techniques of amplification offer the best single means of combating most such handicaps. Third, since people move from one environment to another, the wearable hearing aid brings particularly versatile help. For this reason, a great deal of attention has been given this past third of a century to the development of good, wearable hearing aids and to refining the art of finding hearing aids that are well suited to individual users. Now there is need for a clear summary of what we have learned. This book gives such a summary. It draws together the experiences of three decades in a way that makes those experiences useful to the student of hearing, to the clinical audiologist, and to the interested layman. In this sense the book is a guide to the selection and use of hearing aids.

While the book contains much positive information, there is still a great deal to

AMPLIFICATION FOR THE HEARING-IMPAIRED, THIRD EDITION   ISBN 0-8089-1886-9

learn about how best to use amplification, including wearable hearing aids, with auditorily impaired children and adults. This fact also permeates the focus of the chapters that follow. These chapters review current knowledge while recognizing need for further progress. The book starts with a history of hearing aid development. It next examines how hearing aids are constructed, how they work, how their performance is measured, and how they are coupled to the ear. There then follow discussions on practical and philosophical considerations in choosing a hearing aid, on selection procedures for adults, on selection procedures for preverbal children, and on special hearing aid applications. The book terminates by considering the problems of counseling and by orienting the user to the hearing aids, as well as the relationships between audiologists and other groups who also serve the hard-of-hearing population.

Described in another way, this book focuses heavily on clinical procedures and concerns. In this sense it is a "how to do it" volume. One of its advantages is that a number of authors have contributed chapters. This fact increases the scope of the experience on which the book is based. In general, these writers agree. However, they also express differences of opinion, as is necessary and expected in a field that is still evolving. The reader must recognize at the outset that some of the basic questions about hearing aids are still unresolved and therefore remain the subject of controversy. This fact means that the book is dealing with a maturing, expanding field that promises us a richer future than its present.

A good illustration of a question that is as yet unresolved centers around the issue of selective amplification. This issue emerged in its simplest form with the advent of the wearable vacuum tube hearing aid. A little known anecdote from the late 1930s highlights the controversy neatly. Walter Huth, a conscientious hearing aid engineer, decided to produce a wearable instrument with as high fidelity as he could achieve. With pride, he showed his hearing aid to C. C. Bunch, who was the most experienced audiometrist of that time. Bunch's reaction was negative. He said, "Your hearing aid is designed for normal listeners rather than hard of hearing persons." "See how their hearing deficits slope in different directions." "You should build a whole family of hearing aids each of which is the reverse of one of the characteristic slopes in hearing loss." Huth took Bunch's advice. Because of the encounter, Huth reversed his philosophy, and the companies with which he was associated marketed instruments designed to compensate for several distinctive hearing loss contours.

Bunch's ideas of compensating for each patient's audiometric contour soon lost popularity for two reasons. Large programs for rehabilitation of hearing-impaired service personnel were organized during World War II. The workers in these programs were unable to demonstrate that superior performance with hearing aids was linked uniquely to selective amplification. Concurrently, an experimental study at Harvard (Davis et al. 1946) showed that patients with different contours of loss tended to do better with a system having a frequency response slope that ranged between being flat and a 6 dB per octave rise. Highly comparable results were obtained at about the same time in Great Britain (Medical Research Council 1947).

Thus it would seem that the issue had been settled: that other aspects of hearing aid performance were the more critical ones once a standard frequency response that would be suitable for most patients was achieved.

Clinical audiologists today are consciously modifying frequency responses of hearing aids to meet special needs, and for many clinicians the ultimate goal is prescription fittings. Mentions of the role of selective amplification are found in Chapters 2 through 6. To generalize, we have moved from an era where selective amplification was unpopular to a philosophy where many audiologists remain alert to the patterns of hearing loss exhibited by their patients and keep in mind a variety of ways for modifying the frequency pattern of the amplification the patient is receiving. Thus, the art of selective frequency modification has become a commonly used tool of the clinical audiologist. However, the fact is that the procedures involved are still in the realm of a poorly understood "art." Clinical audiology has not yet formulated any systematic general theory as to the role and proper applications of selective amplification. We operate by rule of thumb rather than by scientifically confirmed principle. The task ahead is to develop a new level of sophistication. There already are a number of indications that research with insight will move us rapidly in this direction.

For example, consider a recent finding that awaits practical application. Clinicians have not currently become adept at utilizing the results that Thomas and Pfannebecker (1974) obtained; namely, that discrimination in quiet is clearly improved for many persons with sensorineural loss by substantially filtering out low frequencies. Since these investigators found large variations in performance from one subject to another and since these variations are not clearly related to audiometric configuration, no clinically applicable generalization is as yet possible. Moreover, there is a need to discover whether the advantages of high pass filtering also apply to noisy environments. These are questions that a future investigation must answer. Once these matters are clarified, it may be possible to specify much more wisely which hearing aid a patient should have.

Or again consider experimentation that is being carried out at Central Institute for the Deaf (Pasco 1974). Here a variety of systematically differentiated response characteristics is being tried with selected hearing-impaired subjects. The limited information available to date suggests that there may soon emerge principles stating much more definitively what modifications in aided frequency response will most enhance speech understanding, although we must recognize that these principles may not call for a different selective amplification for each patient.

There also are hints that proper control of other dimensions of performance will add importantly to more successful hearing aid use in ordinary life situations. As mentioned in Chapter 6, Villchur (1973) reported using a two-channel amplitude compressor to improve the intelligibility for speech sounds achieved by six subjects with sensorineural loss. He adjusted the compression in each channel to compensate for abnormalities in the loudness scale of each subject. Another possibility, which is radical by contemporary opinions, regarding the detrimental role of harmonic distortion is that a combination of frequency shaping and peak clipping may benefit some hearing-impaired persons. The rationale for this statement comes from the work of Thomas and Sparks (1971). They found that subjects with sensorineural loss experienced improved intelligibility for monosyllables in background noise if the incoming signals underwent high pass filtering and infinite amplitude clipping. The clinical applicability of this and other combinations of filtering and amplitude limiting await careful exploration, but the point brought forth by these examples is clear. There is a real probability that we are emerging into a new era of understanding as to which characteristics of hearing aids are clinically desirable. The performance features of future instruments and the method by which they are selected for a patient may be very different five or ten years hence than they are now. Consider as a final thought in this regard the fact that contemporary expertise in microcircuitry allows highly sophisticated signal filtering and manipulation to be achieved, so that frequency and amplitude responses could be adjusted independently at third-octave intervals or less. The technology for processing signals in much more sophisticated ways is here. The only unanswered requirement is that audiology must learn enough about the needs of individual patients to specify what it wishes this sophisticated technology to achieve in the way of hearing aid design. For example, studies on speech perception by the hearing-impaired, such as urged by Bode (Chapter 9), are essential to this achievement.

The foregoing comments must be interpreted properly. They emphasize that we can expect substantial progress in the future. Of course, such developments will not, in the meantime, lessen the capabilities we already have, and it is with these capabilities that the present book is concerned. Thus, in the context just expressed the present book becomes a needed and highly practical progress report. It deals with a contemporary situation that may be expected to last for considerable time and to change through evolution rather than through abrupt reorganization. Moreover, the contemporary situation is beset by issues and interactions that are not exclusively investigative or clinical. Practical forces and conflicts modify contemporary circumstances and therefore must also be considered.

One issue that stands out involves the conflicts among audiologists as to how hearing aids should be selected for patients. Let us look backward briefly. During World War II clinical audiology assumed the responsibility for guiding hard-of-hearing persons in selection of hearing aids. It added the responsibility to carry out these services in environments free from commercial pressure and business interest. Such services were first offered extensively in military programs for aural rehabilitation, but they soon spread to nonmilitary centers, too. A major decision, which had to be made at this point in time, was the choice of the techniques on which to base selection of the preferred hearing aid for a given patient. Two major philosophies emerged that are relevant today. Each had its proponents and these proponents tended to form camps, which too often expended their energies in argument with one another rather than in resolution of basic research issues. Many subviews emerged, as the reader will encounter in such chapters as 4, 5, and 10. The end result, as discussions throughout the book either state or hint, is that an uneasy truce exists. For example, in Chapter 5 various procedures for hearing aid selection are outlined, but then the reader is left to choose the clinical course to follow. The reader cannot help but emerge with the feeling that clinical audiology does not have a positive stand, but that any method for which an audiologist can present a thoughtful argument is probably as good as any dissimilar method for which another audiologist can present a comparably thoughtful argument. The implication is that the two methods are of equal merit. Such indecisiveness cannot be considered the mark of maturity in the profession. Clinical research of sufficient rigor and extent must be conducted to resolve the underlying issues. Clinical audiology must assume responsibility for dealing directly and positively, and as a total profession with the issue of the relative merits of alternative methods for hearing aid selection.

In this regard, we must remind ourselves that intensive research into problems of hearing aid efficiency cannot be carried on merely as an adjunct to the routine management of clinical cases. Systematic attack on a research question requires a scope and control of observation that goes beyond the practical constraints existing in most clinical situations. When a patient is being studied clinically, there are restrictions on the number and variety of amplification characteristics with which that patient can be tested. Moreover, the patient's needs must take precedence over the scientific curiosity of the clinician, so that the characteristics of hearing aids tested must be controlled primarily by contemporary knowledge as to how to meet that patient's needs. Full evaluation of the subtleties of interaction between the details of hearing impairment and the variabilities of hearing aid performance must be sacrificed to the exigencies of the patient's immediate requirements. Do not misunderstand. The competent clinical audiologist, as is apparent later in this book, has developed to a high degree the art of guiding patients in selection of effective hearing aids. However, practicing the contemporary art of hearing aid selection involves taking shortcuts and making intuitive decisions that preclude obtaining the full array of information needed to generate the science of hearing aid selection. Clinical audiology must develop new investigative methods capable of generating such a science and must employ these methods vigorously.

Despite the arguments and disagreements just mentioned, the art of hearing aid selection rests on several stalwart principles. There is a series of clinical goals to be reached provided these goals are obtainable within the constraints of contemporary technology and the patient's hearing disorder. Most clinicians recognize four achievements as the minimum to be sought, namely: (1) restore an adequate sensitivity for the levels of speech and environmental sounds the user finds too faint to hear unaided; (2) restore, retain, or make acquirable the clarity (intelligibility and recognizability) of speech and other special sounds occurring in ordinary, relatively quiet environments; (3) achieve the same potential insofar as possible when these same sounds occur in noisier environments; and (4) keep the higher intensity sounds that reach the hearing aid from being amplified to intolerable levels. There are children and adults whose auditory impairments are so severe that they preclude these individuals from fully reaching these goals; but the goals themselves stand as appropriate clinical aspirations and the recognition of their importance permeates many parts of this book.

These minimum goals can be achieved for many hard-of-hearing persons if they wear single hearing aids. But the goals do not represent full restoration of auditory efficiency. There are other dimensions of hearing that are desirable to recapture. The question is how to do so. Many clinicians feel that binaural hearing aids offer the answer. However, as one can deduce from the resume on binaural hearing aids in Chapter 8, the situation is not that simple. There is relatively little definitive information regarding the benefits of binaural aids. Here we have another instance where the art of guiding hard-of-hearing patients must currently proceed on the basis of clinical intuition and limited experimental evidence. Again, the task that lies ahead for clinical audiology is to isolate clearly each of the several dimensions of binaural efficiency that are disturbed by hearing losses and then to determine the effect that the wearing of two hearing aids has on each of these dimensions. In other words, there are principles underlying each dimension that must be defined more precisely, so that each facet of binaural function can be employed to the individual hearing aid user's best advantage.

Let us pursue this topic further, because the complexities of aided binaural hearing exemplify intricacies that exist in other realms as well. We will concern ourselves for the moment with ear-level hearing aids. In such a case, the role of the "head shadow" emerges as one preeminent determinant of efficiency. We know that a person wearing only one hearing aid will encounter many everyday situations in which that person's head is between the microphone of the hearing aid and the source of the sound. The head blocks the sound and reduces its intensity at the microphone. Sometimes the effect is great enough to make it harder to hear even in a quiet environment. However, the situation is made worse when there is also background sound and this sound is not similarly "shadowed" by the head because it comes from the side nearer the microphone. Since at such a moment the background sound is not also reduced in level, the ratio of wanted sound to background sound is momentarily made less favorable. Extra masking occurs because the single hearing aid is on the wrong side of the head. The situation may be reversed an instant later, but meanwhile, a temporary hardship has occurred. A second hearing aid eliminates such unpredictable disadvantages. Now, one of the two hearing aids will always be advantageously placed. This aid will be free from sound shadow and will temporarily give the superior reception. In the presence of competing sounds, the advantage thus gained in signal-to-competition ratio can be as much as 13 dB (Tillman et al. 1963; Carhart 1970).

Not everyone recognizes that it must still be demonstrated as to how and to what degree the other presumed advantages of binaural hearing are achievable with contemporary hearing aids. Unfortunate interactions between a patient's hearing loss, the nature of the acoustic environment, and the characteristics of hearing aids may erase for some patients the presumed benefits of binaural aids. Nabelek and Picket (1974), for example, found that normal hearers got a 3-dB binaural gain when listening through two hearing aids to test words said against a background babble. Five hard-of-hearing subjects averaged only half as much binaural gain because some did not receive any binaural help while others received the normal benefit. Moreover, we must remember that there are limits to the amount of binaural gain even normal hearers may expect. This gain depends on the masking level differences achieved at those frequencies that are most important to the speech sample of the moment (Carhart et al. 1967; Levitt and Rabiner 1967). The threshold for intelligibility of connected speech is improved for normal listeners in the presence of competition only about 7 dB by optimal binaural conditions. Precise discrimination of consonants benefits 2 or 3 dB less, even though the threshold for mere detection of a single sentence said repeatedly may be increased by about 13 dB (Kock 1950). These benefits are not large but their importance for normal unaided hearers is not to be discounted. Unfortunately, these benefits represent boundaries that only a fraction of the hard-of-hearing population can fully reach with binaural instruments.

Furthermore, there are a number of other questions that must be clarified about each person who seems, on the basis of conventional audiometry, to be a good candidate for two hearing aids. For example, "Can this person fuse the signals received at the two ears via hearing aids into a single wound image and, if so, can this fused image be retained over a satisfactory range of sound intensities?" The work of Wright and Carhart (1960) would indicate that such a fusion of images is sometimes a transient and ephemeral phenomenon for hard-of-hearing subjects listening via two aids.

Another question is, "Can a binaural hearing aid user experience true localization of sound sources as do normal hearers, and, if not, what impressions of directionality can be attained?" Data reported by Bergman and his associates (1965) illustrate the problem. They had hearing-impaired subjects balance two hearing aids so that a loudspeaker in front of the listener was perceived "somewhere along the midplane either directly in front of him, in his head, or directly behind him . . ." (p 36). A person who perceived the image "in his head" was obviously not localizing it fully. Neither was a person who experienced any external projection of the image that seemed very close to the head rather than at the proper distance from it. One must conclude that some of Bergman's subjects experienced crudely lateralized images as opposed to fully localized ones. My point here is not to criticize the Bergman study, but rather to stress that clinicians must not assume that binaural hearing aid users are achieving greater benefits than they actually are. In this regard, still other questions are "Can the binaural hearing aid user obtain as much escape from masking in multisource environments as do normal two-eared listeners?" "Can such a user achieve normal efficiency in fluctuating sound backgrounds, and, if not, what is the scope of the deficit?" "Can such a person resist the degradation of an acoustic environment produced by reverberation as effectively as can a normal hearer, and, if not, how serious is the added problem?" And so on.

We have pursued the topic of binaural hearing aids far enough to realize our limitations of understanding. Considering the fact that this book deals with contemporary practices and knowledge, however, it is somewhat unjust to point out these limitations. The way to eliminate the limitations is to glean new information through research. But this demand for research is in a sense unfair to practicing clinicians. They are bedeviled each day by the specter of imperativeness in a way that even the clinical researcher is not. The researcher can gather fact after fact at leisure until a sufficient edifice of evidence answers the question with surety. How different the clinician's task. The clinician is an investigator, too, but the question is, "What can I do *now* about the needs of the person who is seeking my help at this moment?" The clinician proceeds to gather as much data about the client as can be done in a clinically reasonable time. The luxury of waiting several months or years for other facts to appear is not an option. The decisions of the clinician are more daring than the decisions of the researcher because human needs that require attention today impel clinical decisions to be made more rapidly and on the basis of less evidence than do research decisions. Dedicated and conscientious clinicians should bear this fact in mind proudly. Theirs is the greater courage.

Remembering that the clinical responsibility of today must be met today, this book offers an inclusive guide to the highly diverse array of issues that converge on contemporary audiology. It offers the student excellent coverage of present day opinion, information, and practice. It is thus a very suitable medium for launching the advanced student into the mazes and vicissitudes of the current hearing aid field. But as the student proceeds into this maze, there are cautions to keep in mind.

For example, there is a subtle imbalance in this book. It is more oriented to the problems of adults than to those of children. Only Chapter 6 deals directly with children's needs. This imbalance of emphasis merely recapitulates past history. Adults have always comprised the major segment of the hearing aid market. Therefore, design objectives of engineers have primarily pointed toward the needs of adults. It has become an implicit assumption, accepted by almost everyone, that the potential psychoacoustic capabilities of a child with a hearing loss can be deduced from what is known about adults with comparable loss. This presumption needs confirmation. Do clinicians typically ask whether children who have congenital deafness of the Mondini variety, with consequent gross malformation of the inner ears, might also have important disturbances of psychoacoustic functions within their remaining range of audibility? Or again, is a wider frequency response needed to learn to understand speech than that required to continue to understand it once it has been learned? In other words, the point at issue insofar as children are concerned is that clinical audiology has not attacked many aspects of their needs incisively. There are, of course, notable exceptions, one of which is to be found in the excellent presentation on hearing aids for preverbal children in Chapter 6 of this book. But the plea at this point is that, while we have learned to use hearing aids on children with results that are often acceptable, we can do our best for children only if we change our basic focus and stop defining what we think hearing aids should do for them largely in terms of the needs and responses of hearing-impaired adults.

Another subject requiring careful thought is the relation of the actual hearing aid performance achieved in living situations to that of the physical measurements obtained in anechoic chambers and acoustic test boxes. This topic is discussed at the end of Chapter 2, but it warrants additional comment here.

To explain, it has long been traditional to determine the sound output of a hearing aid earphone in a standardized 2-cc coupler. Many clinicians react to the resultant record as though it were an accurate description of the relative responsiveness of the hearing aid when worn by a listener. However, for several reasons the response in the 2-cc coupler gives an imperfect estimate of the frequency response when the instrument is in actual use (see Chapter 2). First, the hearing aid output measured in a closed 2-cc coupler is not the same as the output in a closed human ear canal (Nichols et al. 1945; Martin 1971). Another factor that modifies frequency response appears when measurements are obtained while the aid is not worn on the head or body, as it would be in real life. In these latter circumstances, diffraction effects and so-called baffle effects (see Chapter 2) occur that change the sound intensity at the hearing aid microphone (Nicholas et al. 1947; Olsen and Carhart 1975). Such effects modify hearing aid output and the meaning of measurements, which are made when such effects are not included, such as occurs in a standard "test box."

Another variable that is often ignored in the clinical world is ear canal resonance, with the consequence that compensation for loss of this resonance is frequently not taken into account when defining the effective frequency response of a hearing aid. To explain, the normally open ear canal functions as a tube that increases the effective sound pressure at the eardrum relative to the pressure at the entrance to the ear canal. This enhancement extends over a substantial band of higher frequencies in the speech range and can reach about 20 dB in the neighborhood of 3000 Hz (Wiener and Ross 1946). *Since plugging the canal with a hearing aid earpiece disturbs this resonance, accurate plotting of the effective frequency response requires compensating for the resulting disruption of ear canal resonance.* Enough data relating to the variables involved have been gathered so that an estimate of total correction needed to compute the true sound pressure levels at the eardrum can be made from frequency response curves obtained via 2-cc coupler. Any clinician, however, who fails to make this correction, but still presumes that the equivalent of open ear reception is being reproduced on the basis of responses measured in a 2-cc coupler, is misguided (Knowles and Burkhard 1975). Moreover, the degree of this inaccuracy will depend on many variables that may be difficult to assess, a point that is touched in a somewhat different way in Chapter 4. The concept of canal resonance effects is discussed at length in Chapter 2.

Stated conversely, the clinical audiologist must continuously remember that *traditionally obtained frequency response curves do not accurately describe the performance of the hearing aid while in use.* Failure to keep this principle in mind may be one of the reasons that the risk of reaching solid generalizations about the relationship between frequency response and clinical effectiveness has been so slow.

A somewhat similar caution is necessary when considering the interpretation of other electroacoustic measurements. The following example will illustrate this point. During World War II excellent data on the technical performances of contemporary hearing aids became available from the Harvard Electroacoustic Laboratory (Nichols et al. 1945). These hearing aids were much larger than the instruments of today, but their electroacoustic excellence was sufficiently comparable for our example still to be pertinent. During 1945, a study was conducted at Harvard's Psychoacoustic Laboratory. This study used hearing aids on which data from the Electroacoustic Laboratory were available. The study demonstrated how much gain persons with normal hearing, when temporarily masked to simulate a prespecified degree of sensorineural hearing loss, could achieve with each of a number of the aforementioned hearing aids (Hudgins et al. 1945). It so happened that the rehabilitation program at Deshon General Hospital was concurrently using these same hearing aids with quite a number of its patients. The Deshon staff was able to assemble groups of patients who had been tested with exactly the same fittings as had been used in the Harvard study. The startling fact that emerged was that the clinical patients achieved notably less gain with these aids, hearing loss for hearing loss, than did the masked normal hearers. There clearly were detrimental interactions that made the benefits of using a hearing aid less when suffering a true hearing loss than when simulating a comparable sensorineural impairment through masking. The point is that if clinicians are not aware that such detrimental effects can occur, they will fail to use with fullest insight the laboratory data available to them.

A serious deficiency of contemporary clinical audiology is the inadequacy of its methods of speech audiometry. This topic per se is not given much attention in this book, although the role of speech audiometry as a help in hearing aid selection is mentioned often. The fact is that speech audiometry, as practiced clinically for hearing aid selection, is relatively archaic and unrevealing. It needs improvement in several ways if its results are to be of greatest help to hearing aid users. For one thing, we are still awaiting a definitive validational study of the relationship between formal scores obtained via speech audiometry and work-a-day hearing aid efficiency. Some attempts, beginning with those of Davis (1948), have been made to correlate performance in life situation with formal test results, but the relations between test scores and efficiencies in the work-a-day world still await adequate description. Furthermore, although there has been a substantial proliferation of speech tests since 1950, this proliferation has often tended to preserve existing weaknesses in test design rather than to eradicate them.

Consider one example of clinical inefficiency in measuring speech discrimination. The W-22 test, which is widely used, contains many test words that are easily discriminated by most patients (Carhart 1965). Time is therefore wasted on these items, and patients' scores tend to cluster at the high end of the scale. Elpern (1961) suggested that the waste in time could be reduced if the test were shortened to half its original length. In many clinics this procedure is now followed. However, Elpern's approach was to cut the total number of items in half rather than to discard the easiest 50 percent of them. The final effect is to reduce the precision (reliability) of the test without expanding significantly the range over which scores distribute themselves. When applied to evaluating a person's performance with hearing aids, the half-list procedure importantly lessens the credence that can be given to each score obtained and hence reduces the confidence with which a clinician can advise a potential hearing aid user.

Another criticism of speech audiometry is that as currently practiced in many places it does not adequately simulate everyday listening situations. This criticism is probably particularly telling when it comes to the evaluation of hearing aids. Tests administered in quiet or in a steady-state noise can fail to reveal detrimental interactions that can occur between hearing loss, hearing aid, and acoustic environment (see Chapter 9). There is now substantial evidence that such unfavorable interactions can occur (Tillman et al. 1970). Moreover, a review of considerable data from several laboratories suggests that the adverse interaction is most pronounced if the background is composed of human speech. It would thus seem that conscientious clinical practice would require selecting a hearing aid in part on the basis of performance in such a speech background. Certainly, the impressions we have gained from observations of aided performance in white noise, in speech spectrum noise, or in quiet are not fully applicable.

One of the relatively unpublicized paradoxes in the field of aural rehabilitation is that the transition from military audiology to civilian audiology brought about a sharp, but still somewhat incompletely recognized, change in the philosophy of patient management.

Early American hearing aid programs emerged as crash ventures. The armed forces established comprehensive rehabilitation centers for deafened service personnel. A point that is often forgotten is that each patient was in the rehabilitation program much longer than is practical today, except for those in a few military and Veterans Administration hospitals. Thus, the selection of a hearing aid in the early days could be made part of an intensive sequence in rehabilitation that could last two or more months. At Deshon General Hospital (Carhart 1946), for example, the rehabilitation procedures accomplished two goals that we usually fail to achieve today. First, patients became sophisticated in what to expect from hearing aids as a class, because they were required to wear a number of different instruments in daily life before their final instruments were issued. They learned what problems hearing aids could pose, with the outcome that they would no longer blame the final instruments as individually defective in these regards. Second, they discarded through everyday use those instruments obviously unsuited to their needs. Eventually three or four aids emerged as particularly good for each patient. The final hearing aid was then chosen from among these instruments. Formal tests were used at this point, but the important thing to remember is that these formal tests were merely the last stage in a long procedure of winnowing out undesirable aids and of habituating the patient to wearable amplification.

The captive thousands of patients for whom weeks and months of training in military hospitals could be ordered disappeared after World War II, even among the main core of veterans with service-connected hearing impairment. These veterans and patients from the civilian sector were seldom willing to accept the prolonged and intensive regimens developed in military rehabilitation centers. In many locations the typical patient now had to be processed in hours rather than weeks. Clinicians, facing this pressure for accelerated procedures, drifted toward the view that hearing aid selection was a relatively independent function. Even though audiologists continued to claim that the hearing aid must be integrated into a total rehabilitation program, this integration very often took place poorly. No one can do extensive rehabilitation on a patient who will not agree to participate as often or as long as the program requires. Therefore, shortcuts and compromises were necessary. A new goal emerged: namely, to access the patient's needs for amplification rapidly, and, if found to need amplification, to discover a good hearing aid also quickly. Associated with this new goal came the necessity to shorten and thus greatly weaken the rehabilitational procedures for adjusting patients to hearing aids.

The future will certainly modify the views and practices of clinical audiology in sociological and economic areas, as well as in the realms of technology and patient management. Moreover, it is well to remember that such changes may possibly come very fast because critical issues are currently under controversy. Chapter 12 is in part concerned with matters of this type. For one thing, the attitudes of clinical audiologists regarding themselves and the field they represent are of prime importance. One sometimes gets the sense that clinical audiologists are willing to settle for the classification of second class professionals. It may be reassuring in this time of conflict to consider the American Speech and Hearing Association as a haven and rallying point. It may be essential to preserve this rallying point in order to win legal privileges and to protect professional territory. But careful evaluation of the scientific and educational issues involved makes clear that the person who has achieved certification in audiology from ASHA has emerged as a professional whose recognized competency is defined by the Master's degree and a moderate amount of supervised clinical experience. There are historical reasons for this situation. However, the point is that as long as either ASHA or clinical audiology are satisfied to accept only this definition as describing competence in clinical audiology, the field cannot expect to be recognized as equal to professions that hold the doctorate as one of their inviolate requirements. This situation is particularly unfortunate when one recalls the caliber of the tasks and responsibilities inherent in top notch clinical audiology.

One effect of the tendency of audiologists to define their field largely in clinical terms is that by so doing they have functioned primarily as consumers of the research performed by others. There is a handicap in being a consumer of scientific information rather than a producer of it. The consumer does not greatly determine the direction of progress, but works with what is at hand, that is, with what others have made available. As some of our earlier comments implied, such a limitation seems to have existed in the technology of wearable hearing aids. The fact that audiologists have not seriously researched hearing aid needs has probably restricted the variety of hearing aid characteristics that have been commercially available. It has been the manufacturing industry whose major spurs to action have consisted of intra-industry competition and feedback from dealer experience that has supplied the variety of hearing aids available in the United States. Clinical opinions have had sporadic impact, but these opinions themselves have not always been consistent. Thus, although one can point to a few examples of effective interaction between manufacturing and clinical groups, as in the case of the early development of CROS and its companion systems (see Chapter 8), clinical audiologists have been forced to "make do" with whatever hearing aid stock was contemporarily available. Even now, as is subtly apparent at points in this book, clinicians do not have the feeling of being even partially in control of this aspect of the situation.

Just a word now about the boundary between hearing aid dealers and clinical audiologists. Many persons of integrity, compassion, experience, and competence are found in each group. These individuals have strong motivations to help hard-of-hearing people. Consequently, we should expect coordination and cooperation between the two groups. Unfortunately, positive interactions develop on a person-to-person basis rather than permeating group attitudes. At this writing, tensions between the commercial and the clinical camps are fairly high. The problem appears on the surface to be largely jurisdictional. However, there is an underlying philosophical cleavage that gives the two groups conflicting frames of reference.

What, then, is the philosophical disparity?

There are two premises from which clinical audiologists ordinarily start. First, they see their main task as coping with the full array of communicational problems brought about by impaired hearing. Without going into detail, this task requires the following steps: (1) assessing communicational capacity thoroughly; (2) determining what communicational, educational, and/or rehabilitational needs must be met; (3) planning programs to do so; (4) participating in the appropriate phases of these programs; and (5) arranging for whatever other forms of help are needed. The tasks of assessing the role of a hearing aid for an individual and of helping this person find a suitable instrument are only part of the work to be accomplished in the first two of the aforementioned five steps. The recognition that the clinical audiologist has five major responsibilities clearly leads to the premise that the total endeavor is of sufficient complexity and diversity, and therefore requires a large amount of formal training and clinical experience in order for it to be carried out competently. There is too much to be learned to presume that it can be mastered by informal study and undirected contact with hearing-impaired persons.

Individuals in the hearing aid business often have a different outlook. Their rehabilitative goal is more restricted, aimed primarily at finding effective wearable amplifiers for persons with hearing impairments, helping these persons in the initial adjustments to their instruments, and supplying the follow-up services that will keep the instruments functioning well. Although there are a few individuals in the business who have embarked on broader approaches, the fact remains that the hearing aid business has not seen its task as that of requiring extensive formal academic preparation. In general, its philosophy has been that field training with supplementation from correspondence work, company workshops, and other short courses can ensure competence. Where licensure of hearing aid dealers is involved, the ground rules may be laid down fairly precisely by state law, but the basic approach still seems to be that hearing aid dealers are business people who must have some special knowledge so that the public will be protected as they go about their business.

Finally, we must mention a less well known, but extremely important, recent development that will probably greatly affect everyone involved with hearing aids.

This development potentially can have a massive influence on both the availability of hearing aids and on their performance characteristics. For instance, it is possible that forthcoming legislation will place hearing aids under the jurisdiction of the Federal Food and Drug Administration. If so, a series of regulations governing the specifications and tolerances that manufacturers must meet will probably go into effect. It does not now appear that specific performance characteristics will be required, except for a few boundaries of electroacoustic response that will be designated. Thus, manufacturers can probably continue to select their own design objectives. Once they have done so, however, all the instruments of that particular model will probably have to fall within relatively narrow tolerances. In this sense they will have to manufacture to tight specifications.

It is hard to foresee the impact that will occur if the aforementioned regulations are promulgated. Past experience with the quality control that has existed in the hearing aid industry suggests that the new regulations may be very hard to meet on a mass production basis. Each new instrument may need to be given rather extensive tests and substantially greater care may need to be taken in matching components. Such factors will drive up the cost of hearing aids. Furthermore, manufacturers may choose to produce fewer types of instruments. They may be slow to incorporate innovative components as these appear. Manufacturers will probably also be constrained from developing highly unconventional hearing aids.

The development just described is only one example of the way in which the hearing aid business may be curtailed by increasing government regulation in the years ahead. Remember that the Federal Trade Commission has been concerned with practices in the hearing aid field for a number of years. Now, hearing aid manufacturers are on the verge of being supervised and held to externally imposed standards by a second regulatory agency. The point at issue is not whether the public should be protected. Of course, it should be protected. The point at issue is that regulation may make it very hard for businesses to continue producing improved hearing aids at acceptable prices. Such difficulties could eventually affect detrimentally the array and versatility of the hearing aids that are clinically available. The end result could be to reduce the help that can be given the hard-of-hearing public via wearable amplification.

Such a turn of events must challenge audiology to pick up the gauntlet that has been lying at its feet for years. During these years clinical audiology should have been developing more definitive methods for using amplification to the best advantage of hearing-impaired children and adults. The record to date is not a proud one. Now other forces are emerging that have the power of final decision as to what hearing aids shall or shall not be. These forces may not have either the clinical experience or the audiological orientation to exercise the best judgment in regards to the needs of the hearing-impaired population. Clinical audiology can remain a viable force in the hearing aid field only if it accepts the responsibility for initiating the research needed to clarify the many unanswered issues that are threaded through this book. The interests and endeavors of many investigators must be enlisted. Substantial funding, some of which has already been committed, must be available.

After clinical needs and requirements have been clarified through such research, the other persons involved will undoubtedly be easily persuaded to support these needs and requirements—whether such persons be manufacturers, the promulgators of regulations, or other individuals who are both interested and influential.

This introduction comes to a close by emphasizing again the paradoxes before us. Hearing aids are now of great benefit to a great many people. Proper clinical insight and management can enhance that benefit. This book is a knowledgeable guide to the current practices and procedures for doing so. But the book also bares the contemporary controversies and unresolved clinical uncertainties that will affect the future. It will be interesting to see whether this book becomes an epitaph to a profession's inability to marshall its intellectual capabilities or the prelude to a manifesto of that profession's capabilities to meet its challenges fully.

REFERENCES

Bergman M, Rusalem H, Malles I, et al: Auditory rehabilitation for hearing-impaired blind persons. ASHA Monographs 12:1–46, 1965

Carhart R: A practical approach to the selection of hearing aids. Transactions American Academy Opthalmology Otolaryngology Jan–Feb, 123–131, 1946

Carhart R: Problems in the measurement of speech discrimination. Arch Otolaryngol 82:253–260, 1965

Carhart R: Problems of the hearing impaired in noisy social gatherings. Oto-Rhino-Laryngology, Excerpta Medica International Congress Series No. 206, 564–568, 1970

Carhart R, Tillman TW, Johnson R: Release of masking for speech through interaural time delay. J Acoust Soc Am 42:124–138, 1967

Davis H: The articulation area and the social adequacy for hearing. Laryngoscope 58: 761–778, 1948

Davis H, Hudgins CV, Marquis RJ, et al: The selection of hearing aids. Laryngoscope 56:84–115, 135–163, 1946

Elpern BS: The relative stability of half-list and full-list discrimination tests. Laryngoscope 71:30–36, 1961

Hudgins CV, Peterson GE, Hawkins JE, et al: Performance tests of hearing aids. Section II of Evaluation of Hearing Aids, Office of Scientific Research and Development, Division 17, Section 17.3, OSRD Report 4666, 1945

Knowles HS, Burkhard MD: Hearing aids on KEMAR. Hearing Instruments 26:19–21, 41, 1975

Kock WE: Binaural localization and masking. J Acoust Soc Am 22:801–804, 1950

Levitt H, Rabiner LR: Predicting binaural gain in intelligibility and release from masking for speech. J Acoust Soc Am 42:820–829, 1967

Martin MC: Are frequency characteristics important? Scand Audiol 1 (suppl):93–98, 1971

Medical Research Council. Hearing Aids and Audiometers. Report of the Committee on Electroacoustics. London, Her Majesty's Stationery Office, Special Report Series, No. 261, 1947

Nabelek AK, Pickett JM: Reception of consonants in a classroom as affected by monaural and binaural listening, noise, reverberation, and hearing aids. J Acoust Soc Am 56:628–639, 1974

Nichols RH Jr, Marquis RJ, Wiklund WG, et al: Electro-acoustic characteristics of hearing aids. Section I of Evaluation of Hearing Aids, Office of Scientific Research and Development, Division 17, Section 17.3, OSRD Report 4666, 1945

Nichols RH Jr, Marquis RJ, Wiklund WG, et al: The influence of body-baffle effects on the performance of hearing aids. J Acoust Soc Am 19:943–951, 1947

Olsen WO, Carhart R: Head diffraction effects of ear-level hearing aids. International Audiology 3:244–258, 1975

Pascoe DP: Frequency responses of hearing aids and their relation to word discrimination by hard-of-hearing subjects. J Acoust Soc Am 56:S46A, 1974

Thomas IB, Pfannebecker GB: Effects of spectral weighting of speech in hearing-impaired subjects. J Audio Engineering Society 22:690–693, 1974

Thomas I, Sparks DW: Discrimination of filtered/clipped speech by hearing-impaired subjects. J Acoust Soc Am 49:1881–1887, 1971

Tillman TW, Carhart R, Olsen WO: Hearing efficiency in a competing speech situation. J Speech Hearing Res 13:789–811, 1970

Tillman TW, Kasten RN, Horner JS: Effect of head shadow on reception of speech. ASHA 5:778–779, 1963

Villchur E: Signal processing to improve speech intelligibility in perceptive deafness. J Acoust Soc Am 53:1646–1657, 1973

Wiener FM, Ross DA: The pressure distribution in the auditory canal in a progressive sound field. J Acoust Soc Am 18:401–408, 1946

Wright HN, Carhart R: The efficiency of binaural listening among the hearing-impaired. Arch Otolaryngol 72:789–797, 1960

Kenneth W. Berger

1

History and Development of Hearing Aids

In terms of the length of time there has been any interest in disorders of hearing, electric hearing aids are relatively new, having been available commercially only since the early 1900s. Prior to the introduction of electric amplification, the hearing-impaired individual had to rely on mechanical devices, some of which were quite bizarre by today's standards. In this chapter, Ken Berger traces the development of mechanical and electrical amplification devices, putting a good deal of emphasis on the evolution of the electric hearing aid. Of particular interest is the chronology of hearing aid "firsts" that is included.

The primary importance of this chapter, in my opinion, is that by becoming familiar with the past, one can develop a better appreciation for the present level of hearing aid technology and can more reliably judge the strengths and weaknesses of today's hearing aids.

MCP

The history of electric hearing aids is not yet a century old. Yet, historic data about and references to early electric hearing aids are scarce. Even more rare are historic facts about pre-electric hearing devices, their manufacture, and their acoustic characteristics.

A number of authors make the statement that the first hearing "aid" for humans was the hand cupped behind the ear. Although the statement is made only on the basis of guessing, without supporting evidence, it might well be true. Then

AMPLIFICATION FOR THE HEARING-IMPAIRED, THIRD EDITION
Copyright © 1988 by Grune & Stratton, Inc.

we might suppose that at some still prehistoric time someone with either normal hearing or with a hearing loss found that an animal horn or a broken seashell served to better focus sound into the external auditory canal. The earliest historic references to hearing aids suggest that the animal horn and seashell were the first hearing devices.

In attempting to determine the early history and development of hearing aids, one is faced with a number of hurdles. First, patient records do not date back to the early development of hearing aids, and some of the earliest patents on nonelectric hearing aids clearly suggest that these were refinements from older basic models. Second, the history of the education of the deaf might be expected to offer some insights into the development of hearing aids, but until the advent of electronic instruments there were few, if any, that greatly benefited the deaf. Therefore, education of the deaf was largely concerned with speechreading or manual communication, and teaching the deaf child to talk. Third, the few very early printed references to hearing instruments are generally within philosophical or medical discussions rather than in published articles or books about the instruments themselves. Thus, the history of pre-electric hearing aids is, at best, sketchy and incomplete. More recent developments in hearing aids are largely unheralded.

SOUND COLLECTORS

As suggested above, the first historic references to aids for hearing were sound collectors. Animal horns appeared to be the most common devices used. These were hollowed and the tip end placed toward the ear, so as to better collect sound and direct it into the external ear. A lesser number of references to the history of hearing aids mention seashells as serving the same purpose.

Curiously, the first published scientific communications on hearing instruments were concerned with *speaking trumpets* and *hearing trumpets* for use by persons with normal hearing. Only later did it become obvious to persons working with the hearing-impaired individual that the same principles could be applied as an aid to hearing impairments. Thus, large ear trumpets were used by ship captains to receive oral messages transmitted from shore or from another ship, and speaking trumpets were merely the same ear trumpets used in reverse. That is, the speaker used the small end to speak into, similar to the way a cheerleader at a football game uses a megaphone. These early speaking and listening trumpets were made of metal or glass. Ear trumpets for people with hearing impairments were commonly made of thin metal or tortoise shell, although a few economy models were mere cardboard cones or tubes. Rather soon in their development, ear trumpets were made collapsible and could be carried more easily; one may also note early efforts to disguise the trumpets.

It may be surmised that gradually a number of instrument makers developed the art of manufacturing speaking and listening trumpets. A few of these artisans, perhaps encouraged or assisted by physicians, surely specialized in such instruments for the deaf. Most of the early manufacturers of "deaf aids" seem to be individuals or firms that manufactured surgical instruments. The earliest firm known to have manufactured hearing aids on a commercial basis was established in London about 1800 by F. C. Rein and Son. Rein manufactured hundreds of different nonelectric hearing instruments, most of them in limited quantities (Berger 1984).

The well-known *acoustic throne* was made by Rein in 1819 for King Goa (John) of Portugal. This instrument is shown in a number of books on hearing aids, and is now on display at the Amplivox factory north of London. The throne consists of hollowed armrests, carved into lion's heads at the front. The armrest cavities lead to a resonant box located in the seat of the throne, and the sound is then heard via a hearing tube connected to the resonator. In addition to the more common type of ear trumpet, the Rein firm also manufactured acoustic urns, ear trumpets with large silver resonators, acoustic devices hidden in the hat or by the beard, and speaking tubes for churches.

Before the twentieth century a number of firms in Europe and the United States began to manufacture an assortment of hearing aids and to innovate them. Still, pre-electric hearing aids had extremely limited effects in helping those with hearing impairments. Small, quite flat metal or tortoise shell trumpets were popular and were usually referred to as ear cornets. Other writers use the terms trumpets and cornets as synonyms. Ear trumpets and cornets provided amplification in a narrow frequency range, which assisted the hard-of-hearing user to some extent.

Figure 1-1 shows the acoustic gain of several ear trumpets that were popular in the pre-electric hearing aid era. These curves are based on free-field unaided versus aided test comparisons (Sabine 1921). The responses shown are for a funnel-shaped trumpet that collapsed from two sections and a longer funnel trumpet that collapsed

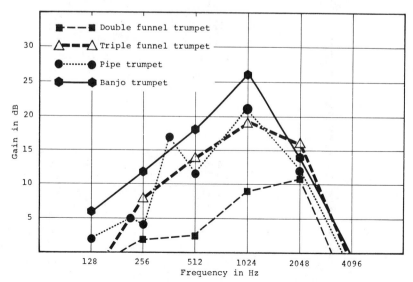

Fig. 1-1. Acoustic gain of ear trumpets.

from three sections. The banjo trumpet was a conical instrument with a rather small cross section that had a scoop or dish-like collector attached to it. The pipe trumpet resembled a large tobacco pipe. It consisted of a conical section that bent and expanded to a large collector area. The frequency responses shown in Figure 1-1 are considerably smoother than those actually produced by ear trumpets, since relatively few frequency points were used in the testing.

BONE CONDUCTORS

Bone conduction hearing devices are mentioned occasionally and appeared rather early in hearing aid development. Most of these were little more than strips of wood or rods of iron. One end of the strip or rod was often held between or touching the teeth of the speaker, and the other end was held in the same manner by the person with a conductive hearing loss.

Numerous individuals over a long period of time "discovered" the usefulness of these rods, sticks, and similar objects as bone conduction hearing devices. Figure 1-2 shows an interesting modification of the rod device that was made by Giovanni

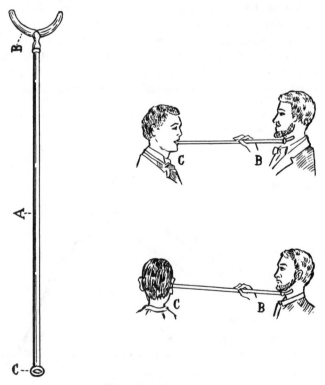

Fig. 1-2. The Fonifero.

Paladino (1842–1917) in 1876. He called this a *Fonifero*. At one end of the rod is a curved portion, almost a complete semicircle, that was rested against the throat of the speaker. The listener's end of the Fonifero was placed against the teeth, the forehead, or the mastoid area. This end of the rod was similar to a small cup. In cases of conductive hearing loss this and similar devices were quite effective but cumbersome. In Paladino's instrument the speaker and listener had to maintain a specific distance from each other. The original illustration of the Fonifero was not clear, which may explain why the drawing of the device in the otolaryngology handbook of Politzer (1878) shows the listener's end shaped like a hook rather than a cup. Several subsequent articles and books evidently used Politzer's illustration as a model and also incorrectly showed the listener's end of the device (Berger 1976c).

In 1879 Richard Rhodes, of Chicago, invented and patented a hearing fan, which he called Rhodes Audiphone. This device consisted of a thin piece of pliable material shaped like a fan. The upper edge of the fan was held against the user's upper teeth or clasped between the teeth. A system of cords permitted the user to increase or decrease the tension on the fan itself, thereby allowing for some adjustment in sound pickup. For approximately the following 5 years, many individuals obtained similar patents for hearing fans of various sizes, shapes, or materials. They also incorporated ideas for folding the fan when it was not in use. These hearing fans did collect sound, and they evidently served their purpose for those with a mild to moderate conductive hearing loss, provided that the user had a good set of teeth! (Berger 1984).

Since women frequently carried fans before the turn of the last century, hearing aids built into or resembling partially collapsed fans were in vogue. The bone conduction fan was discussed above. Another popular version of it had a small ear trumpet built into a half-open fan. Figure 1-3 shows a fan with an ear trumpet built into it. Still another model was made of metal and was merely held behind the ear to direct sound into the ear.

EAR INSERTS

A large number of types, styles, and sizes of ear inserts have been designed in an effort to aid hearing. Some of these ear inserts were much like the metal ear specula used by otologists. Others were more expanded at the external end, so as to collect sound a little better. Most of the ear inserts provided little or no amplification, and it is apparent that their sole value was for individuals who had a collapsed external auditory canal.

Adam Politzer (1835–1920), who gained world renown as head of the Vienna ear clinic, designed an interesting ear insert device. This is shown in Figure 1-4. Politzer's device was made of vulcanite and was shaped like a tiny alpine horn. The circular opening was directed to the rear. Several sizes were available, the largest being 2.5 cm long with a 12-mm-diameter mouth opening and a 5-mm-diameter insert end. In the late 1870s Politzer modified this device by removing the material

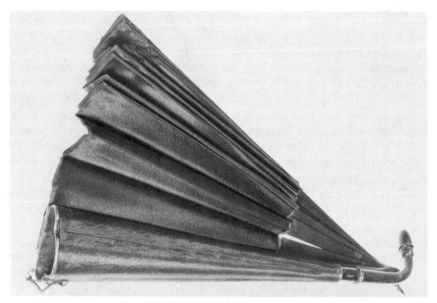

Fig. 1-3.   Hearing fan (courtesy of the Smithsonian Institution).

from the inner angle. This resulted in an L-shaped instrument with a trough. In his book on diseases of the ear, nose, and throat, written in 1891, the noted New York otolaryngologist St. John Roosa stated that he had not found any marked benefit from this Politzer device.

THE CARBON TRANSMITTER

The invention of the telephone in 1876 by Alexander Graham Bell spurred the interest of many toward the development of a device that would not merely collect sound but also amplify it. If speech could be transported across considerable distance, could not the same speech be amplified for the deaf individual?

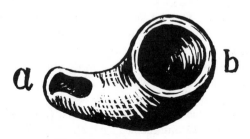

Fig. 1-4.   Politzer ear insert.

In many discussions about the history of hearing aids Alexander Graham Bell is credited with inventing the electric hearing aid for his mother (or his sweetheart, both of whom had a hearing loss) but he gave up the effort to use the ideas to invent the telephone. The facts cast doubt on all such statements, since the electric hearing aid did not appear until almost a quarter of a century after the telephone was invented (Berger 1976a).

Rather than working on an electric amplifier for the deaf, Bell was actually attempting to refine and modify the "singing flame" or manometric flame of König, hoping that this would give the deaf a visual indication of their own speech efforts. Bell, it may be recalled, was a speech teacher. A statement by Bell at the twenty-fifth anniversary celebration of the Horace Mann School for the Deaf, in Boston in 1894, clearly indicates his efforts during the early 1870s regarding an instrument to assist the deaf:

> My original skepticism concerning the possibility of speech reading had one good result; it led me to devise an apparatus that might help the children . . . a machine that should render visible to the eyes of the deaf the vibrations of the air that affect our ears as sound. . . . It was a failure, but the apparatus in the process of time became the telephone of today.

In his classic textbook on otolaryngology, published in 1945, Chevalier Jackson credits Dr. Ferdinand Alt with producing the first electric hearing device in 1900. Alt was an assistant at the Politzer Clinic in Vienna. The instrument is said to have consisted of a carbon microphone, a magnetic earphone, and a battery. Jackson was evidently quoting Max Goldstein, who in his book *Problems of the Deaf,* published in 1933, pictures this instrument. Alt noted that his instrument was of little use if the speaker was more than 2 feet away. It might also be argued that the illustration in Goldstein's book shows an instrument of more recent vintage than 1900, as witness the size, wiring, and connectors (Berger 1970). My own belief is that the 1900 date is an incorrect reading by Goldstein or a misprint for 1906.

Even accepting the year 1900 for Alt's instrument, I have recently uncovered good evidence that the first electric hearing aid was publicly shown in 1898, or at the latest in 1899, and may have been made in an experimental version as early as 1895. This was a table model instrument with a carbon microphone and up to three pairs of earphones. The apparatus was called an *Akoulallion* (coined from the Greek verbs "to hear" and "to speak") and was manufactured in limited quantities by the Akouphone Co., of Alabama. The inventive genius behind the instrument was Miller Reese Hutchison, perhaps better known to most people by his invention of the klaxon horn.

About 1900 the Akoullallion was modified in somewhat smaller dimensions as the Akouphone, and is pictured in the article by Berger (1970). Several articles in the literature on the education of the deaf at that time noted that neither instrument had sufficient power to help those with severe hearing loss. Thus, like the nonelectric hearing instruments, the first electric hearing aids, as made by Alt and by Hutchison, helped only those with a mild to moderate hearing loss.

The Miller Reese Hutchison patents for several hearing aid devices were manufactured and marketed by a series of firms that, with a number of reorganizations, ultimately became the Dictograph Products Company and used the Acousticon tradename. The third generation hearing aid made by Hutchison was called the *Acousticon.* A factor that contributed to popularizing Hutchison's inventions was the use of one of his instruments by Queen Alexandra of England at her coronation in 1902 (Berger 1984).

Within a decade, a number of hearing aid manufacturers began making carbon-type hearing aids: C. W. Harper, of Boston, made an "Oriphone" beginning late in 1902; Mears Radio-Hearing Device Corporation was inaugurated in 1904 by Willard Mears, who had previously been associated with Miller R. Hutchison; Globe Ear-Phone Company began a long and successful business in 1908; the Williams Articulator Company, of Chicago, was established in 1909; Deutsche Akustik Gesellschaft, of Germany, was established in 1910; Siemens & Halske, of Germany, began hearing aid manufacture on a limited basis in 1910; and the Gem Ear Phone Company, of New York City, was established in 1912. Still other manufacturers of hearing aids were established and were successful for a brief span of years.

Of the various hearing aid firms mentioned above, it may be noted that only Acousticon and Siemens are still making hearing aids. In tracing hearing aid history, one can readily note older firms disappearing and new ones forming as each major change in technology transpired: nonelectric to carbon, carbon to vacuum tube, and vacuum tube to transistor.

The carbon hearing aid consisted of a carbon granule or carbon shot microphone—more properly called a carbon transmitter—an earphone, and a battery. Beginning about 1930, a bone vibrator was used in place of the earphone with some models. Also, the earphone was later reduced dramatically in size and an eartip was used to direct the sound to the ear canal, at which point in time it became appropriate to use the term *hearing aid receiver.* Soon thereafter the eartip was replaced with stock vulcanite earmolds, and then with custom-made vulcanite ones, and finally with plastic earmolds (Berger 1976b).

Carbon hearing aids with single microphones and without boosters produced limited gain. A strong resonant peak is seen in the frequency responses. Figure 1-5 shows responses from a Globe carbon aid that was popular around 1916 (Sabine 1921). Like the frequency responses of ear trumpets shown earlier, those for a carbon aid are a comparison of free-field aided and unaided responses. For comparison purposes Figure 1-5 also includes gain data for the same subject, with the hand behind the ear. The carbon aid response is shown for the instrument with the volume control (a sliding resistance) set at both medium and full gain. Like the responses shown for ear trumpets, those for the carbon aid were sampled at a limited number of test frequencies, which obscured the many peaks and valleys of the actual response.

Carbon hearing aids were available in table models or as wearable instruments. The former often had multiple microphones and often included large collecting cones and resonant cavities. The size and shape of the microphones varied, and the

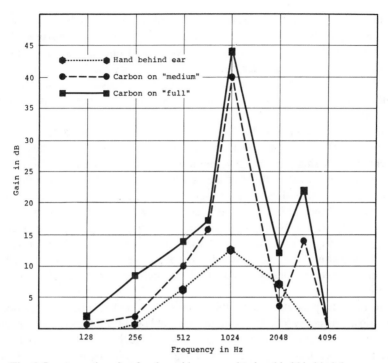

Fig. 1-5. Acoustic gain of carbon aid compared to hand held behind the ear.

instruments designed for persons with a greater hearing loss usually employed two or more microphones united electrically and often physically. A sliding resistance volume control was an early addition to the basic instrument, and later a booster (or amplifier) was available. Essentially, the booster was an enclosed double diaphragm that permitted some additional gain for the instrument, but usually at the expense of greater distortion.

Carbon microphones were somewhat temperamental, and efficiency was easily reduced in humid and dusty environments. The microphone, and particularly the booster, would often operate imperfectly if the wearer made any gross body movements. The instruments were relatively inexpensive, however, and with proper care they lasted a long time. Carbon hearing aids were popular from the first decade of the present century through the early 1940s.

VACUUM TUBE INSTRUMENTS

The major problem with carbon hearing aids was that the amount of acoustic gain possible with them was limited and the frequency response was narrow. What was needed was a device that could greatly raise the power of the speech signal. The vacuum tube amplifier accomplished this goal very well.

In much of the world the vacuum tube is called a *valve,* and in its simplest form it does act as a valve, much like a resistor operating in one direction only. With the invention of the triode vacuum tube in 1906, Lee DeForest added a grid to the cathode and plate of the older diode. The small wire mesh, or grid, permitted control of the electrons from the cathode to the plate. This control, so important in the design of amplifiers, permitted the development of the first electronic hearing aids.

The first vacuum tube hearing aid was developed by Earl C. Hanson and patented in 1921. The instrument, larger than a box camera, was battery-powered and employed a single triode. It is unfortunate that discussions of the history of hearing aids almost uniformly give credit to persons other than Hanson for the first vacuum tube hearing aid. Soon large vacuum tube hearing aids were marketed by L. Gaumont of France, Marconi of England, the Western Electric Company, and Radioear Corporation (Berger 1972). All of these instruments tended to be cumbersome, and were quite expensive. In addition, the triode was notorious for its lack of stability. Because of the size, cost, and difficulties with the amplifier, these earliest vacuum tube hearing aids were not much competition for the carbon instruments available at the time.

In 1931 the pentode vacuum tube, which consisted of a plate, a cathode, and three grids, was perfected. The pentode was stable in performance, had a relatively long life, and readily permitted amplifier stages to be coupled so as to obtain virtually as much increase in power as was desirable. Thus, the first practical and popular vacuum tube hearing aids began to appear in the mid-1930s. These earliest vacuum tube hearing aids, which were wearable, were later referred to as two-piece instruments since typically there was a microphone-amplifier portion and, separately, a battery pack. Most of the two-piece vacuum tube hearing aids were larger and heavier than the existing carbon hearing aids, but they permitted substantially more gain in the signal than did the carbon instruments.

It should be clearly recognized that the first hearing aids that were powerful enough to assist those with a severe to profound hearing loss did not appear on the market until around 1936. Since hearing aids powerful enough to assist the deaf (as opposed to the hard of hearing) did not appear until relatively recent years, it is understandable that oral programs for the deaf did not generally become oral-aural until the 1940s or later.

That the vacuum tube hearing aid did not quickly replace the carbon model can be seen from numerous statements in the professional literature. Weille and Billings, in their 1937 electroacoustic study of hearing aids, employed only carbon instruments "because the average patient wears only a carbon microphone aid." It was estimated that in 1937 approximately 95 percent of the hearing aids in use were carbon instruments (Hayden 1938). Writing in 1940, Hayden still questioned whether vacuum tube aids "will supplant the carbon type hearing aid or vice versa, or whether each will eventually occupy its own definite field."

Soon after the introduction of two-piece vacuum tube hearing aids, hearing aid manufacturers were able to miniaturize their instruments so as to allow for one-piece wearable hearing aids. Miniature vacuum tube technology was pioneered in

England and wearable electronic hearing aids, manufactured by Amplivox, Multitone, and other British firms, first made their appearance there. Arthur M. Wengel of Madison, Wisconsin is credited with manufacturing the first wearable vacuum tube hearing aid in the United States. Early one-piece, or monopack, hearing aids were made in the United States by Beltone, Vacolite, Paravox, and Mears.

Crystal Microphone and Receiver

The purpose of a microphone is to transduce the acoustic signal into an electric signal as faithfully as possible. The carbon microphone was more correctly a transmitter in that it transduced the acoustic signal but could not generate a signal. The crystal microphone, so useful with the vacuum tube hearing aid, actually generates a voltage when pressure is applied to the crystal; this action is known as the piezoelectric effect.

The typical crystal microphone consists of two small slices of crystal cemented together. A small rod connects the diaphragm to the crystals. When changes in sound pressure move the diaphragm, this movement is transmitted to the crystals through the connecting rod and causes the crystals to generate an electric signal that fairly faithfully follows the original acoustic signal. This electric signal is led to the amplifier proper for amplification.

The crystal microphone responds to a larger frequency range than did the carbon microphone and is not as easily damaged by dust or dirt. Nor do position changes of the wearer affect its response. However, the crystal microphone, like the carbon microphone, performs poorly in extreme temperature and humidity conditions.

Once the amplifier in the hearing aid has performed its work, the electric signal needs to be transduced back to acoustic energy. This transduction is accomplished by the earphone or receiver. It has been common practice in the hearing aid industry to use the term receiver to refer to a small earphone (about 1.0 inch or smaller in diameter) to which an earmold is attached.

A receiver is essentially a microphone in reverse. In the case of the crystal receiver, the amplified electronic signal is fed to the crystal. When electric impulses are passed through the crystal, it will vibrate mechanically, setting up airborne sounds that are sent on to the ear.

Magnetic microphones and receivers were also used with vacuum tube hearing aids, particularly later in the vacuum tube hearing aid era. The magnetic microphone is not as fragile as the crystal one. In addition, bone conduction vibrators for hearing aids have been of the magnetic variety in the carbon, vacuum tube, and transistor eras.

Batteries

Carbon hearing aids used one or several batteries, in series. Vacuum tube hearing aids required an "A" battery to warm up the filament of the tube and a "B" battery (plate battery) to achieve amplification. As noted above, the first wearable vacuum tube hearing aids required a separate battery pack. The battery pack was either carried in the pocket or fastened to the underclothing. Persons wearing two-piece vacuum tube instruments can truthfully be said to have been wired for sound.

The cost of batteries for vacuum tube hearing aid users was rather high. To lengthen the life of a battery it was recommended that their use be rotated to allow time for recuperation. Storage of batteries required a cool dry place for best savings. It was possible to recharge the battery, but this did not seem to have been a common practice with vacuum tube hearing aid users.

TRANSISTOR INSTRUMENTS

Hearing aid technology has undergone dramatic changes in a relatively brief span of years. The carbon hearing aid was little more than 25 years old when the much-improved and acoustically more flexible vacuum tube hearing aids appeared on the market in wearable versions. The vacuum tube hearing aid was only about 25 years old when the transistor appeared on the scene.

The transistor was invented at the Bell Telephone Laboratories in December 1947 by J. Bardeen, W. H. Brattain, and W. B. Shockley. The inventors were later awarded the Nobel prize for their work. The first transistors were the point-contact type and were not useful in hearing aids. A refinement, the *geranium junction transistor,* soon appeared, and its first commercial use was in hearing aids. Beginning in 1952 a few hearing aid manufacturers began using junction transistors in place of the output vacuum tube in hearing aids, which required a minimum of circuit change. These were the so-called hybrid transistor hearing aids. Even this slight change, however, resulted in substantial battery savings to the hearing aid user.

Soon all-transistor hearing aids appeared on the market, and within a year or two the vacuum tube wearable hearing aid disappeared entirely. It will be recalled from previous discussion that the vacuum tube gradually replaced the carbon hearing aid, over a period of some years. In the case of the *transistor,* however, it completely replaced the vacuum tube in hearing aids within 2 or 3 years. In comparison with the vacuum tube, the transistor is smaller, more sturdy, requires virtually no warm-up period, and operates well on a single battery of small size. The smaller transistor size and lower battery voltage requirements permitted dramatic miniaturization in the size of the hearing aid.

The body style (or conventional, or pocket aid) could now be made substantially smaller than the older vacuum tube hearing aid. The transistor also permitted other styles of hearing aids to be introduced, such as the behind-the-ear and the hearing aid built within eyeglass temples. Patents for these styles antedate the transistor by many years, but reducing the size of the hearing aid could not be achieved so that the design could not be made practical until the transistor was perfected.

A number of claims for "firsts" in the hearing aid industry have been made by various manufacturers. Dating these firsts depends to some extent on fixing the date a certain instrument or feature was patented, when it was introduced to the manufacturer's dealers, when it was first advertised, and when it was first placed on sale. Early all-transistor hearing aids were placed on the market by Microtone, Maico, Unex, and Radioear. These appeared in January and February of 1953. The first transistor hearing aids were somewhat more expensive than the latest vacuum tube models, and initial difficulties were encountered in the quality of the transistors themselves. In a short period, transistor quality control was achieved, and the dramatic savings in batteries in the transistor instruments quickly spelled the end of the vacuum tube era.

By late 1954 the first eyeglass hearing aids, with the amplifier and microphone enclosed in the temples, made their appearance. Akumed of Germany and Otarion of the United States were the first to market such instruments. Because hearing aid technology at that time did not permit ideal miniaturization, the eyeglass hearing aids contained a microphone and part of the amplifier in one temple. Wiring ran forward and around the lens frame to the other side, and the remainder of the amplifier, leading to a receiver, was in the opposite temple. Barrettes that were marketed during the vacuum tube and transistor eras had much the same arrangement, with the wire leading across the headband.

Within several years, it was possible to house the microphone, amplifier, and internal receiver in a single temple, which permitted binaural ear-level hearing aid fitting. Although the early eyeglass hearing aid wiring arrangements had no special name, it should be noted that, in the 1960s, for special fittings this arrangement was essentially reverted to under the name CROS (contralateral routing of signal). For further discussion of CROS and other across-head routing arrangements, see Chapter 8.

Another hearing aid style permitted by the transistor and smaller battery requirements was the *behind-the-ear model*. This has also been called the *postauricle* and *over-the-ear* style. The behind-the-ear style readily permitted binaural fitting, and the acoustic power of these instruments is now sufficient to reach almost all hearing losses.

A fourth, and currently the most popular hearing aid style is the in-the-ear hearing aid. These instruments began appearing in the latter part of the 1950s in rather large dimensions, and might be better described as at-the-ear rather than in-the-ear. In-the-ear hearing aids are presently available built either within a custom earmold or merely as a small device with a canal portion. Further miniaturization has permitted the in-the-ear hearing aid to be placed in the ear canal, virtually out of sight. This most recent type is called a *canal aid*.

In-ear hearing aids have been made practical by the latest development in amplifiers, *the integrated circuit*. The integrated circuit is a refinement and development of the silicon planar transistor. The integrated circuit consists of transistors, resistors, and "wiring," all on a tiny wafer of silicon or similar material. The integrated circuit has permitted further miniaturization of hearing aids, and is inherently low in power needs as well as being relatively robust. The first hearing aid with an integrated circuit, however, was not an in-ear model but rather appeared in a behind-the-ear style made by Zenith and introduced in 1964. It may be expected that further miniaturization and improvement in the hearing aid amplifier will follow, since the brief history of electronic hearing aids has largely been directed toward miniaturization.

Presently the most space-occupying part of the hearing aid is not the amplifier but the power supply, microphone, and receiver. A number of experimental designs have been tried in reference to transducers and power supplies, but none has appeared to be practical as of this writing. Research in this direction and in the area of implanted hearing aids continues.

Microphones

The crystal microphone was popular with vacuum tube hearing aids. With the advent of the transistor instruments, a microphone of lower impedance was needed. The magnetic microphone, which made its appearance with some vacuum tube instruments, became the one of choice with transistor hearing aids. The magnetic microphone has a rather ideal frequency response over the range of frequencies most important for speech. Very high and very low frequencies, however, need to be sacrificed, particularly when the magnetic microphone is made in extremely small dimensions.

With research and development, a version of the crystal microphone, the ceramic microphone, was perfected. The high-impedance problem of the ceramic microphone was solved by employing the field-effect transistor (FET). The ceramic microphone offered some of the advantages of the older crystal microphone, but unlike the crystal microphone, it is virtually free of humidity and temperature problems. The ceramic microphone permitted extended low-frequency amplification of hearing aids.

Condenser microphones have long been the standard of excellence in the broadcast and recording industry. Unfortunately, condenser microphones have a large voltage need and do not permit miniaturization. The perfection of the FET for ceramic microphones and the discovery of electret-like characteristics of some thin-film plastic materials permitted the development of the electret condenser microphone. An electret is a permanently electrically polarized material, but I shall follow the convention of referring to the electret microphone rather than the longer and more technically correct name *electret condenser microphone*.

The electret microphone has an extremely broad and quite flat frequency response. Like the ceramic microphone, it is rugged and sensitive. The electret microphone is virtually free of problems associated with mechanical feedback or with clothing rub. The electret microphone has replaced the magnetic and the ceramic microphone in most hearing aids.

The latest development in microphones for hearing aids is the directional microphone. In 1969 Willco, at that time a German affiliate of Maico Electronics, Inc., introduced the first hearing aid with a directional microphone. This microphone has both front and rear openings. Sound impinging from the rear is attenuated a significant number of decibels, sufficient for the wearer to focus on sound coming from the front. Directional electret microphones are employed by a number of hearing aid manufacturers around the world.

Earmolds

Few pre-electric hearing aids employed earmolds. Likewise, the first carbon instruments used earphones and did not involve earmolds. Gradually earphones were reduced in size to diameters of about 1 inch or less and were called *receivers.* From the receiver, sound was directed into the external auditory canal by an eartip. Eartips often were available in assorted sizes (Berger 1976b).

In the 1920s stock earmolds of several sizes appeared on the market and replaced the eartips. These were made of hard rubber. A few years later hard rubber custom-made earmolds were introduced. With custom-made earmolds the amplified sound from the hearing aid was efficiently directed into the external auditory canal.

Power Supply

Technically, a battery consists of two or more cells. The words *battery* and *cell,* however, are used interchangeably in reference to hearing aids. With carbon and vacuum tube hearing aids, the zinc oxide battery was employed. These needed to be fairly large in order to be practical. The zinc cell had a sloping discharge characteristic; that is, with use it gradually produces a smaller and smaller voltage. Users had to turn up the volume control of the hearing aid as voltage was reduced. Earlier it was mentioned that for ideal use these batteries needed time for rest and recuperation, and hot weather reduced their life.

During World War II, the mercury cell was developed by Dr. Samuel Ruben. At the close of that war, mercury cells found a ready market with hearing aid manufacturers and users. Mercury cells as compared to zinc cells are smaller and more robust. More important, for hearing aid use the discharge characteristic is such that the voltage drops significantly only at the very end of the cell's useful life. Furthermore, the mercury cell operates under wider temperature ranges and needs no time for rest and recuperation (that is, *depolarization*). The voltage of mercury cells is also rather ideal for transistor needs. With the introduction of transistor hearing aids, the mercury cell was the one most commonly used. The popular no. 401 mercury cell was introduced in 1952.

With the advent of silicon transistors, a battery with more restricted operating voltages was required. To solve this problem, the silver oxide cell was developed. Soon thereafter *silicon planar transistors* were developed, which operate on either mercury or silver cells. In late 1977, just before increased silver prices made the cost of silver cells unacceptably high, the *air cell* was introduced. Air cells have a long shelf life and about double the active life of mercury cells.

In addition rechargeable cells are available. The rechargeable cell, sometimes referred to as an *accumulator,* is considerably more expensive than other types. However, they may be recharged many times, so that over a long use period the cost per hour of hearing aid wear is somewhat lower than for the mercury or silver cell. Rechargeable cells are more popular in Europe and Asia than in North America. The infamous advertising phrase "no batteries to buy" usually refers to a rechargeable cell. However, the phrase is untruthful because ultimately the cell must be replaced.

Just as continuing research in transducers and amplifiers for hearing aids goes on, so do experiments with different types of batteries. At present, lithium cells seem to offer promise for future use in hearing aids. It is probable that in the future batteries for hearing aids will be made in various shapes so as to fit in the hearing aid case wherever there might be room.

COMMENTS

In this brief review of the history of hearing aids, it can be noted that the overriding goal of the manufacturer appears to be more power and a smaller hearing aid. In the 50-year history of the electronic hearing aid, great progress has been made in both of those directions. At the same time, it is disheartening to note that the acoustic fidelity of the product and flexibility in manipulating the output and frequency response have not received as much attention or publicity.

The hearing aid manufacturer seems to have heeded the desires of the hearing aid wearer for a more readily concealed aid and the request of his local dealers for more power in a smaller package. The audiologist has undoubtedly been remiss in not making known his desires for a more flexible hearing aid amplifier and one with greater fidelity. Much of the remainder of this book discusses problems of hearing aid fitting and attempts to overcome those problems so that the ultimate goal—prescription hearing aid fitting—may be perfected. Until hearing aids can be accurately applied to specific hearing loss needs, hearing aid fitting is likely to remain more of a slipshod art than a science.

REFERENCES

Berger KW: The first electric hearing aids. Hear Dealer 21:23–38, 1970
Berger KW: Western Electric hearing aids. Hear Dealer 23:18–20, 1972
Berger KW: From telephone to electric hearing aid. Volta Rev 78:83–89, 1976a
Berger KW: The earliest known custom earmolds. Hearing Aid J 29:5, 10, 35, 1976b
Berger KW: Early bone conduction hearing aid devices. Arch Otolaryngol 102:315–318, 1976c

Berger KW: The Hearing Aid: Its Operation and Development, ed 3. Livonia, Michigan, National Hearing Aid Society, 1984

Hayden AA: Hearing aids from otologists' audiograms. J Am Med Assoc 111:592–596, 1938

Politzer A: Lehrbuch der Ohrenheilkunde. Stuttgart, Verlag von Ferdinand Enke, 1878

Sabine PE: The efficiency of some artificial aids to hearing. Laryngoscope 31:819–830, 1921

Weille FL, Billings BH: A study of the efficiency of carbon microphone hearing aids. N Engl J Med 216:790–794, 1937

Appendix: Chronology of Hearing Aid Development

1551	Cardano described a bone conduction device consisting of a metal shaft or spear.
1640	Artificial eardrum made by Banzer of Germany.
1657	Hoefer, Germany, mentioned ear trumpets in use in Spain.
1670	Sir Samuel Moreland, England, invented a large speaking trumpet.
1673	Kircher wrote a book in which several hearing instruments are illustrated.
1677	Conyers of England worked on modifying Moreland's speaking trumpet.
1757	Jorrisen of Germany rediscovered the bone conduction rod as a hearing aid.
1790s	Townsend trumpet; a metal cone, developed in London.
1800	The firm F. C. Rein, trumpet makers in London, was established.
1805	F. C. Rein manufactured a speaking tube.
1808	Mälzel of Germany began making ear trumpets, including several for the composer Beethoven.
1812	Itard of France used a wooden rod as a bone conduction device.
1820	Duncker of Germany invented a speaking tube.
1826	Arrowsmith of England rediscovered the bone conduction rod for hearing.
1836	First known British patent for a hearing aid.
1853	Toynbee of England developed an artificial eardrum device.
1855	First patent for a hearing aid issued in the United States.
1869	Hawksley & Son of London is established; still in business.
1876	Telephone invented by Bell.
1879	The Audiphone, a bone conduction hearing fan, was invented by Rhodes of Chicago. Many similar devices were developed between 1880 and 1890.
1887	Ear trumpet with diaphragm earpiece patented by Maloney in the United States.
1890	Kirchner & Wilhelm of Stuttgart is established. Makers of hearing instruments; still in business.
1892	First patent for an electric hearing aid issued in the United States to A. E. Miltimore of Catskill, New York.
1898	(or 1899). First hearing aid made by M. R. Hutchison of Mobile, Alabama, which led to the Acousticon tradename.
1898	Marage compared hearing aid responses using the manometric flame.
1899	First Hutchison patent for a hearing aid.
1900	Electric hearing aid said to have been developed by F. Alt, Vienna.
1902	C. W. Harper of Boston began manufacturing electric hearing aids.

1906	Triode vacuum tube invented by DeForest.
1912	First volume control for an electric hearing aid.
1912	Zwaardemaker of The Netherlands measured hearing aid amplification, using calibrated instrumentation.
1920	First vacuum tube hearing aid patented by E. C. Hanson. Manufactured at the beginning of 1921 by Globe.
1923	Marconi of England and Western-Electric of the United States introduced vacuum tube hearing aids.
1923	First electric bone conduction vibrator. A. G. Pohlmann and F. W. Kranz.
1923	First in-ear electric hearing aid patent, Germany.
1924	Vacuum tube hearing aid manufactured by Radioear.
1926	First patent for a custom earmold.
1931	First electric hearing aid eyeglass patent.
1935	The Selex-A-Phone, introduced by Radioear, the first "master hearing aid."
1936	First AGC in a hearing aid; Multitone of London.
1936	First hearing aid with a telephone coil, United States.
1936	First wearable vacuum tube hearing aids appeared in England.
1937	First wearable vacuum tube hearing aid made in the United States.
1938	First audiometer built to hearing threshold, Maico.
1942–44	First one-piece vacuum tube hearing aids, by Paravox, Mears, and Beltone.
1945	The word audiology was "coined" by Canfield and by Carhart.
1946	The so-called Harvard Report was published.
1947	First electronic "master hearing aid"; introduced by Beltone.
1947	Transistor invented in December at Bell Telephone Laboratories.
1948	First hearing aid with a printed circuit; Solo-Pak.
1948	International Hearing Aid Association organized, which in 1952 became the Society of Hearing Aid Audiologists, and in 1965 the National Hearing Aid Society.
1952	First hearing aid that employed a transistor; vacuum tube and transistor hybrid circuit.
1953	First all-transistor hearing aid: Microtone, in January.
1954	First commercially manufactured electronic hearing aid eyeglasses manufactured, Otarion.
1955	First at-ear hearing aid, Dahlberg.
1958	First known report of an implanted hearing aid, France.
1959	First hearing aid dealer state licensing law passed, Oregon.
1960	ANSI (then ASA) standard for the measurement of electroacoustic characteristics of hearing aids was published.
1961	HAIC standard method for describing hearing aid performance was published.

1962   CROS described by Wullstein and Wigand; reported and actually named in 1965 by Harford and Barry.
1964   First hearing aid with an integrated circuit, Zenith.
1969   First directional microphone in a hearing aid, Willco.
1984   In-the-ear models outsell all other types combined.

Michael C. Pollack

2
Electroacoustic Characteristics

In order to work effectively with hearing aids, it is necessary to understand how they work and how their performance is measured. In this chapter, I present information in a practical manner about the electroacoustic characteristics of hearing aids. Throughout the chapter I have included comments indicative of my biases. Among the newer ideas presented are real-ear response measurements using probe microphones, the latest in compression systems and digital technology. It would be easy to become rigidly caught up in the aspects of hardware. Resist this temptation and carefully consider your patients and their use of that hardware.

MCP

Perhaps the most significant advancement in hearing aid technology has been the development of the transistor. Its small size and versatility, coupled with the development of miniature transducers of high-quality performance capabilities, such as the electret microphone, have permitted the miniaturization of hearing aids. This miniaturization allows the aid to be worn at or in the ear and yet provide the listener with a signal quality equal or superior to that of body-worn instruments.

Today, the countless styles, components, power capabilities, and applications of amplification for the hearing-impaired present a confusing and complex array of options to the many professionals concerned with hearing aids. What are the limitations of the various styles of aids? What are the many basic and optional components of amplification systems? How do they work? How does one measure the

AMPLIFICATION FOR THE HEARING-IMPAIRED, THIRD EDITION   ISBN 0-8089-1886-9

performance of a hearing aid? What do these measurements mean? What can go
wrong?

STYLES OF PERSONAL AMPLIFICATION SYSTEMS

Prior to the introduction of the transistor, hearing aids were, because of their
size, worn only on the body. Since the early 1950s, three other basic configurations
have been introduced in addition to the body aid with locations at (1) ear level, (2)
eyeglass (both air- and bone-conduction versions), (3) in-ear and in-canal. Typical
instruments for some of these styles are presented in Figure 2-1.

Body Aids

Until the mid-1960s, the body aid (also referred to as *conventional, on-the-
body,* or *at-the-body style*) was the most common type of aid available. Today, it is
generally recommended only for the most profound hearing losses or for users who,
because of conditions such as stroke or arthritis, cannot manipulate the controls on
smaller instruments. Body-worn instruments, most often rectangular in shape, are

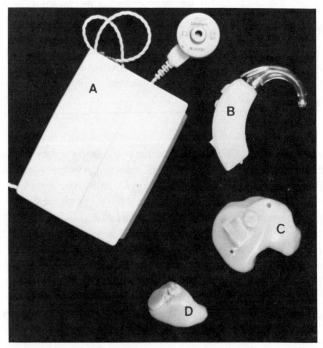

Fig. 2-1. Styles of hearing aids: A = body aid; B = behind-the-
ear aid; C = in-the-ear aid; D = in-the-canal aid.

either worn in a short pocket or special harness, or clipped to the clothing. A wire cord runs from the aid to the air- or bone-conduction receiver at the ear.

Behind-the-Ear Aids

Also known as *over-the-ear, ear-level, at-the-ear,* and *post-auricular* instruments, behind-the-ear (BTE) hearing aids rest behind the pinna, with a plastic "elbow" fitting over the anterior edge of the ear, connecting with a plastic tube that leads to the concha. Table 2-1 presents data from the Hearing Industries Association regarding sales of hearing aids by style from 1963 to 1986. You can see how the percentage of body and BTE aids has decreased dramatically as in-the-ear and in-the-canal aids have gained popularity.

Eyeglass Aids

Many ear-level aid responses were available in comparable eyeglass-temple models. As can be seen in Table 2-1, sales of eyeglass instruments have diminished considerably in recent years.

In-the-Ear Aids

In the past 10 years, there has been a great surge in sales of this type of hearing aid, as noted in Table 2-1. Today, sales of in-the-ear (ITE) hearing aids, including canal instruments, constitute almost 70 percent of the market. With current advances in technology, hearing aid dispensers are now able to successfully fit these styles of instruments to patients who would not have been successful with them a few years ago, especially some high-frequency loss cases.

An important consideration relative to the various styles available is the amplification capability of each. Knowing the style of an instrument tells us very little

Table 2-1
Trends in Hearing Aid Sales

Style	Percent Sold				
	1963	1974	1978	1984	1986
Body aids	20.0	7.1	3.0	0.8	0.8
Eyeglass aids	34.5	22.9	10.0	1.4	0.8
Ear-level aids	43.4	67.4	56.2	39.7	28.5
In-the-ear aids	2.1	2.6	30.8	49.6	58.6
Canal aids				8.3	11.3
CROS-type aids*		4.7	3.0	1.0	0.9

*CROS: Contralateral routing of signal. Includes both ear-level and eyeglass versions. Figures extrapolated from total eyeglass and ear-level figures above.

about its acoustic performance, except that generally, the smaller the aid, the less powerful it is. This concept will be developed at some length later in this chapter.

OPERATIONAL OVERVIEW

Basic Components

Although technological developments have resulted in many styles and applications, all electronic hearing aids operate basically on the same principle. In the broad sense, a hearing aid is any device that more effectively brings sound to the ear. A modern electronic hearing aid, however, is an amplifier whose function is to increase the intensity of sound energy and to deliver it to the ear with as little distortion as possible. Since the acoustic energy of sound cannot be readily amplified directly, it is necessary to convert it to an electrical signal. This signal is amplified and then changed back to acoustical energy.

To do this, any hearing aid contains five basic components (Fig. 2-2): microphone, amplifier, receiver, volume control, and power supply (battery).

MICROPHONE

A microphone is an energy transducer that converts mechanical acoustic energy into an analogous, but weak, electric current. As described in Chapter 1, modern hearing aids use one of two types of microphones: magnetic or electret. A prerequisite for high-quality sound reproduction is the use of a good microphone, because the amplified signal can be no better than the signal received from the microphone. If that signal is of low quality, the output signal will also be of low quality. In other words, a hearing aid is not better than its poorest component, and historically the microphone had been the weakest link in the hearing aid chain. With the advent of the wide spectrum microphones in use today (electret), however, the receiver has now taken on the rather dubious distinction of being the component limiting better hearing aid response.

AMPLIFIER

The weak electric signal generated at the microphone is transmitted to the amplifier, which increases its amplitude (voltage). There are generally several stages to the amplification process. The more stages (transistors and associated circuitry) there are, the greater will be the amount of amplification. Two types of amplifier circuits are used in hearing aids.

A *Class A or single-ended amplifier* consists of three to five amplifier stages and is the most common type used in hearing aids. There is only one output amplifier stage, generally using one output transistor. It has a constant current drain independent of gain control settings and input level. Class A amplifiers are gener-

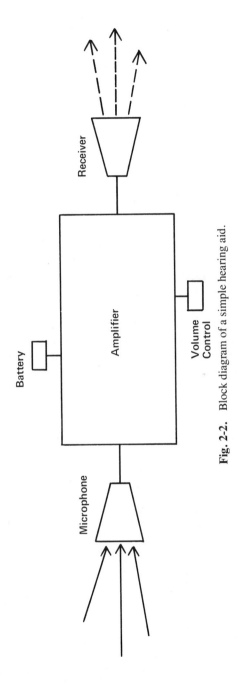

Fig. 2-2. Block diagram of a simple hearing aid.

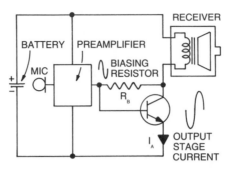

Fig. 2-3. Class A (single-ended) hearing aid amplifier circuit. (Reproduced with permission from Ely WG: Hearing aid battery life. Hearing Instruments 29:12–14, 73, 1978.)

ally used in low and moderate output aids with an average output below 125dB SPL. Figure 2-3 is a schematic diagram of a single-ended amplifier.

The *class B or "push-pull" amplifier* is used in high-output instruments with an average output greater than 125dB SPL. The amplified current is fed into a "phase splitter" that divides it into two signals of opposite phase. These signals are amplified separately by two different output stages and rejoined in the push-pull receiver. Each output stage operates during only about one-half of the signal cycle. Battery current drain is dependent on volume control setting and input level. Because of this, drain is very low in quiet environments. The push-pull amplifier is also characterized by low distortion. Figure 2-4 is a schematic of this type of amplifier.

RECEIVER

In principle a microphone in reverse, the earphone or receiver converts the amplified electric signal into acoustical or sound energy and transmits it to the ear.

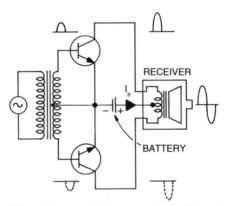

Fig. 2-4. Class B (push-pull) hearing aid amplifier circuit. (Reproduced with permission from Ely WG: Hearing aid battery life. Hearing Instruments 29:12–14, 73, 1978.)

Typically, hearing aid receivers are air-conduction tranducers—presenting sound waves to the external auditory meatus. However, most body-style and some eye-glass aids can be used with bone-conduction receivers. These work in exactly the same way as the bone-conduction vibrator of an audiometer by presenting the signal directly to the mastoid process and, theoretically, bypassing the middle-ear conductive apparatus.

Conventionally, the receiver is located within the enclosure of the ear-level, eyeglass, and ITE aids (internal receivers) but separate from the case of body aids (external receiver).

As I mentioned above, the receiver is now often considered the "weakest link" in a hearing aid. This is because today's electret microphones have a wider and flatter frequency response than do either magnetic or ceramic microphones. One could then assume that the response of electret hearing aids would be greatly extended and flattened. This is not necessarily the case. While electret microphones have widened the low- and high-frequency ends of the spectrum to a great extent, the overall response is very much limited by the response of the receiver. If the receiver has a narrow response, then the overall response of the instrument will reflect this.

Receivers in today's hearing aids are still magnetic and, therefore, have a frequency response considerably narrower than that of the electret microphone. While electret-type receivers are available, they cannot, as of this writing, be used in hearing aids. They require a power supply considerably greater than that provided by conventional hearing aid batteries. Hopefully, within the near future, advances will be made that will allow the use of wider range receivers in hearing aids.

POWER SUPPLY

The battery provides the power for the amplification process. Compared to early vacuum tube batteries, the miniaturized cells used with modern hearing aids are relatively weak (1.3–1.5 V). One of the many advantages of transistors is that they require lower operational voltage for an acoustic output comparable to that of vacuum tube aids. A more detailed discussion of batteries is presented later in this chapter.

VOLUME CONTROL

It is often desirable for a hearing aid user to adjust the sound intensity being received. For example, the user may require less intensity in a very noisy environment. Most hearing aids have a dial or serrated wheel that serves as a volume control. It does not alter the input sound to the aid but adjusts the amount of amplification of the input signal (gain). The volume control is a potentiometer or variable resistor (Fig. 2-5) consisting of a fixed-resistance strip, usually a circular piece of paper or fiber, over which is placed a carbon compound. A sliding contact arm, connected to the external control, moves over this strip and varies resistance to the electrical signal, with a corresponding change in the amount of amplification.

An infrequently considered, but nevertheless important, factor related to vol-

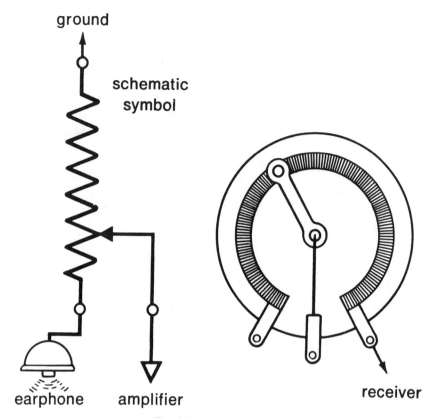

Fig. 2-5. Volume control.

ume controls is their taper characteristic. This refers to the relationship between volume (gain) control rotation and amount of signal attenuation, that is, how much of the maximum amplification is provided at various rotation points (25, 50, 75 percent, and so on).

A study by Kasten and Lotterman (1969) indicated that "the gain control taper does not provide a linear growth in gain." Their examination of 33 different hearing aids revealed a wide range of taper characteristics. Figure 2-6 presents five different tapers from their sample. A number of generalizations can be drawn from these data.

1. Relatively little gain is available once the volume control is beyond 50 percent of its total range. Most of an instrument's gain is delivered in the lower half of the control, while only a limited amount is available in the last half. For example, in Figure 2-6, aid A provides gain to within 5 dB of maximum by the time the control is rotated up to 50 percent, and only an additional 5 dB through the last half of its rotation. The implications of these data are that a user may

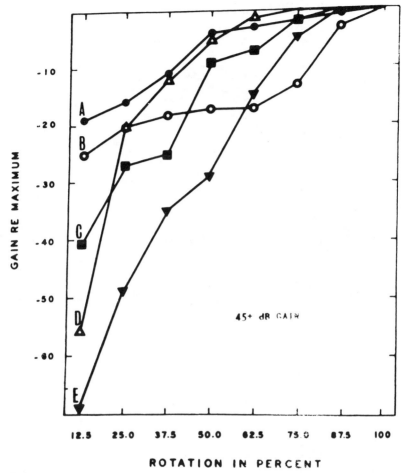

Fig. 2-6. Sample volume control tapers. (Reproduced with permission from Kasten RN, Lotterman SH: Influence of hearing aid gain control rotation on acoustic gain. J Auditory Res 9:35–39, 1969.)

receive some additional amplification by rotating the gain control beyond a 50 percent setting, but may also encounter an unusually high increase in harmonic distortion that could decrease the aided performance (Kasten and Lotterman 1967, Jerger et al 1966, Kasten et al, 1967a).

2. The wide variety of taper characteristics and potentiometer ranges available in modern hearing aids may lead both the aid fitter and the user to overestimate the amount of reserve gain available. For a group of higher power instruments (more than 45-dB average gain) the median value was 60 dB, but only 13 dB of gain remained above 50 percent rotation (Fig. 2-7). Some of the Kasten and Lotterman instruments achieved maximum amplification at or below the 50 percent point, leaving no reserve (Kasten and Lotterman 1967).

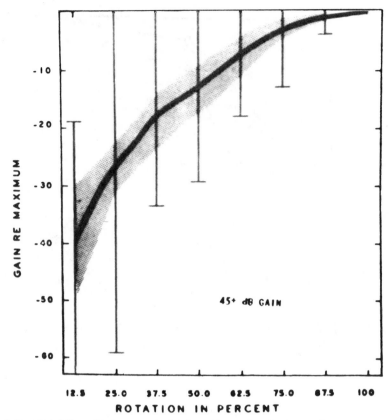

Fig. 2-7. Variability of volume control tapers. (Reproduced with permission from Kasten RN, Lotterman SH: Influence of hearing aid gain control rotation on acoustic gain. J Auditory Res 9:35–39, 1969.)

3. It is important for the clinician to know not only the taper characteristics of the aids being used, but also the potentiometer ranges in order to have some realistic expectations for hearing aids and their performance. It should be noted that hearing aid manufacturers rarely provide this information on model specification sheets.

EARMOLD

The importance of the earmold is discussed in Chapter 3 by McHugh and Morgan. Earmold selection in the hearing aid selection process is discussed in Chapter 5.

TUBING OR CORD

Ear-level and eyeglass hearing aids require some means of delivering the amplified signals to the ear. Plastic tubing, connecting the elbow or receiver nozzle and earmold, is generally used for this purpose. The size, length, and condition of this tube can appreciably affect the signal reaching the ear. These effects are described in the next chapter.

Body-style aids, with the receiver external to the case, require a cord to deliver the amplified electrical signal to the receiver. The condition of this insulated wire and its connections to the aid and receiver are important. The primary concerns are loose connections or a broken wire, which can cause an intermittent or total loss of signal.

Additional Components

While all aids contain the components described above, there are three additional electronic circuits available on most models. All of them (tone control, telecoil, and output limiting control) affect the output signal in some manner.

TONE CONTROL

A tone control is generally regarded as a circuit designed to provide high- or low-frequency emphasis (such as treble and bass adjustments on a stereo). The circuit essentially does this, but by frequency suppression or filtering, rather than by emphasis or additional gain. The tone control is a filter network usually situated between stages of the amplifier. If high-frequency emphasis (HFE) is desired, a high-pass filter network (low frequencies filtered) is used. Conversely, for low-frequency emphasis (LFE), a low-pass filter network is employed.

This is an important concept to keep in mind because tone control labeling can be misleading. Controls are commonly marked H (HFE), N (normal response), and L (LFE), but the circuitry actually performs the opposite of what is suggested; that is, low frequency filtering rather than additional high-frequency gain (Fig. 2-8).

Tone controls can be located on the outside or inside of the case, as a switch or screw adjustment. Some hearing aid manufacturers produce models with no adjustable tone control, but rather a series of different responses with varying degrees of low- or high-frequency filtering. When the aid is ordered, the desired response is specified and appropriate circuitry installed at the factory.

TELEPHONE PICKUP

Many hearing aids are or can be equipped with a special circuit to enhance use with a telephone. The circuit consists of a magnetic induction pickup coil mounted inside the case. The telephone earphone is a magnetic receiver, which, through electromagnetic leakage, generates a magnetic field. If placed next to the telephone receiver, the induction coil picks up the magnetic field and converts it to an electric signal. It is then amplified and again transduced, this time into an acoustic signal. In other words, the telecoil takes the place of a hearing aid microphone as the input component of the aid.

Aids with this component have either a two- or three-position switch that allows use of the microphone alone (M), the telecoil alone (T), or both together

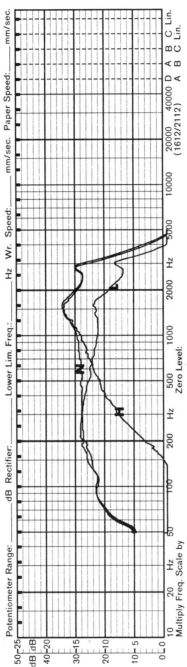

Fig. 2-8. Effect of tone control on hearing aid response.

32

(M/T). If the T position is chosen, the microphone is cut out of the circuit. The advantage of this is the ability to use the aid with a telephone without interference from sounds in the environment. The telecoil can also be used with some induction loop group amplification systems and TV listening devices, as described in Chapter 8.

Newer telephones utilize a microphone-receiver system that allows too little electromagnetic leakage for use with hearing aid telecoils. A variety of permanent and portable amplifiers have been developed in recent years, in part to compensate for this weakness of many conventional phones (refer to Chapter 8 for a discussion of these and other assistive devices).

OUTPUT CONTROL

Many instruments have a screw or lever adjustment to reduce the maximum output intensity that can be generated. The rationales and techniques employed are discussed in the section on output limiting in this chapter.

Feedback

At some time, most of us have experienced a squealing sound from a public-address system, tape recorder, hearing aid, or any other type of amplification system. This is one form of the phenomenon called *feedback*. Feedback can take many forms, both positive and negative, and has been a major engineering consideration in hearing aid design and production. Unfortunately, the professional literature in audiology and hearing aid technology contains little reference to and information about this major problem.

The usable power capability of hearing aids commonly varies according to their size. Body aids are the largest and most powerful. Canal aids are the smallest and provide the least gain and output. BTE and ITE instruments fit between these extremes. There is a very logical rationale for these relationships. Sound waves lose energy as they travel from the source. The further they travel, the greater the intensity loss. If there is any sort of signal leakage (acoustic, mechanical, or magnetic) from the receiver, the coupling system, or both, the escaping sound can be picked up by the microphone and reamplified. The lower the intensity of the leaking sound when it reaches the microphone, the less are the chances that feedback will occur. Therefore, the farther apart the microphone and the receiver are, the greater amount of available output before feedback occurs and the less the energy reaching the microphone. With a body aid, the separation may be as much as 18 inches, so higher amplification levels can be used. ITE transducers may be separated by as little as 0.25 inch, and are therefore the most likely to produce feedback at relatively low output levels. Thus the power of these instruments is severely restricted.

Berger (1974), citing Wanink (1968), has described feedback as a phenomenon that "may be said to be in operation in a system in which a specific output effect results from a specific input signal." For purposes of this discussion, four types of feedback will be considered: acoustical, mechanical, magnetic, and electronic.

ACOUSTICAL FEEDBACK

What is acoustical feedback? To answer this question, we must look at the frequency response of a hearing aid. It is a graphic representation of the amount of amplification provided (gain) as a function of frequency. (This will be discussed at length later in this chapter.) Figure 2-9 shows a typical frequency response curve. Any system has one or more fairly prominent peaks in its response at which it is most sensitive. These peaks are the result of the individual or combined responses of microphone and receiver. If the amplification at that frequency is high enough and sound leakage occurs, the entire circuit may begin to oscillate, with resultant feedback. The fact that different hearing aids have peaks at different frequencies accounts for differences in the perceived pitch of the feedback from aid to aid.

This process is a cyclic one, occurring between the source of the leak and the microphone. Amplified sound escapes and is again picked up by the microphone and reamplified. In cases of low to moderate gain aids, the leaking sound has lost enough energy by the time it reaches the microphone to cause little problem. With high-power instruments, however, a higher-intensity signal reaches the microphone and the cyclic process of reamplification occurs—the sound is amplified again and again until its intensity at the appropriate peak frequency is great enough to set the circuit into oscillation. An interesting sidelight is that if the response of the system were perfectly flat, acoustical feedback would be unlikely because of the absence of resonant peaks. However, no such system exists in hearing aids; there are always peaks and the resultant feedback problem.

As is pointed out in the next chapter, the length and diameter of the tubing used with ear-level and eyeglass aids affect the resonant peaks of the system, either raising or lowering their amplitude and frequency of oscillation and perceived pitch of the feedback. It is possible that length and diameter may determine, to some extent, the presence or absence of acoustical feedback.

Acoustical feedback results from sound propagation through the air from the receiver-earmold coupling to the microphone. Two conditions are generally associated with this type of feedback: (1) direct leak of amplified sound from the medial side of the earmold to the outside and (2) poor acoustic isolation of the receiver, the microphone, or both. This permits the sound to radiate through the case of BTE, ITE, and eyeglass aids and be picked up by the microphone. The latter situation usually occurs only under high-gain conditions. The direct leak can occur in a number of ways:

1. A poorly fitting earmold or ITE shell, allowing sound to escape between the mold and the meatal wall. *Direct sound leakage is the most common cause of acoustical feedback.*
2. Improper connection between the receiver and earmold (body aids) or tubing and earmold (ear-level and eyeglass aids) allowing the sound to leak directly before it is delivered to the ear. This problem can generally be solved by inserting a fabric or plastic washer between the receiver and mold or cord connector in the body aid, or recementing the tubing into the earmold of an ear-

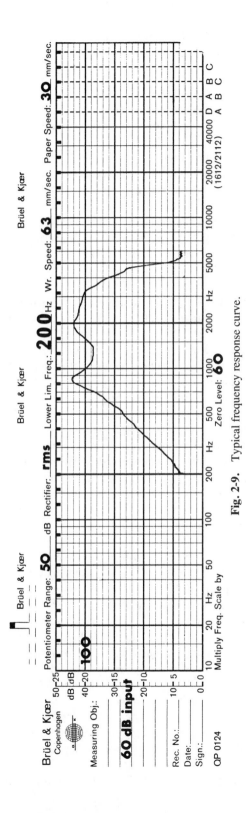

Fig. 2-9. Typical frequency response curve.

35

level aid. More recent receiver designs employ a double seal to prevent leakage through the connector plug holes.

3. A crack in the tubing between the internal receiver and earmold, again allowing a direct leak. The easiest solution is to replace the tubing.
4. A poor fit of the tubing to the elbow or receiver nozzle, allowing the direct leak. The best treatment is new tubing.
5. A poor fitting elbow at the receiver connection of ear-level aids. The cure is to replace the elbow.

A simple way to determine the cause of acoustical feedback is to check each of these factors, beginning with the earmold. First, place a fingertip over the canal opening of the mold, or the receiver port of an ITE or canal aid, and turn the volume control full "on." If no feedback occurs, but has occurred when the aid is worn, the cause is most likely a poorly fitting mold or shell and a new one should be made. If feedback still occurs, check the tubing and its connections to the mold and receiver. In the case of body aids with external receivers, the next step is to insert a washer and repeat the first step. If feedback still is present after all connections have been checked, the problem is probably the result of poor receiver acoustic isolation. In this case, the hearing aid must be returned to the factory for repair.

The second condition noted above is poor acoustic isolation of the receiver or the microphone, or both, within the hearing aid case. Especially at high output levels, the walls of the receiver oscillate mechanically in a "pumping" action. This disturbs the air inside the case, generating a sound wave that travels through the air space to the microphone. Three approaches can be used to solve this problem: (1) maximize the space between microphone and receiver so that the sound pressure reaching the microphone is of lower amplitude, (2) use an interlocking wall between the microphone and receiver to block the sound transmission, and (3) place a rubber tube on the microphone port so that no sound from within the case can reach the microphone diaphragm. The tubing acts to attenuate the sound pressure reaching the microphone from within the case.

An intriguing finding, and one that may open avenues for additional research, is that acoustical feedback is essentially a high-frequency phenomenon. There are two reasons for this: First, peaks in the response curve generally occur within the ranges of 1000–2000 Hz for the primary peak and 3000–4000 Hz for the secondary peak. The former appears to be related to feedback resulting from acoustical radiation through the case, whereas the latter is related to direct sound leakage from the earmold, or tubing, or both. Second, because of their shorter wavelengths, high frequencies can escape around a poorly fitting earmold with greater ease than can low frequencies. Combining this with the above information, we can readily see why acoustical feedback is said to be a *high-frequency phenomenon*.

This has recently presented considerable difficulty to hearing aid engineers. Many manufacturers have been working on designs for extreme high-frequency emphasis instruments but have had to keep gain relatively low because of feedback problems. A possible solution to this might be to use the natural resonant frequency of the external auditory meatus, 2800-3000 Hz. It appears plausible to decrease some high-frequency response in the aid to reduce feedback and still provide high-frequency emphasis by taking advantage of the resonance characteristics of the meatus. This would have the effect of increasing the intensity of higher frequencies reaching the tympanic membrane at a rate of about 3 dB/octave, from 800 Hz upward. Additional research is needed on this question.

Currently, two additional approaches are being used to alleviate acoustical feedback. The first consists of resistance filters in the earhook of BTE aids and the receiver tubing of some ITE instruments. These filters (available in various resistances, from 680 to 3300 Ω) smooth the frequency response by diminishing the primary peak, in the area of 1000 Hz. The other approach, available in only a limited number of hearing aids, is a frequency shifting control, usually referred to as a *feedback reduction control,* that allows the fitter to shift the secondary response peak (around 3000 Hz) to a slightly higher or lower frequency. Depending on the resonant characteristics of the user's external meatus, this slight shift can result in a reduction of acoustical feedback by effectively reducing amplification at the resonant frequency at which the oscillation may occur.

MECHANICAL FEEDBACK

Microphones in all hearing aids, and the receiver in ear-level, eyeglass, and ITE instruments, are mounted inside the case on rubber cushions to isolate them from each other and from the case. These cushions are employed to decrease vibration transmission and to protect the components from shock if the aid is dropped. If these isolators are improperly designed or mounted, or have deteriorated, low-frequency mechanical vibrations (400–500 Hz) from the receiver can vibrate the case. These vibrations will be picked up by the microphone and amplified. A "squeal" is heard that is lower in pitch than that heard because of acoustical feedback. In fact, the distinguishing auditory feature of mechanical feedback is its relatively low pitch. Electret microphones have a low-mass internal construction, which makes them highly resistant to mechanical vibration. Continuing miniaturization of hearing aids has increased the problem of mechanical vibration feedback between the microphone and receiver because of their proximity (Maxwell and Burkhard 1969b). This is another reason for the relatively low gain of some ITE and most canal aids.

This problem can be solved in two ways: (1) more compliant isolation supports for the transducers (better cushioning) are used to achieve high gain without vibrational feedback oscillation (Burkhard 1965, Nordstrom 1974) and (2) microphones and receivers are oriented within the case with their directions of maximum vibration output and sensitivity at right angles to each other to take advantage of directional vibration damping properties (Maxwell and Burkhard 1969a).

MAGNETIC FEEDBACK

Magnetic feedback results from the coupling between the magnetic fields of the receiver and the telephone coil or magnetic microphone. The magnetic field from the receiver can "spill over" to the microphone or telecoil and be transduced to a feedback noise. This problem has been greatly reduced through the use of non-magnetic microphones and improved receiver designs in newer hearing aid models.

ELECTRONIC FEEDBACK

Electronic feedback is often used in amplifier circuits to help control the output of the hearing aid. A portion of the electric signal from the output stage of the amplifier is routed back to the input stage for self-regulatory functions, such as automatic volume control (AVC). Obviously, this is a beneficial form of feedback. Other controlled uses of feedback include giving some condenser microphones directional response characteristics and shaping amplifier response characteristics (Hillman 1974).

There are two forms of electronic feedback that can have a detrimental effect on instrument performance. The first is *electrostatic feedback*. An electrostatic field is caused by a capacitive coupling from the output to the input stages of the amplifier, and becomes a problem when improper techniques are used to attenuate high-frequency amplifier response. The resultant audible sound has a very high pitch, reported as a "hiss."

Electrical oscillation results from inadequate decoupling of battery and amplifier circuits. It is related to battery impedance in that as the usable battery voltage decreases, impedance increases and causes the amplifier circuit to oscillate. This is reflected in a low-frequency "motorboating," which commonly sounds much like the buzz of a sawtooth noise. The cure for electrical oscillation is to replace the battery and improve decoupling, making the circuit impervious to battery voltage changes.

COMBINATION EFFECTS

It is possible for more than one form of feedback to occur simultaneously. These combined effects are overlayed and more than one type of feedback is audible at the same time.

CONCLUSION

As pointed out above, many forms of acoustical feedback can be remedied by the audiologist or hearing aid dispenser by adjusting the earmold, the tubing, or the ITE or canal aid case. If these modifications do not cure the problem, the instrument should be returned to the factory for appropriate repair. This is especially true for mechanical, magnetic, and electronic feedback problems, which ordinarily cannot be remediated outside a repair center.

ELECTROACOUSTIC MEASUREMENTS

History and Rationale

During the early period of electric and electronic instrumentation there was a lack of standardization of performance parameters, including how to measure them and how to report them. Most often, manufacturer's used their own set of "standards" for sales promotion. As Berger (1974) states, "advertising slogans were the rule rather than statements based on scientific fact." Early attempts to achieve industry-wide standards met with little success. Romanow (1942) and Carlisle and Mundel (1944) produced some of the earliest extensive reports on hearing aid electroacoustic measurements. A committee of the American Hearing Aid Association compiled a *Tentative Code for Measurement of Performance of Hearing Aids* (Kranz 1945), but it was neither sufficiently comprehensive nor widely accepted by the industry. For a thorough overview of attempts to standardize hearing aid measurements, the reader should consult Berger (1968 and 1974).

As hearing aid makes and models continued to proliferate, the need became apparent for a method to compare not only the performance of different models but of units of the same model as well. Without being able to describe performance characteristics in detail, a particular aid cannot be compared to others or to published characteristics for that model.

Standards

In 1959 the International Electrotechnical Commission (IEC) published their *Recommended Methods for Measurements of the Electroacoustical Characteristics of Hearing Aids* (IEC 1959). This European standard was slightly modified and adopted by the American National Standards Institute (ANSI, formerly the American Standards Association and United States of America Standards Institute) as American Standard S3.3-1960, *Electroacoustical Characteristics of Hearing Aids* (ANSI 1960). In 1961 the Hearing Aid Industry Conference (HAIC 1961) adopted the *HAIC Standard Method of Expressing Hearing Aid Performance*. It was largely based on S3.3-1960. In the late 1960s, the HAIC standard underwent minor modification and was adopted as ANSI Standard S3.8-1967, *Methods of Expressing Hearing Aid Performance* (ANSI 1967). In essence, the IEC and early ANSI standards describe how to measure performance, while the HAIC and later ANSI standards specify not only how, but what to measure.

In 1976 ANSI adopted a new standard for hearing aids, S3.22-1976, *Specification of Hearing Aid Characteristics* (ANSI 1976). Its latest revision was in 1987. I had planned to include it as an appendix to this edition, as in the first two editions; however, the very high fee charged by the Acoustical Society of America made it economically prohibitive. S3.22-1987 is essentially an update and expansion of the 1967, 1976, and 1982 standards. The main changes include the following: (1) change in the frequencies measured to specify gain and output to 1000, 1600, and 2500 Hz, now called *high-frequency average*; (2) for the first time, the standard includes tolerances on the measured characteristics reported by manufacturers; and (3) also for the first time, an attempt is made to measure some characteristics at a volume control setting approximating a "use" setting referred to as *reference test gain*.

Testing Equipment

Lybarger (1961a,b) described the "typical situation for hearing aid use," as depicted in Figure 2-10. In this situation, the speaker and listener (hearing aid user)

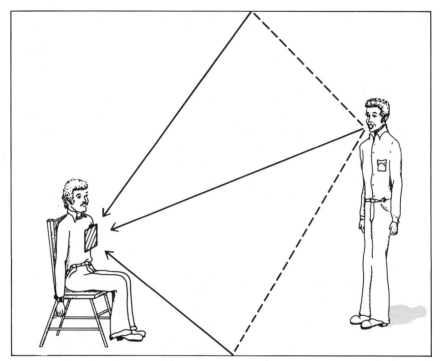

Fig. 2-10. Typical situation for hearing aid use. (Adapted with permission from Lybarger SF: Standardized hearing aid measurements. Audecibel 10:8–10, 1961b.)

are some 3–15 feet apart. The average intensity of conversational speech is about 70 dB SPL at this distance. The speech signal not only reaches the hearing aid microphone through the direct air pathway but is also reflected from the walls, ceiling, and floor of the room in a rather random, uncontrolled manner. Ambient noise in the environment also reaches the microphone and is amplified.

Obviously, this "typical" situation involves far too many uncontrolled variables for standardized measurements. Therefore, the standards specify the use of a free-field environment for testing (implying the use of an anechoic-type chamber) to eliminate reflected and standing waves and to reduce ambient noise levels. To further eliminate variables, the human speaker is replaced with a dynamic loudspeaker, having a "nearly uniform output over the 200–5000 Hz test band ordinarily used for hearing aids" (Lybarger 1961b). Either a discrete or sweep frequency oscillator provides the test signal to the speaker. To ensure a uniform signal to the hearing aid microphone, a monitoring condenser microphone is positioned in the test box enclosure. This microphone and its associated compressor amplifier automatically maintain a constant signal sound pressure within stated tolerances of ± 1.5 dB at 200–3000 Hz and ±2.5 dB at 3000–5000 Hz.

Inside the test enclosure, the sweep or discrete frequency signal is amplified by the hearing aid, the output of which is delivered to a standard 2-cc coupler (artificial

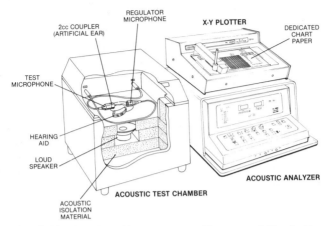

Fig. 2-11. Hearing aid test system. (Courtesy of Phonic Ear, Inc.)

ear) that replaces the human ear for test purposes. From this point, the amplified signal is metered and, in automatic systems, printed out by a graphic level recorder. Figure 2-11 is a block diagram of a complete hearing aid test system. For detailed information regarding the specifications for a test system, the reader is referred to the IEC (1959) or ANSI (1987) standards.

With the added complexity of hearing aids, it has become necessary for every dispenser to have a test system to be sure all new aids perform as specified, to be sure that repaired instruments work properly, to measure response changes made by the dispenser and to measure any deterioration in response over time. The marketing of the less expensive systems has made test arrangements available to most dispensers.

Definitions and Standard Procedures

The performance characteristics most often measured are *Saturation Sound Pressure Level* (HFA-SSPL$_{90}$), *Reference Test Gain* (RTG). *Frequency Response, Equivalent Input Noise Level,* and *Harmonic Distortion.* Additional measures include *Battery Current Drain* and *Automatic Gain Control* (AGC).

FULL-ON GAIN

As defined by ANSI (1987), gain is "the difference between the output sound pressure level in an earphone coupler and the input sound pressure level." This refers to the amount of amplification of the input signal. For example, if the input signal is 60 dB and the output is 115 dB, the gain is 55 dB.

The full-on gain (FOG) is measured with the volume control at its maximum (full-on) position and an input of 60 dB SPL (50 dB for AGC aids). The measurements can be made using either discrete-frequency signals or a sweep-frequency signal. The output is plotted providing a curve describing gain as a function of frequency. From this curve the essential information can be extrapolated to specify the high-frequency average FOG. To do this, the average gain at 1000, 1600, and 2500 Hz is determined.

This provides a limited impression of the amount of amplification through "speech frequencies." While better than the old average of 500, 1000, and 2000 Hz, the HF average can still be misleading, especially if the gain at one of the frequencies is appreciably higher or lower than the others. In this case, one may receive a false impression of how much amplification the aid provides. For example, if the gain is 20 dB at 1000 Hz, 30 dB at 1600 Hz, and 65 dB at 2500 Hz, the HF average would be 45 dB. While this hypothetical instrument might be sufficient for an individual with a high-frequency loss beginning at 1000 Hz, it would most likely not be adequate for someone with a relatively flat loss. This implies the importance of examining the FOG and RTG curves carefully.

In a later section of this chapter, some of the problems inherent in the ANSI standards are discussed, including proposals for considering the use of "speech" or "pink" noise rather than pure tones as the input signal and use of the Zwislocki coupler for a much closer approximation of real-ear hearing aid response.

Another important bit of information, related to the gain curve and the average gain, is the gain-per-octave slope. In the example given above, the gain per octave between 1000 and 1600 Hz is 10 dB, but is 35 dB between 1600 and 2500 Hz. Referring to the discussion of that example, the value of these data is apparent.

Of all hearing aid measurements, only the FOG curve shows the practical maximum gain of the instrument. It is easy to confuse this curve with the "reference test gain frequency response curve" (see below), but by carefully examining the measurement procedure, one can see the differences. Some manufacturers obtain gain information from the frequency response rather than from the gain curve, resulting in a lack of standardized data reporting. Anyone reading hearing aid specifications should be aware of this. It is important to use standardized input levels to obtain data from which comparisons can be made.

REFERENCE TEST GAIN

One of the major changes in the new ANSI standards is the inclusion of *reference test gain* (RTG), which simulates "use" position of the volume control. This is used for certain other measures, including harmonic distortion, frequency response and range, and equivalent input noise level.

To adjust the gain control to RTG position, first determine the HF average SSPL$_{90}$ as described below. Then, using 60 dB input, adjust the control so that the average of the 1000, 1600, and 2500 Hz values is 17 dB less than the HF average SSPL$_{90}$. If the aid does not have enough gain to allow this adjustment, leave the control full-on. For AGC aids, set the control full-on. The rationale for this procedure is that the long-term average SPL for speech at 1 meter is about 65-dB SPL, with peaks typically 12 dB above this value, or 77-dB SPL. Using a 60-dB SPL input and a 17-dB volume control setting back from the $SSPL_{90}$ value gives essentially the same value.

Another way to determine the RTG is to subtract 77-dB from the HF average $SSPL_{90}$. If the aid yields less gain than the value so specified, the RTG is determined with the gain control full-on.

SATURATION SOUND PRESSURE LEVEL

Also referred to as *acoustic output* or *maximum power output (MPO)*, saturation output ($SSPL_{90}$) is the "sound pressure level developed in a 2-cc earphone coupler when the input sound pressure level is 90 dB, with the gain control of the hearing aid full-on" (Ansi 1987). In other words, it is the greatest SPL the aid is capable of producing, regardless of the amount of gain and the intensity of the input signal. Any amplification system can provide only a limited amount of output. A point is reached at which the amplifier cannot amplify further and the receiver cannot transduce a greater signal. If the input increases beyond the level at which saturation occurs, the output will not increase further and, in fact, may decrease, so that the signal will be considerably distorted. We have all experienced this when turning the volume control on a radio or TV to its maximum. Not only is the signal loud, but it is also obviously distorted.

The $SSPL_{90}$ is measured with the gain control at maximum and a 90-dB input. All other controls on the aid are adjusted to give the widest response. Using either a discrete or sweep frequency signal, plot a curve of output as a function of frequency between 200 and 5000 Hz. Using the three frequencies, 1000, 1600, and 2500 Hz, determine the HF average SSPL90. Figure 2-12 shows a typical $SSPL_{90}$ curve.

It is vital to proper fitting to know the maximum output capability of a hearing aid to ensure that (1) the instrument is producing a sound pressure level sufficiently above the user's threshold to be maximally useful and (2) to insure that the aid does not produce a signal that exceeds the user's threshold of discomfort. In other words, the signal must not be too little or too much.

FREQUENCY RESPONSE CURVE

The most common curve on manufacturers' technical sheets is the basic frequency response, describing the relative amount of gain as a function of frequency. It is relative in that the frequency response is not based on maximum gain.

For this measure, the gain control is set at reference test. With the control at this point and the input at a constant 60 dB, the signal frequency is varied and the curve recorded either automatically or manually. The reader is referred to Figure 2-9 for a typical frequency response curve.

To provide a consistent, undistorted graph of the frequency response, it must be plotted on a frequency-by-intensity chart in which the length covered by a 1-octave interval on the frequency abscissa is equal to a 13.5-dB length on the intensity ordinate. This scale is essentially the same as that in which one decade (i.e., 100–1000 Hz) on the abscissa is equal to 50 ± 2 dB on the ordinate, as required in ANSI S3.22-1987.

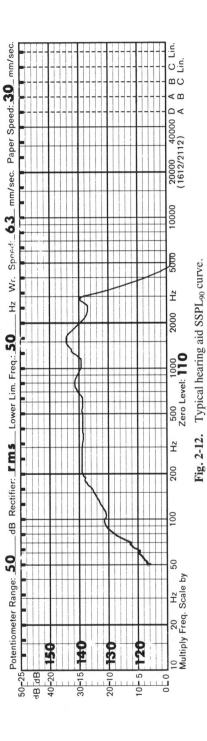

Fig. 2-12. Typical hearing aid SSPL₉₀ curve.

44

The frequency response of any hearing aid depends on the respective responses of all its components: microphone, amplifier, and receiver. As was discussed earlier in this chapter, the amplifier and receiver can process only the signals they receive from the microphone. Therefore, the vital importance of the microphone in the system is evident. By the same token, the overall response of a hearing aid will reflect the characteristics of each component. If the amplifier works on only a restricted frequency range, the aid's response will reflect this, regardless of the characteristics of microphone and receiver. The same analogy holds true for the receiver. With this in mind, along with the difficulties inherent in changing the responses of microphones and internal receivers, most intentional modifications of frequency response are achieved by altering the amplifier (tone control) or tubing-earmold coupling. The latter area is discussed in Chapter 3.

Distortion

An ideal amplification system is one that, among its other characteristics, reproduces an output signal identical to the input signal. However, no such system truly exists. Neither the microphone, amplifier, nor receiver is capable of producing an exact copy of the input signal. *When the acoustic properties of the input signal are not reproduced exactly, the output is said to be distorted in comparison to the input.* This distortion can take the form of resonant peaks or anti-resonant valleys, decreased bandwidth, or nonlinear frequency and/or amplitude reproduction. The ability of an amplification system to accurately reproduce the wave form of the input signal is referred to as *fidelity*—high fidelity for accurate or near accurate reproduction, and low fidelity for poor reproduction. In general, *hearing aids are considered low fidelity systems.*

For the purpose of this discussion, four types of distortion will be considered: nonlinear or amplitude distortion (including harmonic and intermodulation distortion), transient distortion, frequency distortion, and extraneous or noise distortion. The output of a hearing aid is said to be nonlinear when either the amplitude or frequency aspects of the waveform are not in the same relationship as they were in the input signal.

HARMONIC DISTORTION

Other forms of distortion that can affect hearing aid and user performance are often overlooked, making harmonic distortion the type most commonly considered in hearing aid technology. The reasons for this are that harmonic distortion is the easiest to measure and is the only type reported by manufacturers.

Harmonic distortion results when new frequencies are generated that are whole number multiples of the original or fundamental frequency, and that are not part of the input signal. For example, if a hearing aid distorts at 500 Hz, this indicates that in addition to the fundamental tone it amplifies and reproduces, the instrument also generates harmonic frequencies. Thus, in addition to the 500 Hz fundamental, the

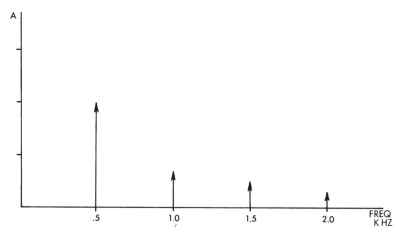

Fig. 2-13. 500-Hz fundamental plus second, third, and fourth harmonics. (Reproduced with permission from Ely WG: A primer of distortion in hearing aids. Hearing Aid J 27:10–11, 34, 1974.)

frequencies of 1000 Hz (second harmonic), 1500 Hz (third harmonic), and so forth, are also present in the output signal (Fig. 2-13).

Generally speaking, the greater the gain setting of an aid, the greater will be the harmonic distortion. Studies have shown high distortion at or near maximum gain in most aids, and lower distortion at reduced settings (Lotterman and Kasten 1967, Kasten et al. 1967). These findings have serious implications in terms of hearing aid selection for the hard-of-hearing. In other words, it would be undesirable to select for an individual an instrument that would have to be set at or near maximum gain in order to achieve a comfort level. In such case, the output signal would contain appreciable distortion, thereby probably lowering both the objective and subjective aspects of aided performance. Harmonic distortion appears to be an important determinant of the degree of success a hearing aid user may achieve with an instrument (Kasten and Lotterman 1967).

If the amount of harmonic distortion is great, the effects can be serious in terms of speech intelligibility; that is, speech will be distorted and intelligibility will be reduced. Various investigations have shown that of all electroacoustic characteristics, harmonic distortion appears to be the one most closely related to aided speech discrimination ability. Results of these studies indicate that speech intelligibility decreases in an inversely proportional function to the level of distortion (Harris et al. 1961, Jerger et al. 1966, Olsen and Carhart 1967, Olsen and Wilbur, 1978). However, these studies used rather severe levels of distortion. It is possible that as the harmonic distortion levels increased, other forms of distortion also increased, thereby reducing listener performance.

Two interesting observations arose from a study of a nonlinear distortion by Kasten and Lotterman (1967). First, there appeared to be an inverse relationship between level of distortion and frequency—as frequency increased, distortion decreased. This finding was supported by Lotterman and Kasten (1967) and Lotterman and Farrar (1965). Second, distortion level appeared to be inversely related to the power category of the aids, that is, greatest distortion in mild gain instruments. Lotterman and Farrar (1965) and Lotterman and Kasten (1967) also found that frequencies at which maximum distortion occurred were higher in ear-level than in body aids.

INTERMODULATION DISTORTION

Intermodulation distortion occurs when the output signal contains frequencies that are arithmetic sums and differences of two or more input frequencies. When two or more signal frequencies (as in speech) are applied simultaneously at the input, it is the result of amplifier nonlinearity. Speech intelligibility can suffer in the presence of intermodulation distortion as a result of unwanted frequencies distorting the primary message signal. When two frequencies are amplified by a nonlinear system, sum and difference tones can be generated. The same nonlinearity that generates harmonic distortion results in intermodulation distortion—harmonic distortion and intermodulation distortion result from the same source, amplifier nonlinearity. Figure 2-14 presents a typical simplified intermodulation distortion example in which are seen the fundamentals (500 and 700 Hz) and the sum (1200 Hz) and difference (200 Hz) frequencies. Figure 2-15 shows the same two fundamentals with the concomitant harmonic and intermodulation distortion frequencies.

TRANSIENT DISTORTION

Transient distortion occurs whenever the hearing aid is unable to duplicate the initial sharp attack (rise time) or the sudden decay (fall time) of a sound. In the latter situation, an alteration or lingering of the waveform often results in what is called

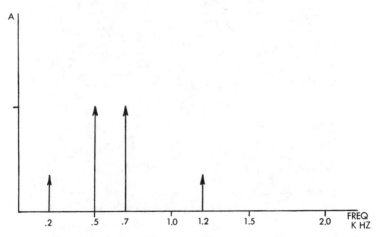

Fig. 2-14. 500- and 700-Hz tones plus sum (1.2-kHz) and difference (0.2-kHz) intermodulation tones. (Reproduced with permission from Ely WG: A primer of distortion in hearing aids. Hearing Aid J 27:10–11, 34, 1974.)

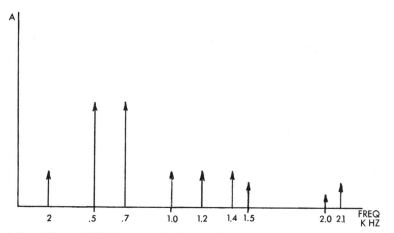

Fig. 2-15. 500- and 700-Hz tones plus harmonic and intermodulation distortion components. (Reproduced with permission from Ely WG: A primer of distortion in hearing aids. Hearing Aid J 27:10–11, 34, 1974.)

"ringing." The way in which the output lags behind the input can be seen in Figure 2-16. This type of distortion appears to be closely related to the presence of sharp resonant peaks in the response of the system. Speech intelligibility can be reduced by transient distortion, since the "ringing" of the output signal interacts with the transient nature of speech. This problem is compounded by the fact that speech is composed of many transients important to discrimination.

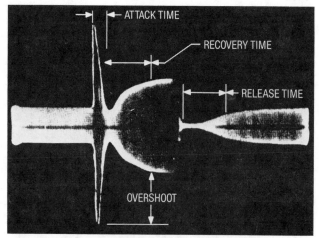

Fig. 2-16. Transient distortion. (Reproduced with permission from Davis H, Silverman SR: Hearing and Deafness. New York, Holt, Rinehart & Winston, 1970.)

FREQUENCY DISTORTION

As considered earlier, the input and output signals are often not the same. If the variations are related to the frequency spectrum of the signal, that is, if the frequency response and bandwidth of the output are different from the input, frequency distortion has occurred. This is related to the concept of fidelity. Because the output signal from a hearing aid is so different from the input, in terms of frequency response and bandwidth, hearing aids can reasonably be called low-fidelity amplification systems.

Curran (1974) points out that we can not reasonably conclude that user performance will be satisfactory simply because published or individually measured harmonic distortion levels are low. As shown above, no clear-cut, consistent relationship has been established between harmonic distortion and speech intelligibility. This may be because harmonic distortion, by itself, may not significantly deteriorate intelligibility. Interaction effects, the appearance of multiple forms of distortion simultaneously, may be more detrimental than any one individual type of distortion. This is an area of much-needed research.

Distortion Measurements

At the time of this writing, the current American National Standard for the *Specification of Hearing Aid Characteristics* (ANSI 1987) does not specify procedures for measuring any type of distortion other than harmonic. Even this procedure is not precise, calling for measurements at 500, 800, and 1600 Hz with a 70-dB SPL input level. However, the standards do not specify provisions or recommendations for methods of reporting distortion levels, that is, at which gain setting distortion should be reported.

Harmonic distortion measurements are expressed in percentages and use the standard formula found in S3.22-1987 for total harmonic distortion (THD). The acceptable amount of distortion in a hearing aid is not standardized, although some investigators have shown that distortion values greater than 10 percent begin to have appreciably negative influences on speech discrimination (Lotterman and Kasten 1967, Jerger et al. 1966, Jirsa and Hodgson 1970, Bode and Kasten 1971). The Veterans Administration and others recommend rejection of any hearing aid with harmonic distortion over 10 percent (Jeffers et al. 1973).

One problem with harmonic distortion measurements is a lack of consistency regarding what is being measured. You can either plot the second harmonic of a number of frequencies (i.e., 500, 800, and 1600 Hz) according to ANSI, or you can add all the harmonics (second, third, fourth, etc.) at one frequency to calculate THD.

Second harmonic distortion alone can be misleading, however, as is shown in Figure 2-17. In this example, we see the frequency response and second and third harmonic curves obtained at three input levels (60, 70, and 80 dB) with the same

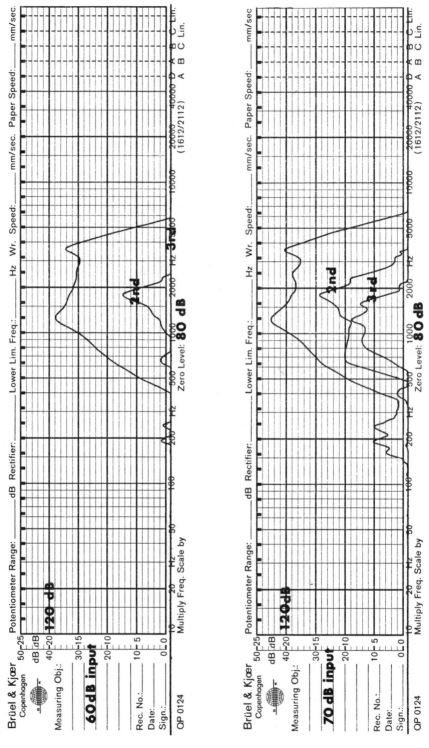

50

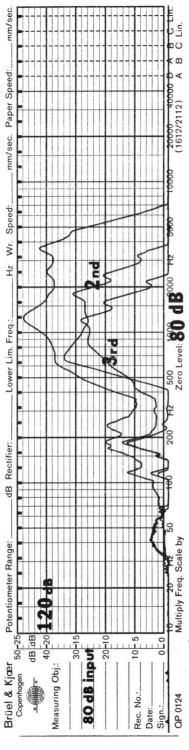

Fig. 2-17. Fundamental, second and third harmonics of the same aid at three different input levels: *top*, 60 dB; *middle*, 70 dB; *bottom*, 80 dB.

aid. As the input level increases, so do both harmonic curves, especially the third. In fact, third harmonic distortion begins to approximate and exceed the second with the 80 dB input. If only second harmonic distortion was measured for the hearing aid used here, this situation could possibly pass unnoticed. THD measurements would pick it up.

Harmonic distortion is measured using a wave analyzer, distortion bridge, or filter set. The procedure involves filtering out the fundamental frequency from the output signal and measuring the intensity level of the remaining second or more harmonics. By use of either the standard formula or conversion table, the intensity difference between the fundamental and harmonics is converted to a percentage value.

This discussion on distortion measurement has been limited to harmonic distortion because, as I mentioned earlier, that is the only type for which there is even a semblance of an adequate and reasonable measurement protocol, much less an agreed-on one. Although frequency distortion is measured as frequency response, there is no means of quantifying it. Intermodulation distortion measurements require two input signals, has a more complex output, and lacks, at present, an acceptable procedure. This is another area ripe for investigation.

Problems with S3.22-1987

The standards specify measurements over the range 200–5000 Hz. Many of today's new aids exceed this range on one or both extremes. One factor that will confound measurements on these instruments is that most commonly used hearing aid test boxes do not meet the need for sound isolation and vibration dampening below 200 Hz. If low-frequency noise levels (below 200 Hz) are high, the test system cannot adequately measure low-frequency amplification of many newer aids. This can give a false impression that these frequencies are not amplified when they are, possibly resulting in misfittings of hearing aids in which low-frequency masking effects could obliterate higher-frequency information necessary for speech intelligibility. The implication here is that even if the standards are revised in this area, existing test chambers will not be adequate for the new measurements.

Another factor is that the 2-cc coupler and microphone systems used in hearing aid measurements are not reliable at and above 5000 Hz, thus presenting obvious difficulties for high frequency measurements.

Another problem with S3.22-1987 is that it still specifies use of the standard 2-cc coupler, which does not and was never intended to reflect real-ear response of a hearing aid. As discussed later in this chapter, there is another system available to measure hearing aid responses that more accurately reflects how the instrument will perform in a human ear.

Nonstandard Measures—Research Needs

The American hearing aid measurement standard ignores several electroacoustic factors related to speech transmission system integrity. Some of these are areas of presumed or demonstrated importance to hearing aid performance that have been completely ignored and/or are in need of further clarification through additional research and standardization. In general, they are self-explanatory:

1. Standardized characteristics of output limiting circuits—peak clipping, input and output compression, signal processing and methods of measuring their performance
2. Measurement and expression methods for transient distortion and intermodulation distortion
3. Frequency response and sensitivity of the hearing aid using a telecoil
4. Standardized expression of volume control taper characteristics
5. Distortion as a function of battery voltage
6. Effect of tone control position on speech intelligibility
7. Measurement of hearing aid signal-to-noise ratios
8. Accountability for head shadow and body baffle effects
9. Clarification of the documented differences in hearing aid performance between the standard 2-cc coupler and the real ear (see the section of this chapter on philosophies and practicalities)

OUTPUT LIMITING AND NOISE REDUCTION

Two of the greatest problems facing hearing aid users are output SPLs exceeding comfort and tolerance levels and reduced speech intelligibility in the presence of competing environmental noise. One of the basic tenets in selecting a hearing aid is to choose an instrument that has sufficient, yet tolerable amplification. Especially for individuals with a reduced dynamic range, such as recruiting ears, it often is necessary to limit the output, at least for high intensity input signals. This situation becomes especially critical when the aids used in locations where ambient noise levels are equal to or exceed the level of the desired speech signal. *The goal is to reduce the level of the noise output while only minimally affecting the speech output.* At the time of this writing, there is a plethora of systems designed to help solve these difficulties. The hearing aid industry is currently in the midst of a name game, with most companies featuring "amazing," "revolutionary," or "remarkable" innovations. In many cases, the names are confusing and/or misleading.

All output limiting systems have as their goals retention of output SPL below uncomfortable loudness (UCL) and improvement of the signal-to-noise ratio. This section will present a discussion of the primary approaches currently employed. It is likely that most, if not all, of them will be obsolete within the next five to ten years, as digital technology is refined to the point where it can be utilized in ear-level and ITE aids.

Linear Amplification and Peak Clipping

Ideally, a hearing aid is a linear amplifier through a significant portion of its input-output range. In a linear system, *for every decibel change in input, there is an*

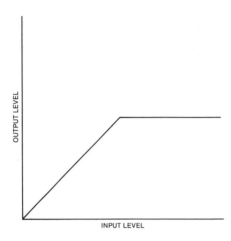

Fig. 2-18. Linear amplification input-output function.

equivalent decibel change in output. This 1:1 ratio is exemplified in Figure 2-18. Graphically, it is represented by a 45 degree angle for the gain function. This continues until the overload or saturation point of the aid is reached, beyond which the amplifier cannot produce greater output.

Beyond saturation, *peak clipping* occurs. This form of output limitation is characteristic of all simple amplifiers. The level at which peak clipping occurs can be either fixed or variable. Some hearing aids still utilize this form of limiting. If variable, the level can be set below the saturation point to prevent output SPLs beyond tolerance limits from reaching the ear.

Figure 2-19 displays the effect of peak clipping upon a sinusoidal waveform. As saturation is reached, the peak amplitude portions of the output signal are "clipped," flattening or squaring the waveform. This results in a physical distortion of the signal because its high-amplitude elements are now restricted relative to its low-amplitude elements.

The effect of this process is the introduction of harmonic distortion and a possible decrease in speech intelligibility. There is some apparent disagreement

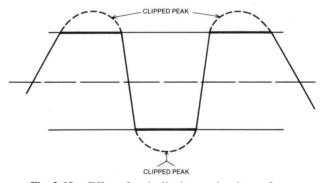

Fig. 2-19. Effect of peak clipping on signal waveform.

about the effect of peak clipping on intelligibility. Older studies (Olsen 1971, Staab 1972) suggest that speech understanding is not appreciably disrupted by clipping and its resultant harmonic and intermodulation distortion. On the other hand, Smriga (1985a) indicates that the introduction of harmonic distortion and the loss of some input information in the output results in a reduced intelligibility. In either case, there is a great reduction in sound quality when peak clipping is used as an output limiting approach, so great that most hearing aid users will complain or reject such an aid.

A brief consideration of acoustic phonetics supports the contention of little loss of intelligibility. In English, vowel sounds are generally lower in frequency and higher in intensity than consonants. Consonants appear to be responsible for carrying the meaning of speech, while vowels carry the intensity. In peak-clipping circuits, only the highest intensity components of the waveform are removed. Lower-intensity elements are unchanged. Since the highest intensities in speech are the vowels, they are reduced, whereas the lower intensity, meaning-carrying consonants are relatively untouched. Therefore, one would not expect speech intelligibility to suffer appreciably but would expect sound quality to decrease.

Nonlinear Amplification

Some amplifier designs avoid reaching saturation by utilizing an amplification ratio of less than 1:1, that is, 1:2 or 1:3. This is depicted in Figure 2-20, which demonstrates that the gain increase diminishes with increased input (less than a 45° gain function). Such a system minimizes peak-clipping effects by delaying or preventing reaching saturation. Essentially, nonlinear amplification is a simple form of compression amplification (described below), which results in more of the input information being present in the output signal.

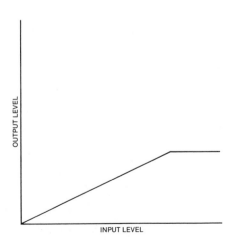

Fig. 2-20. Nonlinear amplifier input-output function.

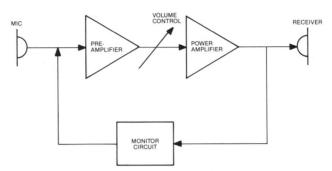

Fig. 2-21. Schematic diagram of an output compression aid.

Compression Amplification

Also referred to as *automatic gain control* (AGC), *automatic volume control* (AVC), and *linear dynamic compression* (LDC), compression amplification is a means of controlling amplifier gain by changing the amplifier characteristics from linear to nonlinear. Its purpose is to both prevent the output from reaching saturation or UCL in the presence of high input levels and to compress the speech signal into the reduced dynamic range of the listener without losing input information.

All compression systems utilize an electronic feedback principle for self-regulation. The circuit monitors the voltage delivered from some point in the system before it reaches the receiver, and activates the compression circuit when appropriate. Figure 2-21 is a schematic drawing of a typical output compression hearing aid. Figure 2-22 presents a typical compression input-output function.

Compression is not a new innovation. Davis et al. (1947) report that as early as 1944 recommendations were made to use compression amplification to limit high output levels as a preferred alternative to peak clipping. The primary advantage of AVC is that none of the signal is lost; the entire signal is compressed. The problem

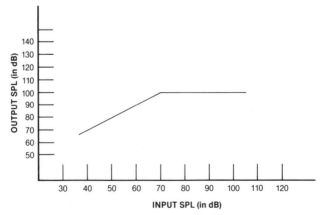

Fig. 2-22. Typical compression input-output function.

was one of size—making the circuit small enough for a wearable hearing aid. Hudgins et al. (1948) demonstrated the feasibility of using AVC in wearable aids. The first commercial wearable aid with it appeared in 1949 (Caraway and Carhart 1967).

VARIABLES

There are four critical variables in any compression system: *limiting level, attack time* (AT), *release time* (RT), and *compression ratio* (CR).

Limiting level, also known as *compression threshold* or *kneepoint,* is the output or input intensity at which the system activates. It is represented by the 100-dB output point in Figure 2-22. The input-output function is linear to the predetermined kneepoint. Above this point, output is restricted because of a gain reduction (increased compression ratio).

The response of a compression system is not instantaneous; some period of time is required for it to operate. This is known as *attack time.* It is the time lapse from the moment signal amplitude (output) exceeds the limiting level to that instant when gain becomes stabilized at a reduced level. Because of the time lag, the output level will momentarily exceed the limiting level and may reach MPO (overshoot) and then immediately decrease as the circuit begins to reduce gain. Because the initial output is so high, the voltage to the AVC system is correspondingly high and, consequently, it may overcompensate to result in a momentary excessively low output (undershoot). After this point, the system stabilizes and continues to operate as long as the input level is high.

To avoid bothersome overshoot and undershoot, and the possibility of the user perceiving a brief period of peak clipping before the attack is completed (a reduction in sound quality), it is generally agreed that AT must be less than 10 msec. The human ear cannot perceive temporal changes of less than 10 msec. Ideally, AT should be as short as possible to prevent sudden loud sounds from being amplified and reaching UCL (Smriga 1985b).

When the input level decreases, it takes a moment for the system to cut off and restore the normal gain function. This time lag is referred to as *release time.* It is defined as the time from the moment input amplitude is decreased to that instant at which gain is again established to within 2 dB of the pre-compressed level. During the lag, the gain remains reduced and, combined with the decreased input, the output momentarily drops. As soon as the appropriate correction is made, output function is restored.

According to Smriga (1986), an ideal RT is difficult to define. If it is too short, the signal-to-noise ratio suffers. A long RT is satisfactory for ongoing signals but not for high intensity, short duration noises. Also, if it is too short, the listener may experience an AGC flutter or "pumping" sensation. Figure 2-16 is an oscilloscopic representation of a compressed signal.

Reference has been made to the time lags involved in AGC operation. As pointed out, a typical AT is less than 10 msec. RT varies between 40 and 150 msec, depending on the circuitry used (Nunley 1973, Berger 1974). These time constants are critical in terms of speech intelligibility. Lynne and Carhart (1963) studied this variable and demonstrated that speech discrimination ability decreased as RT increased. A relatively intense speech component, such as a vowel, can cause the system to operate, with the resulting overshoot. If the circuit is operating, low-intensity consonants can be reproduced too faintly during release, affecting intelligibility.

Most often, RT is longer than AT in order to avoid what is called *AVC flutter*. This condition results when the system reacts to variations in the normal intensity of speech, perhaps even between syllables. Constantly raising and lowering the gain causes a flutter effect. Flutter occurs most often if the RT is too short. An optimal release time is one between the point at which flutter may occur (usually less than 30 msec) and syllables are lost (over about 150 msec).

Advantages Over Peak Clipping

All compression modes have a number of things in common in terms of their advantages over peak clipping. Since none of the amplified signal is lost, as in peak clipping, compressed signals avoid the distortion factor. Output is limited to a level below saturation through a gain reduction to the entire signal. Also, these systems have the effect of expanding the dynamic range for the hearing aid user by providing a wider range of input levels to the ear; yet they do not exceed the tolerance limits of the ear.

Perhaps the most significant benefit in terms of speech intelligibility is that the original signal-to-noise (S/N) ratio of the input signal is maintained. A compressor system decreases the signal and background noise equally. As noted earlier, in a peak clipping circuit only the highest intensity components (usually the primary speech signal vowels) are reduced. For example, consider an instrument with an MPO of 130 dB and a gain of 60 dB being used in an environment with 70 dB of ambient noise and a person speaking at a level of 90 dB (S/N ratio = +20 dB). If this hypothetical aid used peak clipping to avoid reaching MPO, the +20 dB S/N ratio would be lost during amplification. The 70-dB noise would be fully amplified to 130 dB (60-dB gain). On the other hand, the speech would only be amplified 40 dB before it reached MPO and its peak intensities were clipped. The S/N ratio is now 0 dB; the noise is as loud as the speech. If the aid used a compression system, the +20 dB ratio would have been retained, since the gain of the entire input signal would have been reduced.

Output Compression

This type of circuit is the original compression mode and monitors the signal after the power amplifier. It is activated when the output level of the signal reaches a predetermined SPL (system limits or trimpot setting). When the voltage is greater than this preset maximum, the monitor circuit causes a concomitant voltage reduction at the preamplifier. The result is a decrease in the overall circuit voltage and a reduction of the output level. Figure 2-21 is a schematic representation of an output compression (OC) aid.

Note that the monitoring point is *after* the volume control (VC). Therefore, the VC setting will not affect the MPO of the instrument. As a result, the dispenser has direct control over the maximum output of the aid. The advantages are: (1) OC is often the least expensive compression system, (2) the fitter has direct control over the output level, and (3) OC introduces less distortion than peak clipping. The disadvantages are: (1) if the VC is set low, in the presence of higher input levels the preamplifier can saturate, causing peak clipping and its resultant distortion; and (2) since the output ceiling is independent of the volume control setting, higher outputs may not be achievable when desired by the user.

Input Compression

Figure 2-23 is a schematic diagram of an input compression (IC) aid. Note that the monitoring occurs before the power amplifier, being triggered by the voltage output of the preamp. Functionally, that is the only difference between output and input compression systems.

Since the monitoring takes place before the volume control, the VC has a direct effect on the maximum output of the aid. Therefore, the user has control over the MPO. Many IC instruments have trimpot adjustments to set the output maximum in order to avoid exceeding the UCL. The advantages and disadvantages are listed below.

Advantages
1. IC ensures the preamp will not distort.
2. IC introduces less distortion than a peak clipping circuit.
3. The user has control over output SPL.
4. Since the frequency response is not altered, regardless of the input level, IC can prove more effective for speech understanding.

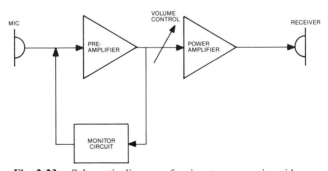

Fig. 2-23.   Schematic diagram of an input compression aid.

Disadvantages
1. The fitter does not have direct control over maximum output levels.
2. Since monitoring occurs before the VC, the user can defeat the purpose of IC by setting the VC at a point where output levels can exceed UCL.

Input-Output Compression

The advantages of both output and input compression (I-O) are generally maintained in systems utilizing both, while the disadvantages of both are reduced or eliminated. Figure 2-24 presents a schematic of this circuit design that utilizes two monitoring points, before and after the volume control. The advantages and disadvantages are listed below.

Advantages
1. It insures that the preamp will not saturate.
2. The fitter has direct control over maximum output.
3. I-O introduces less distortion than any other compression system.

Disadvantages
1. It is more expensive to build, resulting in more costly hearing aids.

Frequency Dependent Compression

One of the potential problems with conventional IC systems is that it is possible for low-frequency noise to activate the compression when higher-frequency speech signals continue to require full linear amplification to be maximally intelligible.

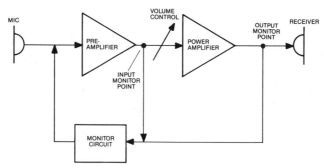

Fig. 2-24. Schematic diagram of an aid utilizing both input and output compression.

Frequency-dependent compression (FDC) designs utilize a higher compression threshold for low-frequency inputs (below 800 to 1600 Hz) than for higher frequencies. The higher threshold for low frequencies prevents premature activation of the circuit, maintaining linear amplification for medium and high-frequency speech sounds when needed. Thus, the circuit activation is determined by both intensity and frequency.

FDC instruments are optimal for individuals who must function in high-noise environments, resulting in an improved signal-to-noise ratio and greater speech intelligibility.

High-Level Compression

As discussed above, if a compression circuit is not frequency-dependent, it may be activated by moderate input levels (below 65 dB), thus possibly degrading speech intelligibility. This is avoided by a high-level compression (HLC) system that utilizes a higher compression threshold, usually above 70 dB SPL. The aid is linear through this input intensity, deferring compressor action until high input levels are reached. Therefore, it provides protection from uncomfortable impulse sounds while providing improved speech understanding via an improved signal-to-noise ratio.

Automatic Signal Processing

One of the most misused and least understood terms concerning hearing aid design and function is *signal processing*. Fundamentally, *any hearing aid that is nonlinear is a signal processor.* If the output signal differs from the input signal in any parameter other than intensity, the hearing aid has functioned as a signal processor. According to Brunved (1985), an automatic signal processor (ASP) is "any device that acoustically, electronically or electrically alters a signal in frequency, intensity or time."

In practice, hearing aids that are designated as ASP instruments perform specific functions to attempt to solve, at least partially, the greatest problem for most hearing aid users—understanding speech in the presence of background noise. Even people with normal hearing or a mild hearing loss, who have little, if any, difficulty understanding speech in quiet, can experience a significant intelligibility decrement in noise.

The problem for any signal processor is to improve speech intelligibility in noise while maintaining performance in quiet. Kates (1986a) defines signal processing as "the manipulation of the signal to enhance or extract the information it contains."

Since there are a variety of operations performed by hearing aids designated as signal processors by their manufacturers, it is understandable that confusion exists regarding what an ASP aid does. Hopefully, manufacturers will soon clearly define the nature of the signal manipulations carried out by instruments they designate as signal processing.

For purposes of this discussion, four operational classifications of signal processing hearing aids are considered here: *loglinear compression, automatic pass-band adjustment, band-splitting amplifiers, and the zeta noise blocker circuit.* The last of these will be described below, under digital processing.

LOGLINEAR COMPRESSION

Figure 2-25 compares the input-output functions of a linear amplifier and a loglinear system. At low-intensity input levels, a loglinear system offers more gain than a linear circuit. As the input level increases, and the limiting level is reached, compression is activated and further increases in gain are reduced relative to the linear amplifier (Smriga 1986).

A loglinear system typically has a low compression threshold and a shallow compression ratio. This approach has been shown to often result in reduced speech understanding in the presence of high noise levels, since the noise activates the compression function of the system, creating a possible foreground/background distortion.

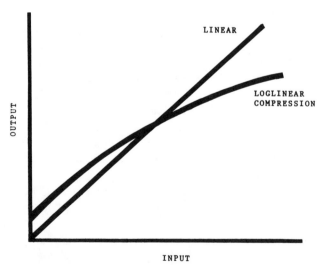

Fig. 2-25. Input-output functions of linear and loglinear amplifiers. (Courtesy of Telex Communications, Inc.)

AUTOMATIC PASSBAND ADJUSTMENT

One of the first hearing aids described as ASP utilized this variation of input frequency-dependent compression. It is a one channel signal processor that has a greater compression range than a typical IC system (as much as a 30–60-dB range). It is frequency dependent in that compression is greater for low frequencies so as to, theoretically, improve the signal-to-noise ratio. For example, in one such system, sounds below 500 Hz and greater than 50 dB that are present for more than 5 msec are considered to be noise and are automatically filtered. In essence, this type of system acts like an automatic high-pass tone control (Heide 1985).

PASSBAND SPLITTING

Another approach to signal processing, presently limited by component size to BTE instruments, is the utilization of a two-channel circuit, one high-pass and the other low-pass. Typically the split occurs at about 800 Hz, although this may be adjustable via a trimpot adjustment. The low-pass channel uses input compression, while the high-pass band is linear. Therefore, as the input level increases, low-frequency amplification decreases. This results in an *automatic passband narrowing,* which enhances the signal-to-noise ratio.

Any automatic signal processing system adjusts itself according to the characteristics of the input signal—it will generally have one frequency response in quiet and a different one as the background noise levels change. The manner in which the signal processor adapts to changes in the auditory environment and modifies its performance parameters defines its function. Keep in mind that ASP is only a *marketing term* with many meanings and without a strict technical definition. It is important to understand the actual function being performed (Kates 1986b).

ADAPTIVE COMPRESSION

One approach to compression amplification (Smriga 1985b) assumes that an "ideal" RT would likely vary from listening situation to listening situation, depending on the duration of the unwanted background noise. Accordingly, one manufacturer adapted technology from the broadcasting industry and developed a compression circuit utilizing an *automatically variable release time.* The monitoring system adjusts the RT in response to the average noise duration. For short duration signals the compression time is reduced and the RT is shorter. For longer duration sounds, the compression time and RT are longer. The RT will vary within a finite range between 50 and 500 msec (Smriga 1986).

Adaptive compression is basically an input-output design, with monitoring occurring both before and after the power amplifier. This is schematically presented in Figure 2-26. Since the frequency response of the instrument does not change, as

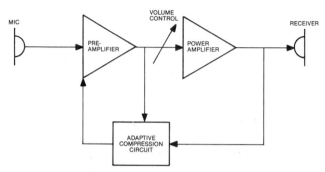

Fig. 2-26. Schematic diagram of an adaptive compression aid.

in FDC, any degradation in speech intelligibility caused by low-frequency noise is likely to remain.

SELECTING A COMPRESSION DESIGN

With the multitude of compression systems available today, a hearing aid fitter has the often difficult task of selecting the optimal design for each user. Dillon and Walker (1983) present three strategies to consider when making these decisions. These considerations are based upon the needs of the patient.

For an individual requiring *low distortion* along with *maximum output limiting,* the optimal system is one that provides: a *high compression threshold* (limiting level) so that the aid functions linearly most of the time and goes into compression just below saturation; a *high compression ratio* so that when the compression is activated, further increases in input intensity will result in little if any increase in output; and *short time constants*, especially RT. The authors suggest that the limiting level should be preset to a fixed value and be independent of the volume control setting. This is best achieved with an *output compression* design with a trimmer set kneepoint.

For cases where *maintenance of the most comfortable loudness (MCL)* in the presence of a reduced dynamic range is of primary importance, we need a system that will keep the output level relatively constant in the presence of ongoing fluctuations of the input signal "without altering the loudness relationships between adjacent individual elements of the speech signal" (Dillon and Walker 1983). *This is the most common reason for using compression amplification.* The optimal system for achieving the goal of keeping the long-term average intensity of the signal at a comfortable level is one that provides a *low compression threshold, high compression ratio*, and *longer time constants* (slow-acting AGC). This can best be achieved by utilizing a *frequency-dependent input compression* instrument. Using a long RT helps to maintain some of the natural intensity fluctuations in speech and to preserve the real-life signal-to-noise ratio.

For true recruiting ears, it is often necessary to alter the relationships between various syllables, referred to by Dillon and Walker (1983), as *whole-range syllable compression.* In such a situation we want all the sounds of interest to the user to be present within the working range of the compressor—every possible input signal is modified to a different output level. To achieve this goal, an optimal system needs a *low compression threshold* so the instrument is in compression for most of its operating cycle, a relatively *low compression ratio* that closely approximates the dynamic range compression characteristics of the recruiting ear, as demonstrated by the *alternate binaural loudness balance* (ABLB) test, and *short time constants* with rapid gain changes, almost syllable by syllable. These goals can best be met with an *IC* system if the intent is only to provide overall range reduction or with an *OC* design if the intent is to closely match the loudness recruitment function of the user. Ideally, an *input-output* design will be used.

Keep in mind that all three sets of considerations and their attendant electronic systems will cause the dynamic range of the output signal to be less than that of the input signal. The decision as to which one to employ can be made only after careful analysis of the reasons for using compression.

All the compression systems described above are *analog* in that they directly utilize acoustical energy. As soon as a true digital processing head-worn hearing aid is available, most, if not all, contemporary compression designs will be obsolete.

DIGITAL HEARING AIDS—NOW AND IN THE FUTURE

In recent years, considerable research has been undertaken to incorporate microprocessor digital technology into hearing aids (Levitt 1982, Nunley et al 1983, Schneuwly 1985, Staab 1985 and 1986, Bartschi 1986, Nielsen 1986). A true digital hearing aid is a *wearable computer* that will allow for software adjustment of a hearing aid's parameters.

Digital signal processing (DSP) will permit the dispenser to customize the performance of the aid for an individual user. It will have the capability of multiple reprogramming as the user's needs change. Optimally, a digital aid will have the flexibility *to adapt its performance in the face of changing environments.* According to Staab (1985), this is the primary goal of a digital instrument.

In performing this task, the greatest difficulty faced by hearing aid users, understanding speech in the presence of background noise, could be practically eliminated. Among the other potential benefits of digital technology in hearing aids are: *elimination of mechanical switches and moving parts* (common sources of breakdown); *greater circuit stability; more precise, variable filtering; programming of earmold acoustics into the aid; elimination of acoustical feedback; smoother frequency responses; frequency transposition; distortion-free compression capability;* and *extracting speech from noise.*

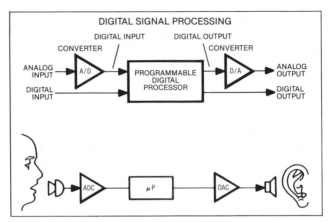

Fig. 2-27. Schematic diagram of a digital hearing aid. (Adapted from Staab WJ: Digital hearing aids. Audiotone Tech Rep 7, 1986. With permission.)

The biggest constraints, so far in the development of digital hearing aids are reduction of component size and a significantly greater power requirement (3 V) than conventional aids. There is no doubt that within the next five to ten years, head-worn digital instruments will be on the market. A body worn prototype has already been developed (Nunley et al. 1983).

Figure 2-27 is a representation of a theoretical digital hearing aid design. It will perform both analog and digital functions. A microphone will convert acoustic energy into electrical energy (analog). An analog-to-digital (A/D) converter will change this analog signal into a digital signal. The signal will pass through a central microprocessing unit that contains the computer programs (digital). A digital-to-analog (D/A) converter will convert the processed digital signal into an analog one that is sent to the receiver.

Zeta Noise Blocker

At the present time (early 1987) there is only one form of digital technology available in hearing aids. The *Zeta Noise Blocker,* which has been incorporated into hearing aids by a few manufacturers, is a combined digital and analog circuit that is designed to analyze an incoming signal and extract unwanted noise from it. It is an integrated circuit and is comprised of four analog filters and a simple digital control unit. *The digital system analyzes the input signal for the presence of noise and automatically adjusts the filters to reduce the background noise.* Its function is similar to some currently available automatic signal processing hearing aids: in the presence of high levels of noise, the bandwidth is restricted adaptively to reduce its interference (Graupe et al. 1986).

These first-generation applications of digital microprocessor technology in

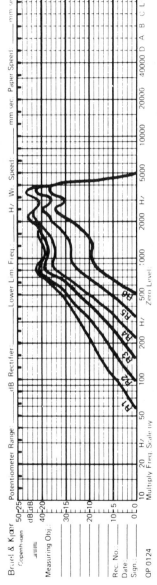

Fig. 2-28. Six different responses available in one hearing aid. (Courtesy of Audiotone.)

67

head-worn hearing aids appear to have several shortcomings (Kates 1986b). Among these are a long AT resulting in a sluggish response, inappropriate filtering resulting from confusing speech for noise or vice versa, high circuit noise, and very short battery life. It is a start, however, and future generations of digital aids will very likely improve dramatically and will certainly cause a drastic change in the entire industry.

ALTERATION OF HEARING AID RESPONSE

There are various methods through which the frequency response of a hearing aid can be altered to meet the specific needs of the user. Modifications of earmolds, tubing, and filter inserts are described in the next chapter.

One method alluded to earlier in this chapter is modification of response through amplifier circuitry. Figure 2-28 presents the various amplification slopes available from one manufacturer. Any one of these slopes is available on many of that company's instruments.

Microphone Placement

Hearing aid microphones can be located in various positions in ear-level (top of ear and bottom behind the ear) and eyeglass instruments (temple piece forward and frame center of head). One factor not often considered is the effect of microphone placement on the frequency response of a hearing aid. Figure 2-29 demonstrates this with four microphone positions, showing the primary effect to be in the 1500–3000-Hz range. The most pertinent observation is the 8–10-dB advantage with the microphone placed at the top rather than at the bottom of the ear in the ear-level case. This can be an effective means of providing additional high-frequency gain.

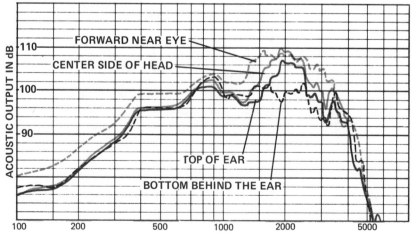

Fig. 2-29. Effect of microphone placement on frequency response. (Courtesy of Zenetron.)

Table 2-2
Battery Life Chart

Battery Drain Current (ma)	675 Battery				13 Battery				312 Battery			
	Mercury Premium 245 mAh		Zinc-Air Premium 520 mAh		Mercury Premium 85 mAh		Zinc-Air Premium 230 mAh		Mercury Premium 45 mAh		Zinc-Air Premium 110 mAh	
	Hours	(Days*)	Hours	(Days*)	Hours	(Days*)	Hours	(Days*)	Hours	(Days*)	Hours	(Days*)
0.4	612	(38)	1300	(81)	213	(13)	575	(36)	113	(7)	275	(17)
0.5	490	(31)	1040	(65)	170	(11)	460	(27)	90	(6)	220	(14)
0.7	350	(22)	743	(46)	121	(8)	329	(21)	64	(4)	157	(10)
1.0	245	(15)	520	(33)	85	(5)	230	(14)	45	(3)	110	(7)
1.4	175	(11)	371	(23)	61	(4)	164	(10)	32	(2)	79	(5)
2.0	123	(8)	260	(16)	43	(3)	115	(7)	23	(1)	55	(3)
2.5	98	(6)	208	(13)	34	(2)	92	(6)	18	(1)	44	(3)
3.0	82	(5)	173	(11)	28	(2)	72	(5)	15	(1)	37	(2)

*Based on 16 hours use per day.

Although efficient from an energy usage point of view, such variance in battery drain makes accurate prediction of battery life almost impossible, because we cannot always predict the user's output needs and actual signal levels. If the manufacturer provides both quiescent and peak drain figures, you can, using the formulas presented on page 70, compute quiescent and peak drain battery life figures. It is safe to assume that the user's average battery life will be somewhere between these two figures.

Another factor to consider is the age of the batteries. As they age over a period of some months, the battery's capacity will diminish. The user may notice a reduced battery life and fault the aid. I counsel my users not to purchase more than one package of batteries, per aid, at a time, and to buy them from us or some other reliable dispenser whose battery stock is fresh. *I discourage buying batteries at drug or discount stores because the age of the batteries is unknown.* This situation is especially relevant for mercury batteries. Zinc-air cells, with the protective tab in place, will have a longer shelf life.

With the development and improvement of zinc-air batteries in the past ten years, most hearing aid users will experience considerably longer battery life at a lower per hour of use cost. Because of the higher and more variable current drain requirements of push-pull amplifier circuits, mercury cells will generally provide longer battery life than zinc-air cells.

PRACTICALITIES AND PHILOSOPHIES

Interpretation of Response Information

Assuming that at least generalized specification sheets and, preferably, individual instrument response characteristics are available from the manufacturer, it takes practice to be able to interpret these data adequately. Most manufacturers use the testing equipment produced by the Bruel and Kjaer (B & K) Company of Copenhagen.

The chart paper has been described in terms of its intensity and frequency scales earlier in this chapter. The left side of Figure 2-32 is a reproduction of the legend area of the graph paper. The information contained therein is vital to accurate interpretation. *Measuring object* identifies the aid being tested and its conditions, specifically, tone control setting, tubing size and length, output control setting, aid model and serial number, AGC setting, input level, and VC setting. The latter two indicate immediately whether the curve is a gain or frequency response function. The differences between these have been described earlier in this chapter. The right side of Figure 2-32 is the frequency response curve obtained with the noted settings.

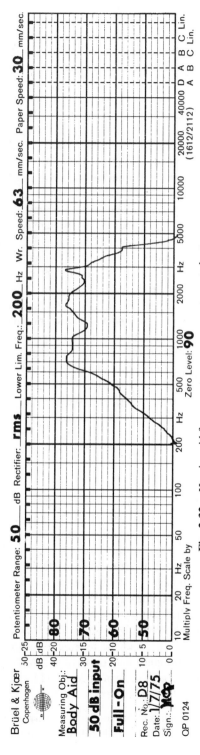

Fig. 2-32. Hearing aid frequency response measurement chart paper.

73

The spaces in the lower section of Figure 2-32 are for information regarding control settings on the test equipment. "Zero level" indicates the intensity value assigned to the "zero" baseline of the graph. This is extremely important, as typical response paper has an intensity (*potentiometer*) range of not more than 50 dB (0–50) on the ordinate. If a hearing aid produces more than 50 dB of gain at any frequency the recording needle will run to the top of the graph and not give complete information. Referring to Figure 2-33, the top of the tracing line is flat, not revealing peaks and valleys in the response. In this example, the zero level was 60 dB, so the potentiometer range was 60–110 dB, but the aid put out a signal greater than 110 dB at some frequencies, resulting in a flattened curve. If the zero level is raised to 70 dB, the range is sufficient to give us the complete information. *Paper speed* (Paper Sp) is the speed with which the graph paper moves through the level recorder, in this case 30 mm/sec. Lower limiting frequency (L Lim Fr) indicates the starting point of the graphic recording, 200 Hz in this example. Potentiometer range (Pot) is either 25 or 50 dB. The latter is most commonly used for hearing aids. Therefore, the interval between horizontal lines on the paper is equal to 2 dB. *Writing speed* (Wr Sp) is the rate of the marking pen movement, 63 mm/sec in this example.

To determine the gain, output, frequency response, or range data from a graph, such as the one in Figure 2-32, one simply follows the procedures outlined for that measure and reads the information off the graph. Note that the intensity scale figures can be read as either gain or output, depending on the reference point. For example, in Figure 2-32 the zero line is 90 dB; therefore, the output at 1000 Hz is 90 + 34 dB (zero level plus graph reading) or 124 dB. Some newer hearing aid test systems provide peak and HFA gain and output data, along with RTG figures.

Practicalities

All manufacturers provide technical specification data sheets for each model of hearing aid they produce. These sheets contain all the required information—gain, output, and frequency response, plus additional information in individual cases. These figures are average responses for the particular model. However, individual aids of that model may vary greatly in terms of gain, output, and frequency range, that is, 10–15-dB variations in gain or output, more or less distortion, and wider or narrower range. Anyone who has measured hearing aid characteristics and compared those measurements to the manufacturer's technical sheets has seen discrepancies. Kasten et al. (1967) demonstrated these differences experimentally.

Therefore, it is to the advantage of the hearing aid dispenser to be provided with or obtain individual performance data on each aid. Many manufacturers now provide these individual data. The American Speech and Hearing Association Conference on Hearing Aid Evaluation Procedures has stated:

Since existing speech tests are often not satisfactorily able to differentiate the performances of various hearing aids, it seems of great importance to know the

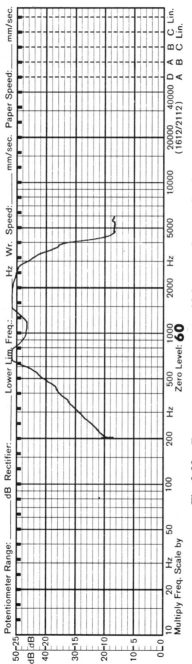

Fig. 2-33. Frequency response curve with inappropriate zero level.

75

electroacoustic characteristics of the various aids . . . knowledge of certain acoustical characteristics of hearing aids is necessary for an evaluation. Therefore the three following considerations should be taken into account: (a) manufacturers' specifications may be incomplete or unavailable; (b) if not available, these specifications must be reported by the centers; and (c) if the center can not determine the characteristics of an aid through its own equipment and personnel, then some arrangement must be made to secure the necessary data.*

What happens to the response of a ear-level aid when the user's head is turned in various directions relative to a sound source? Figure 2-34 shows this relationship. In this example, an ear-level aid with forward-facing microphone was placed on the right ear of KEMAR and a sound source placed to the right of the head. It is obvious that maximum amplification is achieved when the head directly faces the sound source and minimal when it is faced away from the sound. The implication to be drawn from this graph is reinforcement of the concept that a listener should watch the face of a speaker. By doing this, the hearing aid user maximizes the response of the instrument.

Philosophies

While writing this chapter I became aware that the discussions that follow seem to be the most important parts of any consideration of electroacoustic characteristics. If not for the fact that so much background information was necessary to make this section meaningful, I would have included it near the beginning of the chapter.

A close friend of mine is a transactional analyst. I have spoken with him about some of my concerns regarding all the technical aspects of electroacoustic measurements being related to hardware and not to the person who is going to wear the hearing aid. He described the lack of consideration for realistic hearing aid measurements as *bull-kaka*.

That term perfectly described my feelings. All measures of hearing aid function have no meaning unless they can be related to listener behavior. The standard measures do not tell us much, really. They are designed to describe hearing aids in the absence of the listener. If they are to have any meaning, we must be able to predict how they will affect the patient. Until a means of accurately predicting this is found, we have two isolated phenomena—hearing aid performance and listener performance. In Chapter 4, Joe Millin presents some of his ideas on this and related matters. It is an important chapter and should be read carefully.

---

*Reprinted from Castle WE: A conference on hearing aid evaluation procedures. ASHA Reports No. 2, 1967.

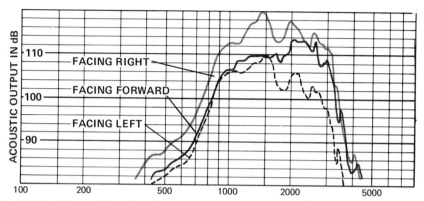

Fig. 2-34. Effect of head turning on frequency response of a BTE aid. (Courtesy of Zenetron.)

KEMAR

When the 2-cc hard-walled coupler was developed some 30 years ago, *it was not designed to yield a response similar to that of the human ear*. The original intent was to provide a means of quality control (comparing the output of one unit of a hearing aid model with that of another unit of the same model) and a consistent electroacoustic measurement standard for the exchange of data between laboratories.

This was true for two reasons: (1) the volume of a typical adult human ear between the medial end of an earmold and the tympanic membrane is about 1.2 cc, not 2 cc; and (2) the hard-walled 2-cc coupler does not approximate the acoustic impedance of the human ear. For these reasons, the acoustical energy transfer functions are significantly different for the 2-cc coupler and a real ear. The effects of these differences will be demonstrated below.

The 2-cc coupler was *never intended for use as a means of selecting a hearing aid* that is appropriate for a particular hearing loss. The typical 2-cc coupler curves provided on manufacturers' specification sheets are not intended to reflect the response of the instrument in a user's ear. Yet, over the years, more and more such use has been made of these curves clinically, as well as in the literature. The various formulas for determining gain by frequency for a hearing loss and non-speech-based hearing aid selection approaches are strongly based on 2 cc rather than real-ear gain and output measurements.

Dalsgaard and Jensen (1976), in discussing the problems with 2-cc coupler measurements, have stated that they "are only of limited value in the clinical practice due to the large difference between the (2-cc) measuring conditions and the actual in-situ (real ear) conditions of use for a hearing aid. . . . These differences are, however, generally overlooked in daily clinical work."

Differences Between 2-cc and Real-Ear Measurements

Sachs and Burkhard (1972a,b) have shown that, generally speaking, *comparisons of hearing aid responses measured in a 2-cc coupler and in a real ear demonstrate a pattern of consistent differences.*

1. Below 800 Hz sound pressure levels in the 2-cc coupler are about 4 dB lower than in the real ear.
2. Between 800 and 8500 Hz, the average real-ear/2-cc ratio increases with frequency at about 3.5 dB/octave. In other words, 2-cc coupler measurements are 5 dB less than real ear measurements at 1000 Hz, 12 dB less at 4000 Hz. The ratio increase is understandable at the higher frequencies because the effective volume of the tympanic membrane, which is a significant portion of the total effective closed volume, decreases. Therefore, the ear impedance does not decrease as rapidly with frequency as does the 2-cc coupler impedance.

The upper two curves of Figure 2-35 show these differences. The top curve is the mean and range measurements of real ear hearing aid gain on 11 ears. The next lower curve is the same hearing aid response as measured in a 2-cc coupler.

Various clinical studies have also demonstrated these differences. As early as 1959, Van Eysbergen and Groen, based on 2-cc/real-ear measurement differences, recommended using the 2-cc coupler only for informational exchanges between

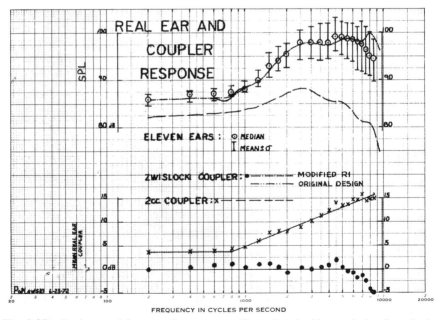

FREQUENCY IN CYCLES PER SECOND

Fig. 2-35. Real-ear and 2-cc coupler response. (Reproduced with permission from Sachs RM, Burkhard MD: Earphone pressure response in ears and couplers. Eighty-third meeting of the Acoustical Society of America, 1972b.)

laboratories. Studebaker and Zachman (1970) and McDonald and Studebaker (1970) showed that the 2-cc coupler is not adequate for either evaluation of hearing aids for clinical purposes or evaluation of earmold modification effects (Chapter 3). The data of these two studies indicate that the measured differences leave many unresolved questions, particularly in higher-frequency regions.

Studies by Tonnison (1975) and Pascoe (1975) provide data again indicating that 2-cc coupler measurements do not adequately reflect real ear hearing aid performance and could lead to erroneous conclusions about hearing aid performance.

Zwislocki Coupler

The documented problems inherent in the use of the 2-cc coupler for clinical hearing aid measurements and a general dissatisfaction with the 2-cc coupler as a basis for predicting sound levels developed by hearing aids at the tympanic membrane led Zwislocki (1971a,b) to develop an alternative coupler. The Zwislocki coupler reproduces the eardrum impedances of a typical adult human ear. Its volume is close to estimates of the volume remaining when the meatus is occluded with an earmold, 1.2 cc.

The coupler has four side-branch resonators that synthesize the acoustic impedance variations in real ears. The "tympanic membrane" is a one-half inch condenser microphone (Fig. 2-36). The four side-branches comprise inertance, resistance, and compliance of the ear canal to create what Zwislocki estimated to be an acoustic impedance approximating that of a normal human adult eardrum.

Referring back to the upper curve in Figure 2-35, it is the response of a hearing aid measured in a Zwislocki coupler. You can see how closely it approximates the means of the measurements taken in real ears. According to Sachs and Burkhard (1972a), between 800 and 7500 Hz, "the mean pressure in real ears and in the Zwislocki coupler differ by no more than 2 dB." Below 800 Hz, "pressure in the Zwislocki coupler is essentially identical to pressure in real ears (with no earmold leaks)."

KEMAR: A Manikin Using the Zwislocki Coupler for Hearing Aid Measurements

One of the major problems with the utilization of electroacoustic measurements in hearing aid fittings is the poor agreement between these measurements and behavioral measurements. The latter include the effect of the user—head diffraction and/or body baffle effects and ear canal resonances interacting with the physical characteristics of the hearing aid to influence the aid's performance on the person. Because of these strong interactions between the hearing aid and the wearer, it is important to include the diffraction and resonance effects in any hearing aid measurements that are to be considered in clinical hearing aid selection procedures. While this idea sounds good on the surface, many inherent problems exist that confound the situation.

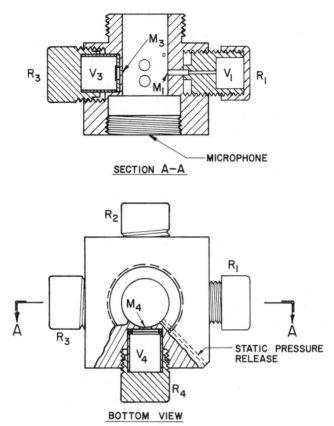

SECTION A-A

BOTTOM VIEW

Fig. 2-36. Schematic diagram of the Zwislocki coupler. (Reproduced with permission from Burkhard MD: Gain technology, in Burkhard MD (ed): Manikin Measurements. Elk Grove Village, Knowles Electronics, 1978.)

As a result of these considerations, Knowles Electronics, Inc., developed an anthropometric manikin to facilitate in situ (on the head) measurements of hearing aid performance (Burkhard and Sachs 1975). Named *KEMAR* (Knowles Electronics Manikin for Acoustic Research), the manikin utilizes the Zwislocki coupler to simulate the acoustic response of a human ear in a free field.

Figure 2-37 is a photograph of the KEMAR manikin in an anechoic chamber. Figure 2-38 shows the Zwislocki coupler inside the head of KEMAR. KEMAR consists of a head and torso, and has the dimensions of an average human adult, including pinnae and ear canals. Using KEMAR it is possible to observe the effects of body and head diffraction on an acoustic signal traveling through a sound field to the ear.

According to Knowles and Burkhard (1975) and Burkhard (1977), a manikin has several other advantages for in situ hearing aid measurements: (1) it is a reproducible test subject that allows for uniformity between laboratories; (2) it can

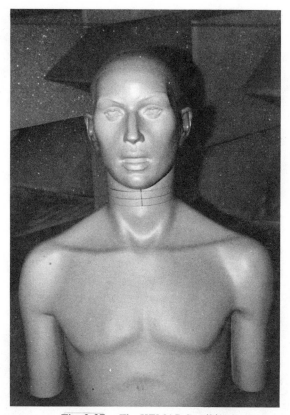

Fig. 2-37. The KEMAR manikin.

be stationary indefinitely for testing; (3) KEMAR can repeatedly be positioned in the same way; and (4) unlike human subjects, the manikin doesn't show response changes as a result of fatigue or other physiologic or psychological changes.

Figure 2-39 depicts the response of the Zwislocki coupler in KEMAR. The input signal for this measurement was an acoustically flat sweep frequency tone at 60 dB SPL. The gain shown demonstrates the effects of diffraction and canal resonance. These data agree with Burkhard's (1977) real-ear measures. We see different gain at the tympanic membrane (coupler microphone) as compared to sound pressure levels at the entrance to the canal, which results from standing-wave resonances in the canal plus the resonances of the pinna and head shadow. It can be referred to as *unaided ear gain.* In other words, to utilize the Zwislocki coupler in hearing aid measurements simulating use on a human ear, it is necessary to use the manikin to obtain the true gain of the instrument.

One difficuly involved in using KEMAR is the need for an anechoic chamber to eliminate sound reflections and standing-wave problems as much as possible. If diffraction effects are to be measured, the chamber must be large enough so that the test point is at least one-quarter wavelength distant from the nearest wedge tip.

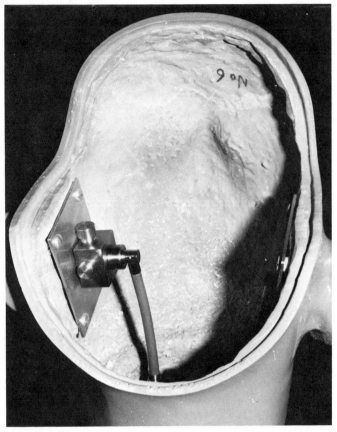

Fig. 2-38. KEMAR with top of head removed to reveal Zwislocki coupler in place.

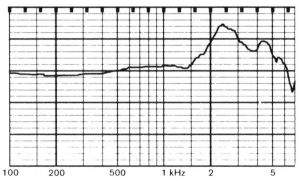

| 100 | 200 | 500 | 1 kHz | 2 | 5 |

Fig. 2-39. Frequency response of Zwislocki coupler in KEMAR.

Therefore, if we want to make measurements to 150 Hz or below, the test point must be at least 22 in from the nearest wedge tip—yielding a chamber that is a minimum of a 6 foot cube. Unfortunately, most of us, clinically, have neither the space nor money for such a room and must therefore depend on data from manufacturers and other research facilities. To date, relatively little of the published KEMAR research has had much clinical applicability. This is discussed in greater depth below.

Another unresolved disagreement concerning KEMAR data is the actual measurement technique to be used. How far should the loudspeaker be from the manikin? Should a compressor control microphone be used during the actual measurements? If so, where should it be located—how far from the speaker and from KEMAR's ear? If not, and the test signal is prerecorded, where should the control microphone be located and should the manikin be present in the field during the recording? Many of these questions have been resolved with the publication of ANSI standard S3.5-1985, the *American National Standard Methods of Measurement of Performance Characteristics of Hearing Aids Under Simulated IN-SITU Working Conditions* (ANSI 1985).

Comparisons of KEMAR and 2-cc Coupler Measurements

How different are response measurements made with KEMAR and with a 2-cc coupler? Figure 2-40 shows such comparisons with two different hearing aids. The upper pairs of curves are SSPL$_{90}$, while the lower pairs are reference test gain.

Studying these curves reveals one of the clinical problems with KEMAR-*variable results*. In the upper curves, KEMAR demonstrates more gain in the mid-frequency range. In the lower set, KEMAR shows greater gain across almost the

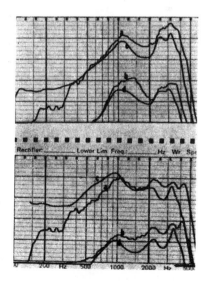

Fig. 2-40. Comparison of responses of two hearing aids measured on KEMAR and in a 2-cc coupler: a = SSPL$_{90}$ on KEMAR; b = RTG on KEMAR; c = SSPL$_{90}$ in 2-cc coupler; d = RTG in 2-cc coupler.

entire range. Helle (1978) studied this and other questions and found no consistent degree pattern of differences for different hearing aid types, although he found the same direction pattern discussed above.

These and other comparative measurements lead to the safe conclusion that 2-cc coupler measurements can seriously underestimate hearing aid gain and output. The problem, as can be seen from these figures, is that *KEMAR/2-cc differences are not constant*. Depending on measurement setup, microphone location, and receiver impedance, the degree of difference will vary. For this reason, *it may not be possible to generate a consistent correction curve, as some manufacturers have attempted, to convert 2-cc curves to KEMAR/real ear curves.*

Cautions

While the Zwislocki coupler and KEMAR have given us much needed information about hearing aid responses, almost as many problems and questions have arisen as have been answered. Some of these, such as inconsistency in degree of change, variables due to microphone placement and receiver impedance, the need for an anechoic chamber, and differences in measurement techniques, have already been discussed above. Because of these factors, caution must be taken in applying KEMAR data to clinical work.

In addition, there is a major caution that we need to consider. However precise KEMAR measurements are, and however similar to average real-ear measurements they are, such data are not absolute. *KEMAR is only an average system,* and many variables need to be taken into account for each patient, as there are no apparent constant factors among real people. Their ears vary in volume, dimensions, impedance, pinna size, and head size (among other differences), all of which will alter the response of the hearing aid on any one particular person. Add to this the response changes possible with earmold modifications (Chapter 3), and many new questions should come to each of us.

At the present time, using KEMAR data we can, at best, begin to make more concrete general predictions about how the aid will function on the ear, up to the tympanic membrane. I hope that future research into meatus volume, pliability of meatus, and pinna tissues and their effect on aid response, along with answers to some of the other questions noted above, will give us data with which we can become much more accurate in our predictions and selections.

In the Meantime. . . .

Until researchers give us this much-needed information, I believe it is becoming highly incumbent upon hearing aid manufacturers to provide us with much more comprehensive technical data about each model they produce. Specifically, I would like to see the following: (1) KEMAR measurements at all aid control settings; (2) specification of measurement procedures; (3) KEMAR versus 2-cc coupler measurements; (4) comprehensive KEMAR curves demonstrating the effects of earmold modifications; and (5) complete data on the standard KEMAR/Zwislocki coupler configuration, as well as data on a modified system that would simulate smaller people, such as children.

REAL-EAR PROBE MICROPHONE MEASUREMENTS*

As was noted above, since its development some 40 years ago, hearing aid dispensers have relied on 2-cc coupler measurements to determine the electroacoustic parameters of appropriate amplification systems for the hearing-impaired. This has occurred despite the injunctions of the developer of the 2-cc coupler (Romanow 1942) that it is not a real-ear simulator and differs from the real ear because of differences in impedance, volume, and diffraction. I will not repeat here the data that is presented above, demonstrating that 2-cc coupler measurements understate low- and midfrequency gain and exaggerate high-frequency measurements, above 2000 Hz, by 10–12 dB/octave.

Despite all of these data, hearing aid fitters, audiologists, and hearing aid dealers alike are only now beginning to acknowledge that 2-cc coupler measurements are not appropriate for describing the sound levels and spectrum delivered to the ear of the hearing aid user.

Realism in Hearing Aid Measurement Techniques

Over the years there has been an extensive search for a quick and reliable clinical procedure for selecting and monitoring optimal amplification. A number of techniques have been developed and implemented for measuring the performance of hearing aids. These methods cross a wide continuum of realism in terms of their accuracy in predicting real-ear performance. Figure 2-41 presents a number of these approaches on a continuum from least realistic to most realistic. As can be seen, the original 2-cc coupler, with its earmold simulator, is the least accurate method, while probe microphone procedures are the most accurate for predicting hearing aid performance on an individual hearing-impaired patient.

CONVERSION FORMULAS

Various researchers have presented data to convert 2-cc coupler data to approximations of real-ear performance (Sachs and Burkhard 1972b; Killion and Monser 1980; Libby 1985, 1986a). Probe microphone measurements eliminate the need for conversion figures in most cases. Libby (1986b) presents updated conversion factors to compute insertion gain from 2-cc coupler measurements. They may be useful when making initial hearing aid preselection, prior to measuring the performance of

---

*I would like to acknowledge Rastronics USA, Inc., for providing the equipment and technical assistance required to gather much of the data reported in this section.

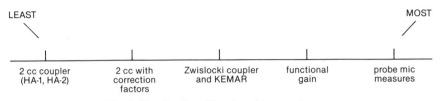

Fig. 2-41.   Reality of hearing aid measurements.

the hearing aid on the user. These figures are presented in Table 2-3 and should be added to the ideal insertion gain figures you have determined for the individual, to compensate for such factors as microphone location, head diffraction, and body baffle and errors in 2-cc coupler measurements. In other words, you are working from insertion gain toward 2-cc coupler data in order to select a hearing aid that, based on its 2-cc coupler response, will most closely produce the insertion gain desired.

FITTING FORMULAS

Whether we admit the fact or not, every hearing aid fitter uses some form of formula approach to selecting an appropriate hearing aid for a patient. Some use the formal prescriptive formulas, such as those described by Berger in Chapter 7. Others use a "seat of the pants" approach that entails eyeballing specification sheet frequency response curves and comparing them to the patient's audiogram. Most of these approaches, formal or informal, are based on some variation of Lybarger's (1944) so-called half-gain rule.

REAL-EAR SIMULATING COUPLER

As described above, the Zwislocki coupler and the KEMAR manikin represent an average normal ear. This system has been used extensively in recent years as an

Table 2-3
Insertion Gain to 2-cc Coupler Conversion Factors

Type of Aid	250	500	1000	2000	3000	4000	6000
ITE (unvented)	−4	−4	−4	+1	+3	−3	−8
BTE (unvented)	−4	−4	−3	+6	+10	+5	+3
Vented*	−13	+2	0	0	0	0	0
IROS†/CROS*	−36	−24	−12	0	+3	0	0
3-mm Libby horn*	−1	−2	−3	0	+6	+8	+2

*Corrections added to those for ITE a BTE fitting.
†IROS: ipsilateral routing of signal.
Adapted from Libby ER: State-of-the-art of hearing aid selection procedures. Hearing Instruments 36:30–38 62, 1985, and Libby ER: The 1/3–2/3 insertion gain hearing aid selection guide. Hearing Instrument 37: 27–28, 1986b.

approximation of real-ear measurements. KEMAR is not an actual hearing-impaired person, however, and does not take into consideration the considerable variations from person to person that will affect the performance of a hearing aid in the individual's ear.

FUNCTIONAL GAIN

Comparison of unaided and aided soundfield thresholds for warble tones, narrow bands of noise, or some other stimulus, is utilized to give a reasonably close approximation of the gain provided by the hearing aid in the user's ear. Sound field audiometry (functional gain) is, obviously, the closest approximation to reality without probe microphone measurements. However, functional gain measures are plagued by a number of variables related to the reliability of the signal and the patient. Among these are subject threshold variability, measurements at only a limited number of discreet frequencies, the necessity for a sound booth or sound treated room, and excessive testing time.

None of these methods has received universal acceptance since most are based on inferences from behavioral tests or dependent on the conversion of laboratory data to real ears.

It is necessary that we finally acknowledge the fact that, for an amplification system to work optimally, we must consider the various factors that influence the signal that reaches the user's tympanic membrane. Figure 2-42 describes a variety of these variables, ranging from sound source and environmental noise to baffle and diffraction effects to earmold acoustics and canal effects. Although this figure presents a BTE hearing aid, these variables are very similar for ITE and canal fittings.

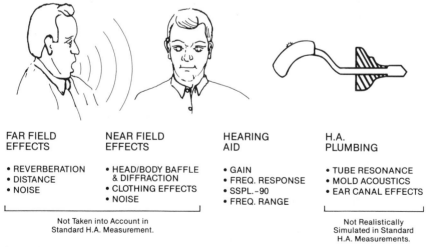

FAR FIELD EFFECTS	NEAR FIELD EFFECTS	HEARING AID	H.A. PLUMBING
• REVERBERATION	• HEAD/BODY BAFFLE	• GAIN	• TUBE RESONANCE
• DISTANCE	& DIFFRACTION	• FREQ. RESPONSE	• MOLD ACOUSTICS
• NOISE	• CLOTHING EFFECTS	• SSPL.–90	• EAR CANAL EFFECTS
	• NOISE	• FREQ. RANGE	

Not Taken into Account in
Standard H.A. Measurement.

Not Realistically
Simulated in Standard
H.A. Measurements.

Fig. 2-42. Variables affecting the spectrum and level of an auditory signal from source (hearing aid) to tympanic membrane.

Historical Perspective

Attempts at obtaining real-ear measurements are not new. Weiner and Ross (1946) published the first report of such endeavors. This was followed by the work of Ewertsen et al. (1957) and Kraup and Scott-Nielsen (1965). Most of these studies attempted to gather information regarding the resonance characteristics of the human ear canal.

All of these studies culminated in the classic report of Shaw (1974), in which he summarized data from some eleven other studies with his own real-ear data to present the first concrete analysis of pinna and canal resonance effects. This was the first study that concretely demonstrated the high-frequency natural amplification of the ear canal, peaking at approximately 17 dB in the range of 2700–2800 Hz. Dalsgaard and Jensen (1976) replicated Shaw's study, verifying his mean resonance curve, but pointing out the variability from subject to subject. These intersubject differences involve both the amplitude of the resonance peak and the frequency at which it occurs. For example, I have measured open ear canal resonance on otoscopically normal ears that have demonstrated resonance peaks ranging from 16 dB at 2400 Hz to 23 dB at 2500 Hz to 15 dB at 3500 Hz. I have also seen cases that demonstrate considerably less canal resonance than any of these examples. Figure 2-43 shows canal resonance curves on three otoscopically normal left ears. While subject A demonstrates an essentially flat resonance peak at about 13 dB from 2000 to above 3000 Hz, subject B demonstrates a peak of 15 dB at 3000 Hz, and subject C exhibits a peak of 23 dB at about 2500 Hz. These examples, along with the data of Dalsgaard and Jensen, support the view that simulations of average normal ear response (KEMAR) and conversion formulas could result in misleading indications

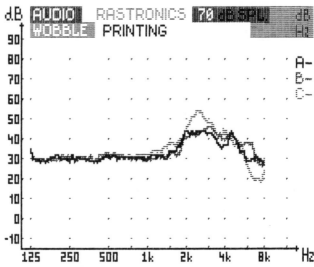

Fig. 2-43. Open-ear resonance curves on three otoscopically normal ears.

of the spectrum and intensity of the signal reaching an individual user's tympanic membrane. Also to be considered are surgically altered ears, especially those that have undergone fenestration and mastoidectomy. Both of these procedures dramatically alter the size and shape of the canal, resulting in a myriad of resonance patterns, ranging from a near absence of canal resonance to a resonance curve that can demonstrate multiple peaks. All of this strongly suggests the need for real-ear measurements on each patient.

The early probe microphone systems had severe limitations for clinical use, especially time of operation, possible tissue damage, and the need for an additional probe bore in the earmold (Nielsen 1985). Harford (1980) was among the first to propose the use of real-ear measurements for the verification of hearing aid performance in a clinical setting. He utilized a popular, commercially available hearing aid test box and customized tiny electret microphones, substituting the patient's ears for the test box.

In more recent years, a number of clinical probe microphone systems have been introduced, utilizing a subminiature electret microphone and a soft silicone probe tube to reduce the chances of physical damage. As Harford (1980, 1981, 1984), Schwartz (1986), and Preves (1986) have indicated, there are a number of desirable features that are or should be present in any clinically useful system to verify hearing aid selection on the user. Among these features are:

1. Quick, simple, reliable, and repeatable testing procedures and results.
2. General applicability across the entire age and gender spectrum of the population.
3. Requires no special test environment.
4. The computer system is menu-driven for ease of operation.
5. Provides both insertion gain and in situ response (see below).
6. Allows for variable input levels.
7. Has both video screen and hardcopy capability for presentation of results.
8. Has the ability to store, recall, and erase data.
9. Has a choice of stimuli, both wide and narrow in frequency bands.

In other words, the system should be easy to operate, be fast, and provide reliable data. Such a system removes the guesswork and mystique from the hearing and selection and verification process, and removes the fatigue factor from the comparative hearing aid evaluation procedures that we have used for so long.

Terminology

At the time of this writing, efforts are under way to establish a national standard for probe microphone measurements. Preves and Sullivan (1987) have proposed modifying the definitions in ANSI S3.35-1985 (ANSI 1985) "by simply substituting 'wearer' for 'manikin' and omitting 'simulated.'" Realizing that some terms may be altered when a national standard is adopted, I will utilize the Preves and Sullivan format throughout this discussion.

INSERTION GAIN

Also known as *orthotelephonic gain* and *etymotic gain, insertion gain* is the *difference between the SPL produced by the hearing aid in the wearer's ear and the SPL in the wearer's ear with the hearing aid absent.* In other words, it is the difference between the aided and unaided (open ear) sound pressure level measured at or near the tympanic membrane. It is a relative measure of the real-ear gain of the hearing aid, and correlates well up to 4000–5000 Hz with soundfield functional gain measurements obtained in a typical hearing aid evaluation (Harford 1984, Preves 1985, Dillon and Murray 1987). In other words, insertion gain is the increase in the sound pressure level measured at the tympanic membrane, with the hearing aid operating on the ear, compared to the sound pressure level at the same point without a hearing aid present and with the ear canal occluded. According to Killion (1985), insertion gain is an indication of the amplification the hearing aid is providing for the patient to compensate for the hearing loss.

As will be discussed below, when an ear is occluded with an earmold or ITE hearing aid, the open-ear canal resonance will be reduced, eliminated or distorted, depending on the degree to which the ear is occluded. For this reason, open-ear canal resonance is not included in insertion gain measurements, as can be seen in Figure 2-44. A full explanation of this figure will be undertakened below.

IN SITU RESPONSE

In situ response is considered to be an absolute measurement of the total response of the hearing aid system, including the anatomy of the user's ear. It is the *difference between the SPL produced by the hearing aid in the wearer's ear and a reference SPL at a defined point in a free field.* It is a measurement of the total hearing aid response, including the head and body diffraction effects. Studies by Schwartz (1986) have shown the in situ measurements correlate well with KEMAR hearing aid measurements.

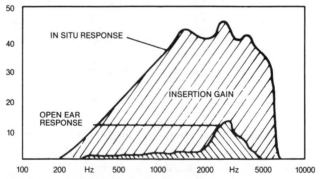

Fig. 2-44. Insertion gain and in situ response. (Reproduced from Nielsen HB: Hearing aid fitting based on insertion gain measurements. Audecibel 34:16–19, 1985.)

There is disagreement concerning whether insertion gain or in situ response is the more important measurement for hearing aid selection and validation. Harford (1985, 1986) and Schwartz (1986) state that in situ is the more important because it is an indication of what signal is reaching the tympanic membrane, including byproducts of the interaction between the output of the aid, the anatomy of the ear, and the head and body effects, including the open ear canal resonance. On the other hand, Preves and Sullivan (1987) quote from ANSI S3.35, "The in situ frequency response does not represent the acoustical assistance provided by the hearing aid because the wearer's unoccluded ear gain frequency response is included. Consequently, the use of in situ frequency response without an accompanying insertion gain frequency response can be misleading and is strongly discouraged." In addition, if one were to compare insertion gain and in situ response measures of real-ear response, it appears that insertion gain is more easily reproducible and freer from artifacts than is the in situ data. As was noted above, a strong correlation exists between probe microphone insertion gain and behavioral functional gain data.

Figure 2-44 presents the open-ear canal resonance and in situ response for an individual. By definition, the in situ response is the total response of the hearing aid system, while the insertion gain is the difference between the open-ear response and the in situ response. Figure 2-45 is another presentation of the same concepts. These measurements were obtained from an otoscopically normal ear using a canal hearing aid. The A curve is the insertion gain for the hearing aid, while the B curve is the open ear canal resonance, and the C curve is the in situ response. As can be seen, if you subtract the insertion gain curve from the in situ gain curve, the result will be an approximation of the open-ear canal resonance.

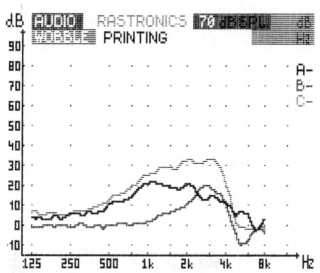

Fig. 2-45. Real-ear measurements (canal aid) depicting insertion gain (A), open-ear resonance (B), and in situ response (C).

INSERTION LOSS

Various authors (Petersen et al. 1982, Libby 1985) have demonstrated a decrease in unaided sound pressure level at the tympanic membrane when the ear canal is occluded. *The insertion of an earmold or hearing aid in the ear canal will change the resonance pattern of the ear.* Primarily, this occurs for two reasons: (1) the loss of head/body baffle and pinna effects, and (2) a change occurs in the resonance characteristics of the canal by occluding and shortening it. The resonance frequency of a cavity is, in part, related to its length and volume. Shortening the canal with an earmold or hearing aid results in an upward shift of the resonance frequency, at least an octave or more in most cases. The result of this is effectively eliminating the natural resonance amplification of the ear. This is a loss of as much as 15–20 dB of resonance between 2500 to 3500 Hz. Figure 2-46 shows the open-ear canal resonance (A curve) for an individual, along with this same measurement with the ear occluded by a nonfunctional canal hearing aid (B curve). Note the dramatic loss of resonance amplification from 2000 Hz to over 4000 Hz.

This loss of natural resonance is alleviated, to some extent, through the use of venting in the earmold or ITE hearing aid. The more the canal is open, the less will be the loss of resonance amplification. For example, Figure 2-47 demonstrates the reduced effects on the resonance pattern with a tube-fit BTE instrument. This figure shows that two different sizes of tubing (3-mm horn and No. 13), leaving the canal relatively open, have less effect on the natural resonance than does a closed earmold or canal hearing aid, as shown in Figure 2-46.

According to Libby (1986), the measurement of insertion loss due to earmold or hearing aid occlusion plays a significant role in determining insertion require-

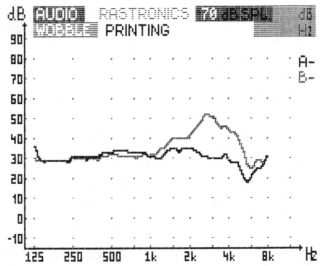

Fig. 2-46. Insertion loss with canal occluded: A = occluded resonance (unaided); B = open-ear resonance.

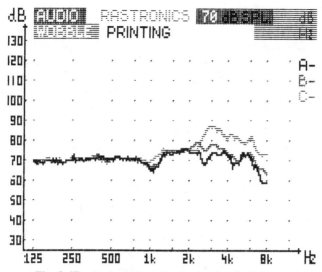

Fig. 2-47.   Reduced insertion loss with tube fitting.

ments for an individual hearing-impaired patient. A mild loss, requiring a nonoccluding mold hearing aid system, with minimum insertion loss, will require little compensation for insertion loss when determining the appropriate insertion gain figures. Conversely, a closed earmold system for a profound loss can create an insertion loss of 20–25 dB or more and may require an insertion gain of up to two-thirds of the unaided hearing threshold levels. *The greater the insertion loss, the greater is the need to compensate for it when determining necessary insertion gain figures for an individual's hearing loss.*

The importance of insertion loss becomes even more significant when we consider the long-term average intensity of the spectrum. Figure 2-48 presents a graphic depiction of this long-term average intensity function. Note how the intensity of speech sounds decreases toward the high frequencies, the range most impor-

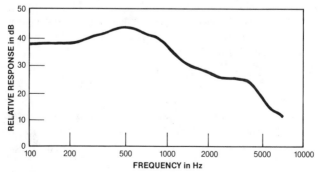

Fig. 2-48.   Long-term average intensity of speech as a function of frequency.

tant for speech perception. The natural open-ear canal resonance helps to partially restore that decrease. If we lose that boost by inserting an earmold or ITE instrument, without compensating for this loss with additional insertion gain, speech perception will likely suffer. This may, at least partially, explain why functional gain measurements typically do not demonstrate the amount of high frequency amplification, especially above 2500 Hz, that would be predicted by most prescriptive formula approaches.

Differences between Insertion Gain and 2-cc Coupler Measurements

Madsen (1986) discusses five reasons for the noted discrepancies between insertion gain and 2-cc coupler measurements: (1) in practice, the hearing aid is mounted on the head of the patient, which changes the gain and spectrum characteristics of the aid as a result of diffraction effects; (2) the size of the sound channel in an earmold or ITE hearing aid will differ from the dimensions of the channel in the earmold simulator of a 2-cc coupler; (3) the earmold or the ITE hearing aid will not always fit snugly in the ear canal. In many cases there will be leakage around the mold or aid that will change the frequency response, especially in the low frequencies; (4) the acoustic impedance of the cavity between the earmold tip and the tympanic membrane, combined with the impedance of the tympanic membrane itself, will not be equal to the impedance of a simple 2-cc cavity; and (5) insertion of an earmold into the canal will change the resonance patterns of the canal.

Clinical Applications of Probe Microphone Measurements

Real-ear measurements reflect the output of the hearing aid interacting with the impedance characteristics of the ear. Because these measurements are physical, they require only passive cooperation by the patient and avoid many of the difficulties associated with functional gain measurements. Such systems finally enable the hearing aid fitter to see, rather than assume or make an educated guess about, the response of the hearing aid in place in the user's ear. Now, when we make adjustments to the trimpots on the aid, modify the earmold, or try various hearing aids on the patient, we are able to objectively view how closely the response of the aid matches the desired frequency response. Invariably, this will result in much more precise and satisfactory hearing aid fittings.

Also, when a patient complains about sound quality, "barrel effect," or tolerance problems, we are able to objectify these reports and visualize the factors in the response of the hearing aid that may be causing these complaints. Probe microphone measurements bring us a major step closer to determining how well the combination of the hearing aid, earmold, and the individual's ear canal is performing in order to provide the user with the kind of electroacoustic characteristics that that person's hearing loss and demands placed on that person's hearing warrant. These measurements are the link between the user's perceptual comments and objective measurement.

I want to stress that *probe measurements are not being presented as a substitute for speech discrimination testing as part of a hearing aid evaluation, but rather as a reliable alternative for functional gain measurements.*

ORDERING CUSTOM AIDS

The use of correction factors, such as those presented in Table 2-3, can assist us greatly in selecting BTE hearing aids for our patients. However, they are not useful when ordering custom ITE or in-the-canal aids. Typically, the manufacturer determines the frequency response of the instrument based on the audiogram and speech testing information that is included with the order. The use of probe microphone measurements may prove to be of assistance in ordering custom aids. First, measure open- and closed-ear canal resonance and send this to the manufacturer along with the order for the instrument. These measurement will approximate the insertion loss that will result from an ITE instrument. When requested, the manufacturer may be able to compensate for this insertion loss when building the aid. Additionally, using a BTE instrument and a stock mold on a patient to simulate the electroacoustic characteristics and venting of an ITE instrument, measure the insertion gain and in-situ gain with this configuration and send it with the other data to the manufacturer. This may also assist them in building a more appropriate instrument for your patient.

"USE" GAIN

Lybarger (1944) presented the classic work that resulted in our adoption of the so-called half-gain rule, which stated that "use" setting for a hearing aid should approximate half of the hearing loss. During the past 35 years, various proposals and studies have suggested that the half-gain rule may not be appropriate for all hearing aid users (Fletcher 1952, Harford 1984, Leijon et al. 1984, Libby 1985, Schwartz 1986). One potential problem with prescriptive formula approaches for hearing aid selection is that most, if not all, of them are based on the half-gain rule. Review of the various studies just cited suggests that a more appropriate guideline for "use" gain would be: *gain equal to approximately one-third of the hearing loss for mild to moderate losses, one-half gain for moderate to severe losses, and gain up to two-thirds of the hearing loss for severe to profound losses.* In part, these differences may be due to the amount of the natural canal resonance that remains with a particular hearing aid fitting. The greater the hearing loss, the greater is the need for the ear canal to be almost completely occluded, resulting in increased insertion loss. Therefore, the hearing aid itself needs to provide greater amplification in the higher frequencies for more severe losses to compensate for this insertion loss.

THE FUTURE

Just as following the introduction and popularization of clinical middle-ear impedance measurements in the early 1970s, as more clinical and research facilities begin using probe microphone measurements, answers will be forthcoming to a variety of research questions. Some of the areas needing additional clarification are:

1. More precise correlational data between functional gain, insertion gain, and in-situ response.
2. Comparison of real-ear measures versus 2-cc coupler measurements on a large subject population in order to generate more accurate correction factors, one set for adult ears and one set for childrens' ears.
3. Additional data on the effect of the length of the external auditory meatus on the resonance frequency of the ear. The average ear canal is a cylinder approximately 7.5 mm in diameter with an average volume of 1 cc and a length of 22–25 mm. Children can have a canal volume as small as .5 cc. It is already known that as the size of the canal decreases, sound pressure levels increase, given the same input SPL.
4. Measurement of use gain on a large population of hearing aid users to determine the reliability of the one-third, one-half, and two-third gain rules.
5. How much high-frequency amplification is best? How much low-frequency amplification is needed?
6. Specification of probe microphone measurement procedures to reduce or eliminate current sources of measurement error such as proper insertion depth of the probe tube into the ear canal, how far beyond the earmold or ITE tip the probe should extend, the optimal location of a reference microphone during measurements, and the standardized distance from signal source to hearing aid microphone.
7. Uniformity of terminology to reduce the confusions resulting from the use of nonstandard terms from laboratory to laboratory.

Answers to these and many other questions will come in time. Real-ear probe microphone measurements will soon become as much a part of our daily clinical activities as the other routine procedures we now employ. I estimate that within 5 years, 50–75 percent of all hearing aid dispensers will utilize some form of probe microphone measurements. When digital hearing aids become a reality, these measurements will become even more important and more critical for an optimal hearing aid fitting. As Teter (in Mahon 1986) says, *"Just as today no audiologist would practice without impedance, probe measurements will become a necessary part of every dispenser's practice."*

REALISTIC GAIN MEASUREMENTS

In introductory audiology courses we are told that SRT and speech discrimination measures are important because pure tone thresholds do not give a realistic indication of hearing handicap. After all, how often are we required to listen to and interpret pure tones in our everyday lives?

We can apply this logic to hearing aid measurements, especially acoustic gain.

All measurement standards call for the use of pure tone input signals. I do not consider this procedure to be realistic in terms of how the aid performs under everyday listening conditions. Of course, running speech is acoustically too variable to be used as an input for electroacoustic measurements. However, couldn't a broadband random noise, such as "speech" noise or "pink" noise, serve a similar function? The Veterans Administration has been using such a random noise (200–5000 Hz) for evaluation of their contract aids for years. I would like to see research in this area.

Related to the input employed for gain measures is the setting of the volume control. All the standards require the control to be set at full-on. While this yields a nice number signifying maximum gain, it is also unrealistic. First, no hearing aid should be worn at full gain because, as I discussed earlier, distortion increases dramatically at gain control settings over about three-fourths rotation. Second, McCandless (1974) has reported on a study of 500 hearing aid users in which it was found that the average "use" gain setting was equal to about half the unaided SRT, that is, if the unaided SRT was 50 dB, the "use" gain was about 25 dB.

While it would be impossible to measure gain at every "use" setting for purposes of specification sheet data, is it necessary to use full-on volume control settings? A more realistic approach would be to measure gain at a volume control setting below maximum, such as reference test level. The Veterans Administration measures gain and frequency response with the control set to give an output 12 dB below maximum. With this type of procedure, gain measures that more closely approximate the aid's performance at use settings would be obtained, and these data could be published on technical sheets.

In addition, it would be ideal if curves could be run on each aid at the individual listener's use settings. Then the actual electroacoustic performance of the aid at these everyday settings would be available. The advantages of this are obvious. Of course, this requires that every dispenser's office have a test box arrangement.

HEARING AID DIRECTIONALITY

In the late 1960s, so-called directional hearing aids came onto the American market. Manufacturer claims for this "revolutionary" innovation included a tremendous reduction of sound from behind the user due to the rear microphone port. When measuring hearing aid directionality in a sound box or in a soundfield without a head, such effects can be seen. When measuring such phenomena on KEMAR, however, greatly different effects are seen. Figure 2-49 is the polar response of a nondirectional hearing aid, and Figure 2-50 is the polar response of a directional aid on KEMAR and in a 2 cc coupler. In the 2 cc coupler, the omnidirectional or nondirectional microphone aid shows no directionality. On KEMAR, however, definite directional characteristics are seen as a result of head shadow and diffraction. For the "directional" instrument, the KEMAR response is very different from

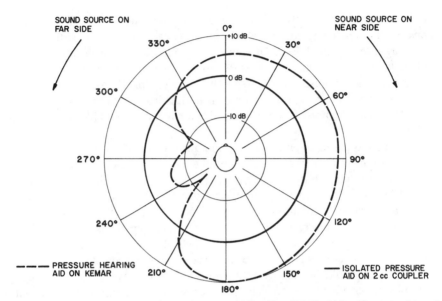

Fig. 2-49. Polar response at 2000 Hz for an omnidirectional BTE aid in a 2 cc coupler and on KEMAR. (Reproduced with permission from Burkhard MD: Gain technology, in Burkhard MD (ed): Manikin Measurements. Elk Grove Village, Knowles Electronics, 1978.)

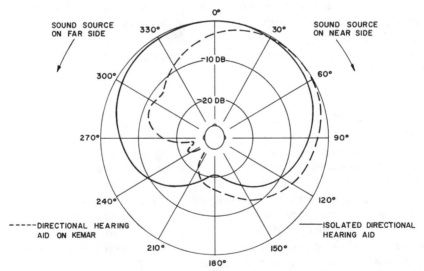

Fig. 2-50. Polar response at 2000 Hz for a directional BTE aid in a 2 cc coupler and on KEMAR. (Reproduced with permission from Burkhard MD: Gain technology, in Burkhard MD (ed): Manikin Measurements. Elk Grove Village, Knowles Electronics, 1978.)

the 2 cc measurement. If you compare the two KEMAR curves, you can see that both aids have substantial directionality, especially for sounds coming from the side of the head opposite the ear on which the aid is worn. The pattern for the directional instrument is somewhat more pronounced for sound sources between 150 degrees and 210 degrees than it is for the other aid.

The conclusion I draw from these data is that, *in use, any hearing aid worn at the ear must be considered a directional instrument.* The "directional" microphones in some aids only alter the details of this directionality.

RESEARCH NEEDS

Throughout this chapter I have alluded to numerous areas within the subject of electroacoustic characteristics that are in need of further extensive research. Rather than elaborate on each of them again, I have listed those that I consider the most important. Beside each is the page of the chapter on which it was first mentioned. In addition, on page 53 I have listed nine areas generally ignored in American standards. Each of them needs more investigation.

1. Tubing length and diameter effects on acoustic feedback (p. 34).
2. Feedback as a high-frequency phenomenon (p. 36).
3. Utilization of external auditory meatus resonance characteristics for high-frequency emphasis amplification (p. 36).
4. Interaction distortion effect (p. 49).
5. Output limiting standard measurements (p. 52).
6. Gain and frequency response measures at use settings (p. 96).
7. Use of "pink" and noise and "speech" noise for electroacoustic measures (p. 96).

REFERENCES

American National Standards Institute: Electroacoustical characteristics of hearing aids. American Standard S3.3-1960. New York, ANSI, 1960

American National Standards Institute: Methods of expressing hearing aid performance. American Standard S3.8-1967. New York, ANSI, 1967

American National Standards Institute: Specification of hearing aid characteristics. American Standard S3.22-1976. New York, ANSI, 1976

American National Standards Institute: Specification of hearing aid characteristics. American Standard S3.22-1987. New York, ANSI, 1987

American National Standards Institute: Methods of measurement of performance characteristics of hearing aids under simulated IN SITU working conditions. American Standard S3.35-1985. New York, ANSI, 1985

Bartschi A: Toward the hearing aid of the future. Hearing J 39:25-27, 1986

Berger KW: Hearing aid evaluative procedures. Natl Hearing Aid J 21:33-36, 1968

Berger KW: The Hearing Aid: Its Operation and Development (ed.2). Detroit, National Hearing Aid Society, 1974

Bode DL, Kasten RN: Hearing aid distortion and consonant identification. J Speech Hearing Res 14:323–331, 1971

Brunved P: Coming to terms with hearing aid technology. Hearing J 38:15–19, 1985

Burkhard MD: Protection against shock and vibration. Meeting of the Audio Engineering Society, New York, 1965

Burkhard MD: KEMAR: A manikin for hearing aid tests. J Audiol Technique 16:102–112, 1977

Burkhard MD: Gain terminology, in Burkhard MD (ed): Manikin Measurements. Elk Grove Village, Knowles Electronics, 1978

Burkhard MD, Sachs RM: Anthropometric manikin for acoustic research. J Acoust Soc Am, 58:214–222, 1978

Caraway BJ, Carhart R: Influence of compressor action on speech intelligibility. J Acoust Soc Am, 41:1424–1433, 1967

Carlisle RW, Mundel AB: Practical hearing aid measurements. J Acoust Soc Am, 16:45–51,1944

Castle WE: A conference on hearing aid evaluation procedures. ASHA Reports No. 2, 1967

Curran JR: Harmonic distortion and intelligibility. Hearing Aid J, 27:39, 1974

Dalsgaard SC, Jensen OD: Measurement of the insertion gain of hearing aids. J Audiol Technique, 15:170–183, 1976

Davis H, Silverman SR: Hearing and Deafness. New York, Holt, Rinehart & Winston, 1970

Davis H, Stevens SS, Nichols RH, et al. Hearing Aids: An experimental Study of Design Objectives. Cambridge, Harvard University Press, 1947

Dillon H, Murray N: Accuracy of twelve methods for estimating the real-ear gain of hearing aids. Ear Hearing, 8:2–11, 1987

Dillon H, Walker G: Compression—input or output control? Hearing Instruments, 34:20–22, 42, 1983

Ely WG: A primer on distortion in hearing aids. Hearing Aid J, 27:10–11, 34, 1974

Ely WG: Hearing aid battery life. Hearing Instruments, 29:12–14, 73, 1978

Erber NP: Body-baffle and real-ear effects in the selection of hearing aids for deaf children. J Speech Hearing Disorders, 38:224–231, 1973

Ewertsen HN, Ipsen JB, Scott-Nielsen S: On acoustical characteristics of the ear mould. Acta Otolaryngologica, 47:312, 1957

Fletcher H: The perception of speech sounds by a deafened person. J Acoust Soc Am, 24:490–497, 1952

Graupe D, Grosspietsch JK, Taylor RT: A self-automatic noise filtering system—Part I: Overview and description. Hearing Instruments 37:29–34, 1986

Harford ER: The use of a probe microphone in the ear canal for the measurement of hearing aid performance. Ear Hearing, 1:329–337, 1980

Harford ER: A new clinical technique for verification of hearing aid response. Arch Otolaryngol, 107:461–468, 1981

Harford ER: The use of real-ear measures for fitting wearable amplification. Hearing, J, 37:20–25, 1984

Harford ER: Personal communication, 1985

Harford ER: Personal communication, 1986

Harris JD, Haines H, Kelsey R, et al.: The relation between speech intelligibility and the electroacoustic characteristics of low fidelity circuitry. J Auditory Res, 1:357–381, 1961

Hearing Aid Industry Conference. HAIC Standard Method of Expressing Hearing Aid Performance. New York, HAIC, 1961

Heide J: Personal communication, 1985

Helle R: Frequency response of behind the ear hearing aids measured on KEMAR, in Burkhard MD (ed): Manikin Measurements. Elk Grove Village, Knowles Electronics, 1978

Hillman NS: Personal communication, 1974

Hudgins CV, Marquis RJ, Nichols RH, et al.: The comparative performance of an experimental hearing aid and two commercial instruments. J Acoust Soc Am, 20:241–258, 1948

International Electrotechnical Commission. *Recommended Methods for Measurements of the Electroacoustical Characteristics of Hearing Aids.* IEC Publication 118. Geneva, IEC, 1959

Jeffers J, Behrens T, Rubin M, et al.: Task force I: Standards for hearing aids. J Acad Rehab Audiol, 6:13–19, 1973

Jerger J, Speaks C, Malmquist C: Hearing aid performance and hearing aid selection. J Speech Hearing Res, 9:136–149, 1966

Jirsa RE, Hodgson WR: Effects of harmonic distortion in hearing aids on speech intelligibility for normals and hypacusics. J Auditory Res, 10:213–217, 1970

Kasten RN, Lotterman SH: A longitudinal examination of harmonic distortion in hearing aids. J Speech Hearing Res, 10:777–781, 1967

Kasten RN, Lotterman SH, Revoile SG: Variability of gain versus frequency characteristics in hearing aids. Acoustica 19:154–160, 1967a

Kasten RN, Lotterman SH, Burnett ED: The influence of nonlinear distortion on hearing aid processed signals. Convention of the American Speech and Hearing Association, Chicago, 1967b

Kasten RN, Lotterman SH: Influence of hearing aid gain control rotation on acoustic gain. J Auditory Res, 9:35–39, 1969

Kates JM: Signal processing for hearing aids. Hearing Instruments, 37:19–22, 1986a

Kates, JM. Signal processing circuits. Siemens Technical Update, November, 1986b.

Killion MC: Personal communication, 1985

Killion MC, & Monser, EL: CORFIG: Coupler response for flat insertion gain, in Studebaker GA, Hochberg I (eds): Acoustical Factors Affecting Hearing Aid Performance. Baltimore, University Park Press, 1980

Knowles HS, Burkhard MD: Hearing aids on KEMAR. Hearing Instruments 26:19–21, 1975

Kranz FW: Tentative code for measurement of performance of hearing aids. J Acoust Soc Am, 17:144–150, 1945

Kraup S, Scott-Nielsen S: Sound pressure measurements in the auditory canal. Nordisk Audiologi 4:90, 1965

Leijon A, Eriksson-Mangold M, Bech-Karlsen A: A preferred hearing aid gain and bass cut in relation to prescriptive fitting. Scand Audiol 13, 1984

Levitt H: An array-processor computer hearing aid (Abstr). ASHA 24, 1982

Libby ER: State-of-the-art of hearing aid selection procedures. Hearing Instruments 36:30–38, 62, 1985

Libby ER: The shift toward real ear measurements, Hearing Instruments, 37:6–7, 50, 1986a

Libby ER: The 1/3-2/3 insertion gain hearing aid selection guide. Hearing Instruments 37:27–28, 1986b

Lotterman SH, Kasten RN: The influence of gain control rotation on nonlinear distortion in hearing aids. J Speech Hearing Res 10:593–599, 1967

Lotterman SH, Farrar NR: Nonlinear distortion in wearable amplification. ASHA 7:364–365, 1965

Lybarger SF: U.S. Patent Application SN 543,278, 1944

Lybarger SF: A new HAIC standard method of expressing hearing aid performance. Hearing Dealer 11:16–17, 1961a

Lybarger SF: Standardized hearing aid measurements. Audecibel 10:8–10, 1961b

Lynne G, Carhart R: Influence of attack and release in compression amplification on understanding of speech by hypoacustics. J Speech Hearing Disorders 28:124–139, 1963

Madsen PB: Insertion gain optimization. Hearing Instruments 37:28–32, 1986

Mahon WJ: Real-ear probe measurements: A procedures comes of age. Hearing J 39:7–11, 1986

Maxwell RJ, Burkhard MD: Vibration isolation of the BL microphone. Knowles Electronics Special Report, 1969a

Maxwell RJ, Burkhard MD: Vibration isolator design. Knowles Electronics Special Report, 1969b

McCandless G: Hearing Aids and Loudness Discomfort. Oticongress III, Copenhagen, Denmark, 1974

McDonald FD, Studebaker G: Earmold alteration effects as measured in the human auditory meatus. J Acoust Soc Am 48:1366–1371, 1970

Nielsen B: Digital hearing aids: Where are they? Hearing Instruments 37:6, 45, 1986

Nielsen HB: Hearing aid fitting based on insertion gain measurements. Audecibel 34:16–19, 1985

Nordstrom D: Personal communication, 1974.

Nunley J: Automatic volume control instrumentation. Hearing Dealer 24:22–24, 1973

Nunley J, Staab W, Steadman J, et al: A wearable digital hearing aid. Hearing J 36:29–31, 34–35, 1983

Olsen WO: Peak clipping and speech intelligibility. Symposium on Amplification for Sensorineural Hearing Loss. Twin Peaks, CA, 1971.

Olsen WO, Carhart R: Development of test procedures for evaluation of binaural hearing aids. Bull Prosthetics Res 10:22–49, 1967

Olsen WO, Wilbur SA: Hearing aid distortion and speech intelligibility. Convention of the American Speech and Hearing Association, Denver, 1978

Pascoe DP: Frequency responses of hearing aids and their effects on the speech perception of hearing-impaired subjects. Ann Otol Rhinol Laryngol 84 (Suppl 23) 1975

Pedersen B, Lauridsen O, Birk-Nielsen H: Clinical measurement of hearing aid insertion gain. Scand Audiol 11:181–186, 1982

Preves D: Personal communication, 1985

Preves D: Probe microphone measurements. Spring meeting of Ohio Hearing Aid Society, 1986

Preves D, Sullivan RF: Sound field equalization for real ear measurements with probe microphones. Hearing Instruments 38:20–26, 64, 1987

Romanow FF: Methods for measuring the performance of hearing aids. J Acoust Soc Am 13:294, 1942

Sachs RM, Burkhard MD: Zwislocki coupler evaluation with insert earphones. Report 20022-1, Knowles Electronics, 1972a

Sachs RM, Burkhard MD: Earphone pressure response in ears and couplers. Eighty-third meeting of the Acoustical Society of America, 1972b

Schneuwly D: Digital technology, the hearing aid and computer fittings. Hearing Instruments 36:16–17, 62, 1985

Schwartz D: Real ear measurements. Madsen Electronics School for Real Ear Measurements, Cincinnati, 1986

Shaw EAG: Transformation of sound pressure level from the free field to the eardrum in the horizontal plane. J Acoust Soc Am 56:1948–1961, 1974

Smriga D: Modern compression technology: Development and applications—Part I. Hearing J 38:28–32, 1985a

Smriga D: Modern compression technology: Development and applications—Part II. Hearing J 38:13–16, 1985b

Smriga D: Modern compression technology, Fall meeting Ohio Hearing Aid Society, 1986

Staab WJ: Hearing aid compression amplification: Fittings. Natl Hearing Aid J 12:34–35, 1972

Staab WJ: Digital hearing aids. Hearing Instruments 36:14–24, 1985

Staab WJ: Digital hearing aids. Audiotone Tech Rep 7, 1986

Studebaker G, Zachman T: Investigation of the acoustics of earmold vents. J Acoust Soc Am 47:1107–1115, 1970

Tonnison W: Measuring in-the-ear gain of hearing aids by the acoustic reflex method. J Speech Hearing Res 18:17–30, 1975

Wanink A: Whistling in hearing aids. Fenestra, 5, 1968

Weiner FM, Ross OA: The pressure distribution in the auditory canal in a progressive sound field. J Acoust Soc Am 18:401–408, 1946

Zwislocki JJ: An acoustic coupler for earphone calibration. Laboratory of Sensory Communication, Syracuse University, Special Report LSC-S-7, 1971a

Zwislocki JJ: An ear-like coupler for earphone calibration. Laboratory of Sensory Communication, Syracuse University, Special Report LSC-S-9, 1971b

Eugene R. McHugh
Randy Morgan

3

Earmold/ITE Shell Technology and Acoustics

In the preceding chapter, I described the various ways in which the electro-acoustic characteristics of a hearing aid can affect user performance and satisfaction. This chapter considers delivery of the amplified signal from the hearing aid receiver to the tympanic membrane. Gene McHugh and Randy Morgan bring a wealth of knowledge and experience to this task. They present a comprehensive overview of the importance of this coupling of aid and ear-mold, and its effect on hearing aid performance. The most important concepts in this chapter, in my view, are: (1) that a mechanical modification of the earmold or in-the-ear (ITE) shell can shape the amplified signal as well as many electronic modifications of the aid without introducing the distortion factors often seen with electronic alterations of the signal; (2) that data gathered from KEMAR and probe microphone measurements of earmold/shell effects differ from classical views; (3) that nonoccluding earmolds/shells can substantially affect user satisfaction; and (4) that coupling effects are not consistent for all aids, but are influenced by hearing aid electronics and mechanics. Everyone working with hearing aids should be thoroughly familiar with the manner in which aid flexibility can be increased and the rather simple means available to mechanically solve many user complaints.

MCP

The primary function of an earmold is to provide a sound channel from the hearing aid's receiver to the eardrum that is free from oscillation (feedback). The second function, when necessary, is to acoustically "shape" the signal once it is

AMPLIFICATION FOR THE HEARING-IMPAIRED, THIRD EDITION ISBN 0-8089-1886-9

transduced by the receiver. The third function is to serve as a comfortable and effective anchor to help keep the hearing aid or earmold inside the ear (Pollack and Morgan 1980).

Since ITE instruments make up the majority of fittings in the United States (Cranmer 1986), we will include them throughout this chapter. Hereafter, the term *hearing aid* should be regarded as either a full-shell, half-shell, or canal style of ITE hearing aid.

HISTORY

Although the first earmold appeared around the turn of the century, earmolds as we know them today were not used until the 1920s. Berger (1974) reported that a dentist in New York postulated that earmolds should be "customized" and subsequently began manufacturing vulcanized custom earmolds. In that time, plaster of paris material was used to make ear impressions. By the 1940s, ethyl methacrylate, which is significantly easier to work with, replaced plaster of paris when an impression of the ear was needed.

In the 1920s, only body aids with external type receivers were in existence. These earmolds had no tubing and were designed mainly to hold an external receiver in the ear. With the development of postauricular hearing aids in the 1950s, other styles of earmolds began to appear on the market. The shell and skeleton styles that are popular today were among the first tube-type earmolds to appear.

Interestingly, dispensers in that era found that certain modifications on the earmold could produce acoustical changes in the hearing aid's response, thus marking the beginning of earmold modification. Lybarger (1958) was among the first to write about their predictable effects. Earmold modifications have become more and more refined, playing an integral part in the fitting of all hearing aids (Killion 1981, Lybarger 1985).

In 1962 the National Association of Earmold Laboratories (NAEL) established a designation of earmold styles, tubing sizes, or earmold materials. NAEL has continued to standardize tubing sizes, adopt standard nomenclature for earmold styles, and assist in the development and introduction of new earmold materials as well as new styles of earmolds.

IMPRESSION TECHNIQUE

Practically every hearing aid fitting requires an impression of the ear be taken. While rudimentary, it is an important procedure that requires more than a casual review of material, impression technique, and general ordering.

To understand the various styles of earmolds, it is important the reader be familiar with the anatomy of the external ear. Figure 3-1A depicts the outer ear and its various parts; figure 3-1B shows a standard earmold. The same numbering system is used to identify the parts of both figures.

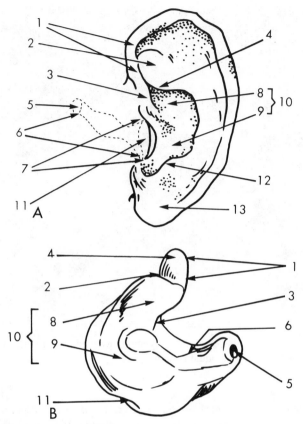

Fig. 3-1. (A) The pinna and its parts: (1) helix; (2) fossa; (3) crus; (4) antihelix; (5) tympanic membrane; (6) auditory meatus (canal); (7) aperture; (8) canba; (9) cavum; (10) concha (bowl); (11) tragus; (12) antitragus; (13) lobule (lobe). (B) Standard earmold with pinna landmarks.

Ear Impression Material

Presently there are two basic types of impression materials most frequently used by hearing aid dispensers. The most popular is the "powder-liquid" material from an ethyl methacrylate polymer. The second material is "silicone" from a silicone-based polymer.

Ethyl methacrylate impression material consists of powder particles (polymer) and liquid (monomer). In mixing the material, pour the liquid into the mixing bowl *first* and then the powder. The polymerization process results in an "ethyl methacrylate" (Fig. 3-2).

Silicone-based impression material consists of a two-paste system with a base material (silano-terminated gum) in one paste and an activator agent in the other. In

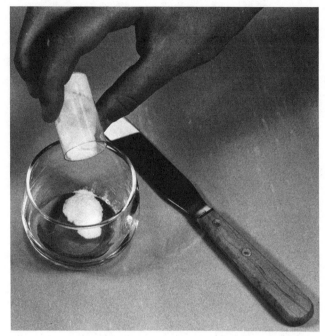

Fig. 3-2. Mixing ethyl methacrylate (powder and liquid) impression material; pour liquid in first.

mixing the material, place the base material on a wax pad and carefully add the activator. Use a spatula to knead the two agents together (Fig. 3-3).

Both materials are excellent for making ear impressions, but not all impression materials are the same. Some have short curing times, some long. Variables such as toughness and heat stability need to be examined.

Little, if any, time has been spent studying the effects of earmold impression materials, and the way they are mixed, on overall stability. Qualitative data by Agnew (1986) have shown that significant dimensional shifts and/or shrinkage is possible in either ethyl methacrylate *or* silicone materials. Other studies have shown that differences primarily occur in the summer months and recommend using silicone-based elastomer impression materials when temperatures exceed 85°F (McHugh and Purinsh 1984).

Ear Impression Equipment

The following instruments are necessary for making an ear impression: (1) otoscope and earlight, (2) otoblock with thread, (3) mixing bowl or wax pad, (4) spatula, (5) tweezers, (6) appropriate syringe, (7) base impression material, and (8) activator.

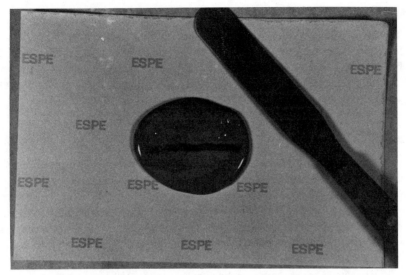

Fig. 3-3. Mixing silicone impression material.

Examination of the Ear

A thorough examination of the ear canals and tympanic membranes should always be made with an otoscope before taking an impression. The examination should include the following steps:

1. Inspect for discharge or infection. Do not take an impression if either of these conditions exist; instead, refer the patient to a physician (preferably ENT).
2. Inspect for excessive wax. If the ear canal is partially or entirely occluded, refer the patient to a physician to have the ear cleaned and irrigated before taking an impression.
3. Determine whether the patient has undergone ear surgery. If so, always obtain a medical clearance first and check whether additional otoblock packing is needed.
4. Inspect pinnae and canals for malformations that would normally be regarded as irregularities by a hearing aid manufacturer or earmold laboratory and note them on their order form.
5. Inspect for a prolapsing canal. If present, use an otoblock large enough to hold the canal open while taking the impression.
6. Vellus hairs in male ear canals may need to be snipped away before attempting an impression.
7. Check the texture of the ear. Is it hard, medium, or very soft? Using normal to dry impression material on a very soft ear may stretch the canal resulting in an overall poor ear impression.

Preparing the Subject

After examining the ear, place an otoblock at the canal opening. Use an earlight to position the block just beyond the isthmus of the ear canal (Fig. 3-4). The otoblock serves two purposes: (1) it allows the impression material to completely fill the canal, thereby providing the best representation; and (2) it helps to protect the eardrum.

Making the Ear Impression

Mix the impression material together and quickly spatulate it into the syringe as shown in Figure 3-5. *Note:* Usually, different syringes are used for powder-liquid and silicone-base impression materials.

As shown in Figure 3-6, push the plunger into the syringe until the material begins to come out the end of the nozzle. Then position the syringe into the canal as deeply as possible and begin to inject the material.

You will notice that as the material begins to flow out the end of the nozzle, it will flow back and cover the top of the nozzle (Fig. 3-7). This is correct. Now, ease the nozzle out a bit and as the material begins to fill the ear, remember to *always keep the end of the nozzle embedded in the impression material.* This serves to limit potential "voids" in the final impression. As the canal is filled, move the nozzle tip to the lower concha and fill the bowl area completely. Work the tip all the way up into the helix area and fill. The impression should provide good definition in the entire canal, concha, and helix areas (Fig. 3-8). Be careful not to inject the material with too much pressure, as this can distort the shape of the ear and result in a poor earmold fit.

Do not apply any finger pressure at all, as it will distort the shape of the ear and/or the impression material.

Let the impression material cure for at least 10 minutes, or until you are unable to make a fingernail indentation in the material. To remove the impression, start by pulling gently around the pinna to break the seal. The impression material in the helix area should then be pulled out and allowed to rest against the ear. Grab the impression and with a slight forward rotation, remove from the ear (Fig. 3-9).

Check the ear for any material that might have remained inside it. Inspect the impression for abnormal voids or folds that might affect fabrication of the custom earmold or hearing aid. Since the impression material continues to cure, leave it in a cool and open place, for instance, a refrigerator, for 30 minutes prior to packaging. Figure 3-10 shows a perfect finished impression.

When shipping powder-liquid impressions, use a cardboard platform and cement the impression to it, using rubber cement. If the fitting is binaural, both ear impressions may be placed into the same box. Shipment of silicone impressions does not require the impression be cemented, as the silicone is much more dimensionally stable (i.e., keeps its shape). Lastly, fold and place the completed order form over the lower half of the box as shown in Figure 3-11 and close it. It's now ready for mailing out to your chosen laboratory.

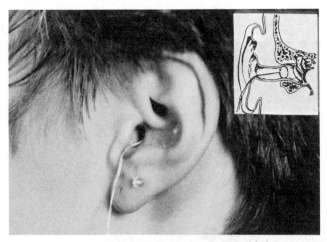

Fig. 3-4. Position otoblock just beyond canal isthmus.

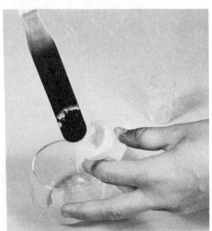

Fig. 3-5. Mix powder liquid together quickly and spatulate into syringe.

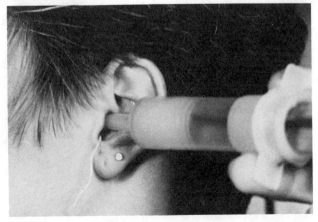

Fig. 3-6. Insert syringe and immediately begin injecting impression material.

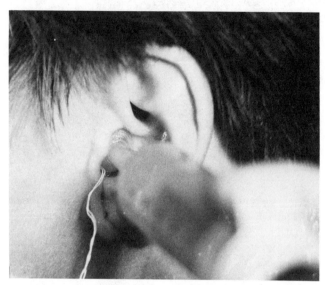

Fig. 3-7. Keep tip of syringe in the impression material to avoid air bubbles.

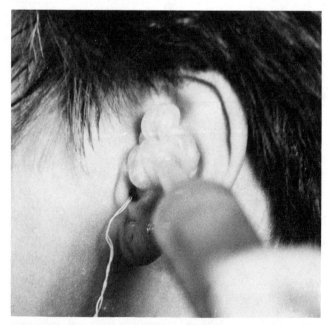

Fig. 3-8. Allow material to fill helix and concha bowl areas.

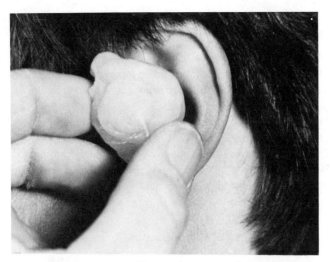

Fig. 3-9. Wait 10 minutes, then remove impression.

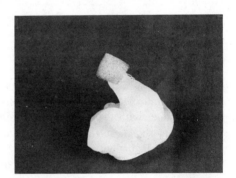

Fig. 3-10. A "perfect" impression.

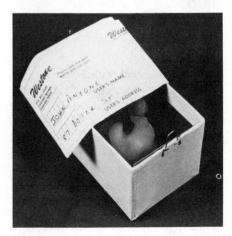

Fig. 3-11. The impression and completed order are ready to be shipped.

Some quality assurance steps to reduce the effects of impression material distortion before and after it has left your office are as follows:

1. Use *premeasured* impression material when possible.
2. Don't change ingredient ratios while mixing.
3. Mix material using method and time recommended by the manufacturer.
4. Always use the syringe method.
5. Don't remove the impression until the recommended curing time has elapsed; perhaps use a belled timer.
6. Protect impression from damage by immediately putting it in the shipping box.
7. Place in refrigerator for 2 hours before shipping.

EARMOLD AND HEARING AID MATERIALS

A number of materials are used in the fabrication of earmolds: They are Lucite (methyl methacrylate), polyvinyl chloride (PVC), silicone, and polyethylene. The two most common however, are *Lucite* and *PVC* materials.

Hard Plastic Molds

Lucite is a relatively hard acrylic plastic that can be manufactured in a variety of shades and colors. Practically any style of earmold can be made from methyl methacrylate, with the usual color of simply "clear" or "transparent." Most ITE hearing aid shells are made from Lucite materials with color being similar to the skin tone of the patient.

Lucite has three properties that make it very popular: (1) it is durable, (2) it can be modified easily when necessary, and (3) it is basically nontoxic (Lybarger, 1978).

Soft Molds

PVC material is the leading soft material used in today's earmolds and tubing. This material is available in various degrees of softness and/or resistance to discoloration. It is pliable and relatively durable. Most importantly, PVC can be modified when necessary (Leavitt 1981). It does harden with age however, thus necessitating more frequent replacement than lucite molds.

Nonallergenic Molds

If a patient presents with a history of pruritus, irritation, or swelling of the ear canal from the use of Lucite or PVC, there are nonallergenic alternatives. *Polyeth-*

ylene material is the counterpart to Lucite (hard mold), whereas *silicone* is the nonallergenic counterpart to PVC.

Neither polyethylene nor silicone are cosmetically appealing, and both have been shown to be very difficult to modify and retube. For this reason, they are used only in the cases where an allergy exists.

When to Use Lucite or PVC Earmolds

It is common for dispensers to develop their own guidelines regarding which earmold material to use with what type of case. For adults, however, *gain requirements* of the hearing aid normally dictate the material to be preferred (Lybarger 1985). On average, when the acoustic gain of an instrument is *less* than 55 dB (re: SPL), *Lucite* is regarded as the material of choice since it is more durable. When the gain of an instrument *exceeds* 55 dB, however, a PVC mold may be necessary to better adhere to the shape of the ear canal, thereby reducing the propensity for acoustic feedback. PVC material is also recommended for young children to protect the concha and meatus tissue in the event the child is hit on the ear (Pollack and Morgan 1980).

EARMOLD STYLES

When choosing the style of an earmold, the priority of selection usually takes on the following order (1) type of hearing aid [body, behind-the-ear (BTE) or ITE], (2) possibility of acoustical feedback, (3) possible acoustic modifications, and (4) comfort. Sullivan (1985) describes four basic fitting classifications that directly relate to these factors: class I fittings, which allow for maximum ventilation; class II fittings, which call for moderate earmold or hearing aid venting; class III fittings, where an unvented earmold or hearing is used which has inadvertent leaks; and class IV fittings, where every attempt is made to prevent all sound leakage.

Table 3-1 and Figures 3-12 through 3-19 describe the common styles in use today, based on the most standardized terminology (NAEL 1970).

ACOUSTIC EFFECTS FROM EARMOLD/SHELL MODIFICATION

While there are a host of advanced modifications that can be made in the plumbing between the hearing aid's receiver and tympanic membrane, the three most basic alterations are through the use of (1) various size vents, (2) filters, and (3) sound bore diameters.

Venting is used to control low-frequency response; *filtering* is used to control mid-frequency response, and *sound-bore diameter* is used to control high-frequency response. By mastering these three precepts, one may solve many problems during routine hearing aid fittings.

Table 3-1
Common Earmold Styles

Earmold Style	Description and Purpose
Regular or receiver	Solid mold with plastic or metal snap ring to accommodate the appropriate size receiver; designed for use primarily with body aids (Fig. 3-12)
Shell	Fills concha completely; in BTE fittings, used mostly for severe losses when higher levels of acoustic gain or output are needed; can be ordered with or without the helix portion; adding the helix enhances retention but may cause discomfort; the shell style is the most common style in ITE fittings (Fig. 3-13)
Skeleton	Similar to the shell style except that the center of the concha bowl is removed leaving a "ring" around the posterior perimeter of the concha for retention; used in BTE fittings only (Fig. 3-14)
3/4 and semiskeleton	These styles are variations of the skeleton mold where portions of the perimeter are removed, usually for reasons of "comfort" (Fig. 3-15)
Half-shell	The name denotes the style; the mold covers the bottom 1/2 of the concha bowl. The helix portion, a common source of tenderness in many users, is removed; used in BTE and ITE fittings (Fig. 3-16)
Canal	Also referred to as the canal hook, designed for mild-moderate losses; this style is popular since it is cosmetically appealing and easy to insert; the retention factor is poor and may result in feedback if too much acoustic gain is required; used in BTE and ITE fittings (Fig. 3-17)
Acoustic modifier	A very popular mold, this skeleton-shaped mold has a very short canal, a large cavity hollowed out at the end of the sound bore, and a variable vent; used in BTE and ITE fittings (Fig. 3-18)
Free-field	This mold is simply a plastic ring to hold the tube in the ear; the purpose is to provide a maximum venting effect; used in BTE and ITE fittings (Fig. 3-19)

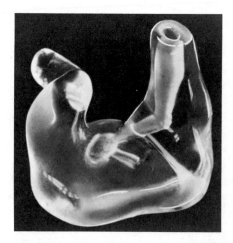

Fig. 3-12. Regular (external receiver) mold.

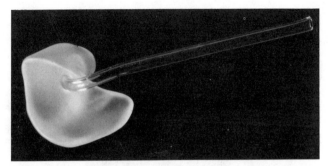

Fig. 3-13 Shell mold.

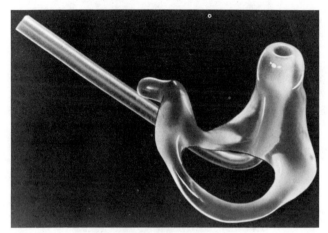

Fig. 3-14. Skeleton mold.

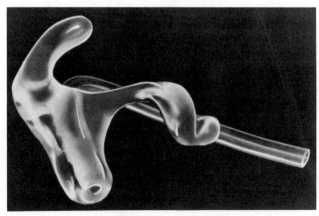

Fig. 3-15. Semiskeleton mold.

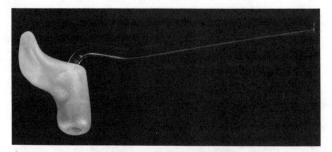

Fig. 3-16. Half-shell mold.

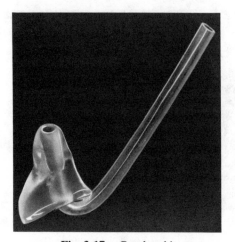

Fig. 3-17. Canal mold.

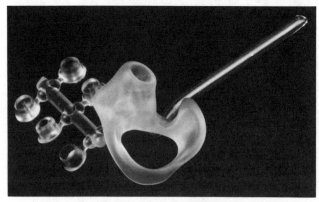

Fig. 3-18. Acoustic modifier mold.

118

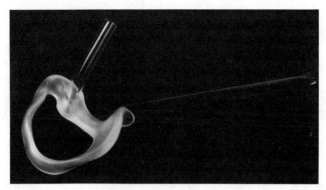

Fig. 3-19. Free-field mold.

Libby (1981) presents these modifications in an easily understood format, and its reading is recommended. Figure 3-20 is from Libby (1981) and graphically depicts the general effects from venting, filters, and soundbore diameter on the frequency response in hearing aids.

Table 3-2 describes all of the effects that can be achieved through various earmold modifications. *Note:* Many of these alterations do not result in *large* changes in the frequency response of the hearing aid, but may result in significant improvement in subjective user comfort. For example, a very small vent (0.5 mm), while not altering the frequency response appreciably, often does provide a release of sound pressure that can alleviate complaints about pressure or fullness in the ear.

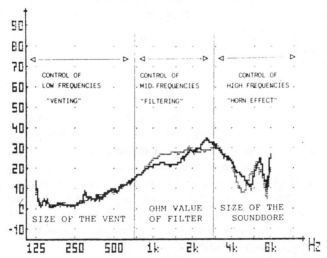

Fig. 3-20. General effects from earmold modifications. (Adapted by E.R. McHugh from Libby ER: Achieving a transparent, smooth, wideband hearing aid response. Hearing Instruments 32:9–12, 1981. With permission)

Table 3-2
Effect of Coupling Modifications on Hearing Aid Response

Modification	Effect on Low Frequencies (< 750 Hz)	Effect on Midfrequencies (0.75–1.5 kHz)	Effect on High Frequencies (> 3000 Hz)
Longer tubing	Increases	Peaks shift to lower frequency	Negligible
Shorter tubing	Slightly decreases	Peaks shift to higher frequency	Slightly increases
Larger-ID* tubing	Negligible	Peaks shift to higher frequency	Slightly increases
Smaller-ID tubing	Negligible	Peaks shift to lower frequency	Slightly decreases
Large-diameter soundbore	Negligible	Peaks shift to higher frequency	Increases
Smaller-diameter soundbore	Negligible	Peaks shift to lower frequency	Decreases
Longer soundbore	Negligible	Peaks shift to lower frequency	Negligible
Shorter soundbore	Negligible	Peaks shift to higher frequency	Negligible
0.5-mm vent†	Negligible	Negligible	Negligible
1.0-mm vent	Slightly decreases	Negligible	Negligible
2.0-mm vent	Decreases	Negligible	Negligible
3.0-mm vent	Decreases	Increases peak height	Negligible
Nonoccluding mold	Strongly decreases	Peaks slightly shift upward	Negligible
Low-ohm filter	Negligible	Peaks slightly rounded	Negligible
High-ohm filter	Slightly decreases	Peaks smoothed	Slightly decreases

*Internal diameter.
†Used primarily for subject comfort by releasing sound pressure

Venting

A "vent" is a hole drilled from the face of an earmold or hearing aid to its sound input channel or parallel to this channel, thereby intentionally producing a sound leak. Depending on its length and diameter, a vent will alter the low-frequency characteristics of the hearing aid response.

There are three circumstances that frequently present themselves where venting should be considered: (1) to relieve fullness or pressure in the ear, referred to as *pressure equalization;* (2) to improve *sound quality;* and (3) to provide a *relative enhancement of the high-frequency response* through attenuating the lows (Pollack and Morgan 1980, Lybarger 1985).

PRESSURE EQUALIZATION

Most earmolds do not provide a completely tight (hermetic) seal, but it may feel that way to the patient. Therefore, a small vent, on the order of 0.5 mm (0.020

inch), can be drilled to let the ear breathe and relieve the feeling of fullness often experienced by hearing aid users. Any dispenser who senses this from the outset should order the earmold or hearing aid with the 0.5-mm vent or order a variable vent, which will be described below.

IMPROVING SOUND QUALITY

New hearing aid users will often experience what has become known as the "barrel effect," which is the enhancement of the hearing aid user's *own voice* while wearing amplification. Complaints such as "It sounds hollow" or "It sounds as though I am talking in a drum" are typical. The complaint stems from amplification below 750 Hz, which causes the user to hear his or her own voice louder and slightly delayed. To alleviate the complaint, a vent may be used to reduce the low-frequency response.

HIGH-FREQUENCY ENHANCEMENT

The majority of hearing aid patients have some degree of sloping sensorineural involvement where attenuation of the low frequencies is a necessary part of creating a high-frequency emphasis system. Vent diameters from 1 to 2 mm (any length) are normally used for "moderate" low-frequency attenuation, while strong low-frequency reduction requires vent diameters of 3 mm and vent lengths of 6.3 mm (Lybarger 1985).

THE PROBLEM OF ACOUSTIC FEEDBACK

The major drawback in creating a vent in the earmold or hearing aid is the problem of amplified sound escaping through the vent and being reamplified by the hearing aid, referred to as "feedback." One normally hears a "whistling," which is at a pitch level near the resonant frequency of the receiver. Reducing the vent diameter, inserting lamb's wool in the vent, or completely plugging up the vent will sometimes alleviate this problem. However, you are often back at square one regarding the patient's "subjective complaint of fullness" and your desire to attenuate the lower frequencies to alleviate the problem. It is a dilemma that every dispenser knows all too well, and it usually ends up as a compromise. Pollack presents more discussion concerning controlling feedback in Chapter 2.

THE IMPORTANCE OF ACOUSTIC VERSUS ELECTRIC VENTING

Cox and Alexander (1983) studied the relative effects of low-frequency attenuation through electrical means (using hearing aid tone controls) versus through acoustical means (using earmold venting). In this study, a group of users were fit with two sets of hearing aids having the same frequency response and asked to make a quality judgment. One frequency response was achieved through the use of electrical filtering (using the tone control on the hearing aid with a closed earmold) and the other through acoustic filtering (using a relatively wideband hearing aid with venting). Clearly, most hearing aid users prefer low-frequency attenuation acoustic venting. In concert with the these results, it is recommended to vent as much as possible, and, insofar as venting applies to feedback, vent as much as you can "get away" with.

DIAGONAL VERSUS PARALLEL VENTING

A diagonal or angle vent is drilled from the face of an earmold into the soundbore, whereas a parallel vent does not intersect the soundbore (Pollack and Morgan 1980, Lybarger 1985). Research by Studebaker and Cox (1977) and Cox (1979) show similar low-frequency attenuation from both parallel and diagonal venting methods, but a slight loss of the higher frequency response with the use of diagonal earmold venting. Unless space is severely limited, most earmolds, and all hearing aids are made with the vent parallel to the soundbore.

VARIABLE VENTING

It is often impossible to know exactly which size vent to use in an earmold or hearing aid. Therefore, earmold manufacturers began offering variable venting methods in the early 1970s (Blue 1972).

Variable venting provides a practical solution to the problems of knowing how much to vent. Two systems in use today are positive venting valves (PVVs) and select-a-vents (SAVs). A PVV has a 3-mm vent through the earmold and a seating ring that holds hard plastic vent inserts (Fig. 3-21). The SAV is similar to the PVV, but there is no seating ring, and the inserts, made from PVC material, range from a total plug to a 0.156-inch vent. In ITE hearing aids, the open vent size is 2 mm. Six short tubes varying in diameter are provided that can be inserted into the vent hole for selective venting capabilities. Whichever system is used, variable venting is both practical and effective. Figure 3-22 shows the relative effect on frequency response using a variable venting system.

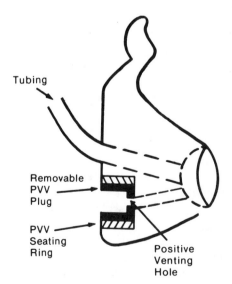

Tubing

Removable
PVV
Plug

PVV
Seating
Ring

Positive
Venting
Hole

Fig. 3-21. Positive venting valve with seating ring that holds variable vent sizes.

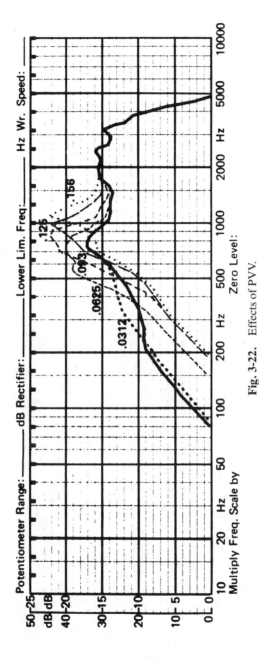

Fig. 3-22.   Effects of PVV.

123

NONOCCLUDING EARMOLDS AND HEARING AIDS

Nonoccluding earmolds have been used since the 1940s, when innovative hearing aid dispensers used only tube fittings in cases of steeply falling high-frequency hearing loss (Payne 1977). Nonoccluding earmolds and hearing aids create a maximum vent for the same benefits as described above, along with providing the benefit of allowing direct sound to enter the ear canal in a relatively normal way.

In their now classic report on CROS (contralateral routing of signal) fittings for persons with unilateral hearing loss, Harford and Barry (1965) described a special kind of nonoccluding earmold for the normal ear that has become known as the *CROS mold* (Fig. 3-23, A and B). When used on the same ear as the hearing aid, the term *IROS mold* is sometimes used meaning ipsilateral routing of signal. The term *free-field* was later popularized by Hewitt (1977) describing a mold with a lucite ring supporting heavy walled tubing (Fig. 3-19).

Filters

Filters are normally used to reduce the mid-frequency response of the hearing aid (Libby 1981). Filters, or "acoustic dampers," are usually placed at the end of

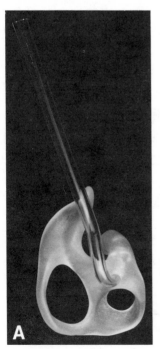
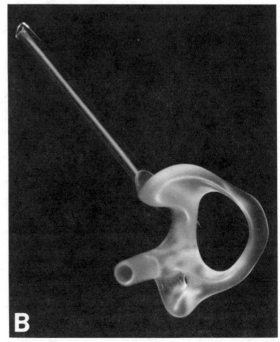

Fig. 3-23. CROS molds showing (A) large-diameter vent and (B) depth into canal and soundbore diameter.

the earhook and are designed merely to provide a smoothening of the response peaks resulting from the effects of the hearing aid and tubing (Carlson 1974, Lybarger 1979). They were not designed to significantly increase or decrease the mid-frequency range, but merely *smooth* the resonant peaks in a hearing aid frequency response, generally around 1000 Hz. Most hearing aid and earmold manufacturers now provide ready-made earhooks with dampers in them for convenience. For sufficient damping, use 680–1500 acoustic ohms; any higher ohmage level tends to reduce the overall mid-frequency response too much, thereby limiting the primary area where the amplification is located (Fig. 3-35).

Increasing or Decreasing the Soundbore Diameter

The understanding of the effects of soundbore diameter have been greatly facilitated through the work of Killion (1976, 1979, 1981). His 1981 treatise is advised reading for details on a special series of earmolds and their acoustic effects typically referred to as the "Killion molds."

Soundbore diameter mostly affects the high-frequency response (Libby 1981). Increasing or decreasing the diameter of the last 10 mm in an earmold system has an appreciable effect on the hearing aid response in the high frequencies. In short, *increasing the diameter enhances the highs and decreasing the diameter decreases the highs.*

Normally, total earmold plumbing from the receiver in a BTE hearing aid to the earmold's tip is 43 mm long × 1.93 mm in diameter. *Doubling the diameter of the last 10 mm to 4 mm tends to increase the response above 3000 Hz by approximately 10 dB.* Conversely, *halving the diameter of the last 10 mm from 1.93 to 1.0 mm tends to reduce the response above 1000 Hz by approximately 10 dB* (Fig. 3-36).

For patients with high-frequency hearing loss, enlarging the soundbore diameter increases the high-frequency response, which may prove extremely beneficial. Oppositely, for patients with a severe reverse-slope curve, ordering an earmold with a soundbore of 0.5–1.0 mm will appreciably attenuate the high-frequency response of the hearing aid and prove an appropriate modification. Therefore, the use of this axiom has been of practical value during our routine hearing aid fittings.

Application of Special Molds

Most specialty earmold ITE styles provide either a specific acoustic or practical advantage over conventional earmold and hearing aid styles. Figures 3-24 through 3-27 describe selected specialty styles and when each is appropriate.

REAL-EAR MEASUREMENT OF EARMOLD MODIFICATION EFFECTS

Probe microphone real-ear analysis is becoming commonplace in today's modern hearing aid office (Libby 1987). This is for good reason; any dispenser who

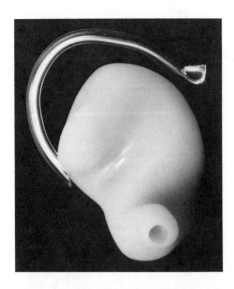

Fig. 3-24. Wire-retainer mold. Often used with children to help keep their BTE aids on.

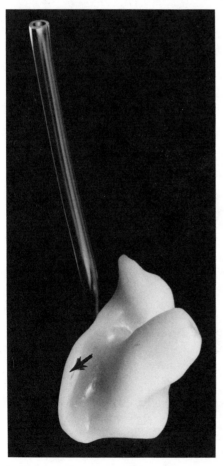

Fig. 3-25. Tragus mold. Used with BTE fittings of 65-dB gain or higher to prevent feedback.

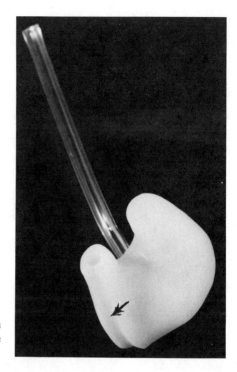

Fig. 3-26. External vent mold. Used with patients having active drainage from the middle ear.

utilizes real-ear measurements is aware of the tremendous patient to patient variability inherent with hearing aid fittings.

Before 1983, most earmold/shell modifications were based on real-ear research, but the factor of variability was rarely addressed. Questions regarding size of the canal (large or small) and/or shape were speculated on. Since 1983, however, the popularity of in-office real-ear measurement devices has made it possible to examine the issue of intersubject variability. Those of us using real-ear analysis have noted that variability due to size and shape is so great that each patient should be examined independently.

While it may be impossible to absolutely predict how an earmold or hearing aid modification will affect a hearing aid's frequency response, knowledge of basic earmold acoustics makes it possible to, at least, move in "the right direction" when a specific problem is presented. To illustrate the effects of earmold modification using real-ear analysis, the following curves (Figs. 3-28 to 3-36, 3-38) were taken on the same person's ear utilizing a BTE hearing aid (Siemens 268D-W) set to a constant volume level by using the same measurement criteria (Hawkins 1987). The purpose of showing these measurements is to demonstrate real-life effects from earmold modifications. Remember that this is one person's ear and may not be representative of most ears because of the extreme variability between ears.

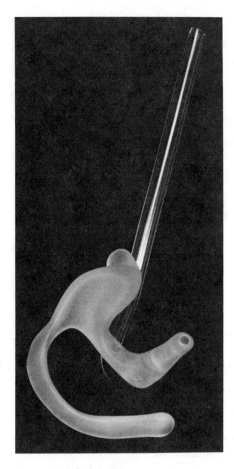

Fig. 3-27. Janssen mold. A convenient alternative to the free-field mold style.

Venting for Low-Frequency Attentuation

Figure 3-28 shows the basic response of a wideband postauricular hearing aid utilizing a standard "closed" earmold. With a 0.5 mm vent drilled parallel to soundbore, essentially no effect is observed in the hearing aid response (Fig. 3-29), although much relief is experienced by the user through pressure equalization. When a 2-mm vent parallel to the soundbore is made, the effects on the frequency response are relatively minor. Indeed, it is interesting that even with a 3-mm vent parallel to the soundbore, the effects in this ear are relatively minimal (Figs. 3-30 and 3-31).

Two popular earmold styles that are designed to provide high-frequency emphasis are the acoustic modifier and the free-field earmolds (Table 3-1). Figure 3-32 shows the response of the postauricular hearing aid with (1) a closed mold, (2) an acoustic modifier mold with an unfiltered 3-mm vent, and (3) a free-field earmold using 18 mm of No. 13 heavy-walled tubing. Once again, the differences between

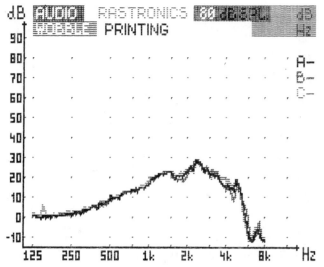

Fig. 3-28. Real-ear response of wideband BTE with closed mold.

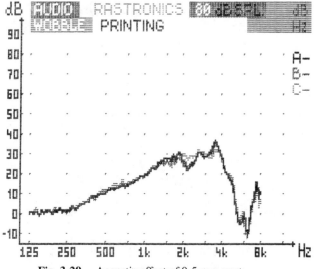

Fig. 3-29. Acoustic effect of 0.5-mm vent.

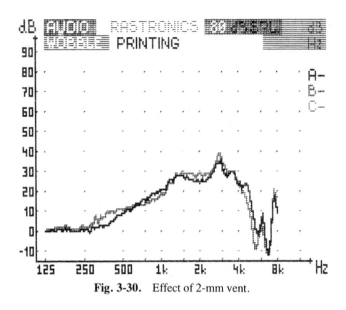

Fig. 3-30. Effect of 2-mm vent.

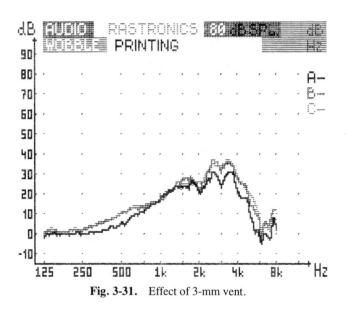

Fig. 3-31. Effect of 3-mm vent.

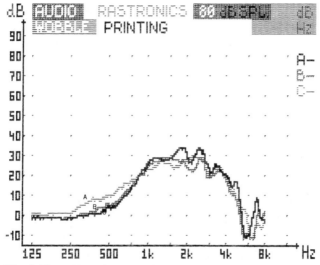

Fig. 3-32.   Effect of (A) closed mold; (B) acoustic modifier (un-filter); (C) "free-field" mold.

curves using real-ear analysis appear to be minimal in this person's ear. Meanwhile, the user reported enhanced subjective improvement in "sound quality."

Substantial difference from venting is evidenced in the comparative analysis between the closed mold and the CROS mold. Figure 3-33 shows the CROS mold curve. Note the relative attentuation in the low frequencies and enhancement of high frequencies utilizing this earmold style.

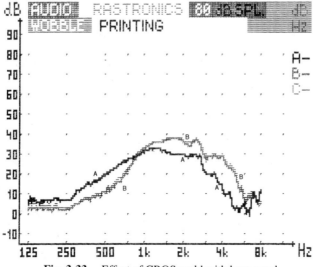

Fig. 3-33.   Effect of CROS mold with long canal.

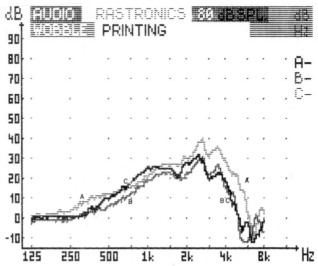

Fig. 3-34. Effect of (A) closed mold versus (B) 2-mm angled vent versus (C) 2-mm parallel vent.

Research (Studebaker and Cox 1977, Cox 1979) suggests that a parallel vent, if compared to the closed-mold response, would affect only the low-frequency response whereas as angled vent would attenuate both ends of the frequency response curve. This postulate could not be replicated in this user's ear (Fig. 3-34), which compares the curves of (1) a closed mold; (2) a 2-mm angled vent, and (3) a 2-mm parallel vent. Indeed, both angled and parallel vents performed similarly, providing low- and high-frequency response attenuation. Please note that this does not disprove the research of Studebaker and Cox, but instead suggests that individual variability must be considered in all hearing aid fittings.

The results of venting in this person's ear revealed the following subjective and objective results: (1) pressure equalization, (2) improvement in sound quality, and (3) low-frequency attenuation (although the amount of reduction was less than expected).

Filtering for Midfrequency Smoothing of Resonance Peaks

Filters or dampers have been traditionally used in earmold plumbing to reduce the height of some or all of the resonant peaks in the hearing aid output. Dampers that are 2 mm wide are usually placed at the end of the earhook for convenience purposes. While locating the damper at other locations in the tubing or earmold has been shown to be more effective acoustically, wax and moisture often interfere (Carlson 1974, Killion 1981, Lybarger 1985).

Figure 3-35 shows the relative influence of damping on the hearing aid response. Curve A shows the hearing aid response with an undamped earhook, while curve B shows the effect of a damped earhook with the damper (Star damper)

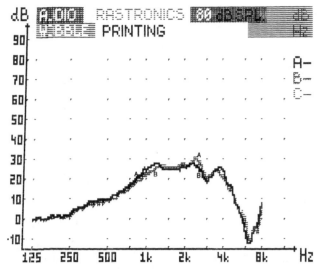

Fig. 3-35. Effect of damping element in the earhook on midfrequency peaks.

located at the juncture of the earhook and tubing. *Note:* In our experience, damping using the Carlson and Mostardo dampers (U.S. Patent No. 4,006,321) of 680 Ω produces similar effects as the Star damper. However, the Carlson-Mostardo dampers tend to "clog up" with moisture faster than the Star damper, requiring more frequent exchanges.

Filters or dampers are beneficial in smoothing hearing aid peaks that are caused by the hearing aid electronics before the earhook. Note that many peaks result from usual, and sometimes unusual, resonances in an individual's ear that may be difficult to control with the use of earmold filters.

Increasing and Decreasing the Soundbore Diameter

The "normal" inside diameter of No. 13 tubing (1.93 mm) usually defines the soundbore diameter. Indeed, most hearing aid responses measured on traditional couplers use 46 mm of tubing 1.93 mm in diameter (Lybarger 1985). Theoretically, increasing this diameter to 4 mm in the last 10 mm enhances the high-frequency response, while decreasing the diameter to 1 mm in the final 10 mm attenuates the high-frequency response.

Figure 3-36 illustrates the relative effects from modifications in the earmold diameter. As is shown, the effects are quite predictable on this individual's ear. Expansion of the soundbore diameter from the standard 1.93 mm (A) to 4 mm (B) enhances the response above 2000 Hz by approximately 10 dB, whereas using an earmold with a soundbore diameter of 1 mm (C) reveals a loss in high-frequency response above 1000 Hz by approximately 10 dB.

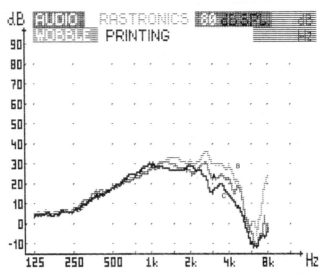

Fig. 3-36. Acoustic effect of soundbore diameter on high-frequency response. (A = 1.93 mm, B = 4 mm, C = 1.0 mm)

This modification is often referred to as the "horn effect" because of its properties as an acoustical transformer for higher frequencies (Mason 1927, Cox 1979). The horn effect is associated with an increase in soundbore diameter, whereas the term *reverse horn* is applied when soundbore diameter is reduced purposely, thus impeding high-frequency transmission (Libby 1981).

Special tubing arrangements such as the "Libby horn" (NAEL 1981) and earmold models such as the continuous flow adapter (CFA) are recommended as a practical alternative to creating the horn effect. For example, to increase the soundbore diameter to 4-mm, a large portion of tubing must be removed to make room for the increased diameter. This weakens the plastic cement bond between mold and tubing and could create a need for periodic retubing. This is beneficial for neither the dispenser nor the patient. Instead, the use of a *complete* tube such as the Libby horn (Fig. 3-37), which has the acoustic properties desired and adheres to the body of the earmold, may be the more practical approach. The principle of the CFA is the same.

The curve for the regular 4-mm Libby horn is similar to the 4-mm curve shown in Figure 3-36. The effect of the 4-mm Libby horn is shown in Figure 3-38.

Often the 4-mm Libby horn is too big for many ear canals, especially children. In these cases the 3-mm-diameter Libby horn is recommended. While the 3-mm Libby horn was not evaluated, the response may be interpolated as falling between the 1.93-mm and 4-mm curves in Figure 3-38.

The "horn" and "reverse horn" effects are predictable and essential in earmold acoustics. Enhancement of word intelligibility for patients with mild to severe sloping sensorineural hearing loss may be achieved through the horn effect (soundbore diameter > 2 mm). Oppositely, an occasional patient presents with rela-

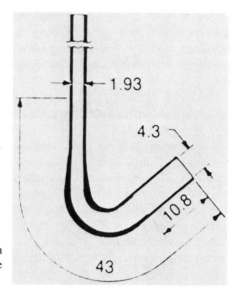

Fig. 3-37. Dimensions of the Libby horn tube. The "horn effect" serves to enhance the high-frequency response.

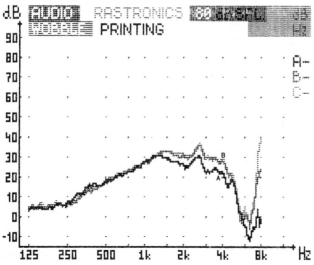

Fig. 3-38. Effect of Libby horn on high-frequency response. (A = No. 13 tubing, B = 4-mm horn)

135

tively normal high-frequency thresholds (3–6 kHz) where reducing the high-frequency output is needed for comfort. Ordering a reverse horn (soundbore diameter = 0.05 mm) or inserting and cementing a piece of No. 18 tubing (1 mm in diameter) may achieve the desired reverse horn effect.

IN-OFFICE MODIFICATIONS OF EARMOLDS AND ITE HEARING AIDS

According to Riess and Cuthier (1986), approximately 25–30 percent of all hearing aid fittings can benefit from some type of modification. This has been our experience as well. Too many variables, including impression technique, impression material, type of mold, or hearing aid are involved to simply blame the laboratory when the fit is not perfect or an undesired acoustic leak occurs when the patient smiles or chews.

It is vitally necessary for today's dispenser to have the equipment and skills required to be proficient in modifying earmolds and ITE hearing aids. Below is our recommended list of tools for a typical in-office repair laboratory:

1. *Bench lathe with quick-change chuck*—two speeds with one end for drilling, sanding, and pumicing and the other for buffing. Normally sanding on Lucite is made on the "high" speed while sanding on PVC is made on "slow" (Fig. 3-39).

2. *Drills*—used to *start* a modification on a vent or soundbore. A small selection is needed; 0.5, 1, 2, and 3 mm (Fig. 3-40).

3. *Burs*—used to *finish up* a modification by cleaning out the vent or soundbore. Again a small selection is needed; 1, 2, 3, and 4 mm (Fig. 3-41).

4. *White-stone sanders*—shaped flat or triangular on lathe for simple modification on canal or for sore spots (Fig. 3-42).

5. *Pumice-impregnated rubber*—on lathe as first step before polishing (Fig. 3-43).

6. *Cotton rag wheels and buffing*—on back of lathe for final polishing process (Fig. 3-44).

When There Is Earmold or Hearing Aid Discomfort

Modification for the purpose of "comfort" is a common in-office procedure. Often, this kind of modification is found to be necessary after the patient has worn the earmold or aid for a week or so. It is important to differentiate between diffuse and localized acute discomfort.

If the problem is acute, inspect the patient's ear(s) for redness; ask the patient where it hurts, to identify specifically where to grind the mold or hearing aid. Usually, acute pain or discomfort occurs in the helix, the valley between the helix and the canal, the intertragal notch, or the end of the canal.

If the discomfort is diffuse, analysis of the problem is more difficult and

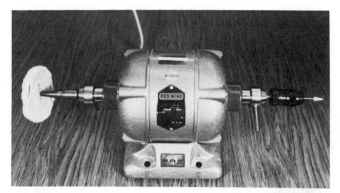

Fig. 3-39. Bench lathe for earmold/hearing aid modifications.

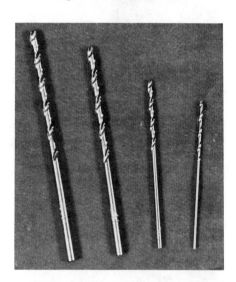

Fig. 3-40. Selection of drills for venting.

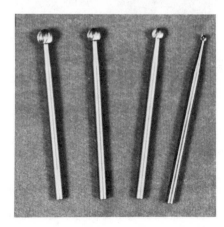

Fig. 3-41. Burs for cleaning vents and soundbore.

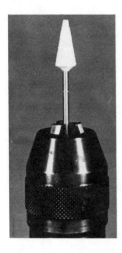

Fig. 3-42. White-stone sanders for grinding.

caution should be taken when modifying the mold or hearing aid without knowing specifically where to grind. Once again, check the ear for redness to obtain as much specific information as possible before *generally* grinding down the earpiece.

When sanding, have the lathe facing you. Hold the mold or hearing aid with both hands, resting them on a block for stability (Fig. 3-45). Hold the earpiece securely and begin sanding in a fluid motion: do not thin too much in any one area. After sanding, change to a pumice-impregnated bit and begin smoothing the modified areas in a similar way. Once these areas look fairly smooth, hold the earpiece under a cotton buff wheel on the back of the lathe for the final finishing touch. Clean off the mold or shell and try it on the patient.

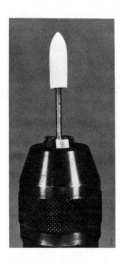

Fig. 3-43. Pumice-impregnated rubber.

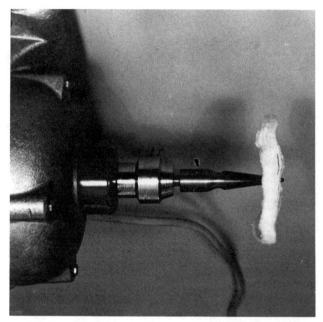

Fig. 3-44. Cotton rag wheel (buffer).

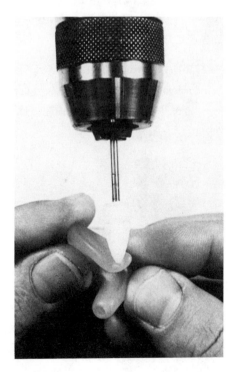

Fig. 3-45. Proper grinding of the earpiece.

In-Office Acoustic Modifications

It is preferable to request any desired modifications *when ordering* a hearing aid or earmold. However, in cases where in-office modification is needed, here are some hints.

CREATING A VENT

Making a vent *is difficult* and often embarrassing since it is not uncommon to drill right out the side of the earpiece. This is why SAVs are so popular. It may be wise to practice on a few unusable earmolds before attempting this with a real person's earmold or hearing aid.

The process for methyl methacrylate molds and hearing aids involves two steps: (1) using a drill to make a path and (2) using a bur for exact diameter and to clean out the vent (Fig. 3-46). Again, have the drill pointing toward you and place a block under your hands for stability. Hold the earpiece with both hands and use a drill slightly smaller than the needed diameter to make the path. Change to a bur that is the exact diameter required and gently clean the vent out, taking care not to penetrate the side of the earpiece.

ENLARGING A VENT

Since the vent is already present, use the desired diameter bur and follow the procedure shown in Figure 3-46. Take your time and be very careful not to pierce the side.

FILTERING OF MIDFREQUENCY PEAKS

In postauricular hearing aids, exchange a *filtered* earhook for the unfiltered one. Filtering of midfrequency peaks in ITE hearing aids is best achieved *out* of the office by having the manufacturer insert a filtered microphone.

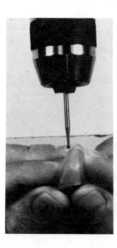

Fig. 3-46. To make a vent, use 1-mm *drill* to create a path and clean out using a bur.

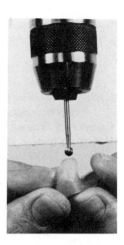

Fig. 3-47. Bur is used to enlarge soundbore diameter.

APPLYING HORN EFFECTS

An easy and effective in-office modification on earmolds involves the expansion of the soundbore diameter for high-frequency enhancement. Figure 3-47 shows the process of using either a 3- or 4-mm bur to create the desired soundbore diameter.

Any in-office modification of an earmold or hearing aid's soundbore or vent will affect the frequency response in some way. In the final analysis, however, it is easier for the earmold or hearing aid laboratory to apply any necessary style or acoustic modification than to do it yourself. Their job is to do it right and, moreover, make it look good.

CONCLUSION

It becomes readily apparent even after minimal hearing aid experience, that the earmold/ITE shell is a significant part of any hearing aid system. Applying advanced knowledge of earmold acoustics can greatly expand an audiologist's fitting potential.

The use of real-ear probe microphone measurement is advocated to measure fitting results when earmold modifications are required. Real-ear analysis provides documentation of the acoustic response between the hearing aid and the eardrum.

Finally, good ear impression technique cannot be overemphasized. Know what a good impression looks like and the effects of the impression material once it's made.

REFERENCES

Agnew J: A study of the stability of ear impression material. Hearing J 39:29–33, 1986
Berger KW: The Hearing Aid: Its Operation and Development (ed 3). Detroit, National Hearing Aid Society, 1974

142   Eugene R. McHugh and Randy Morgan

Blue J: Positive venting valve concept. Hearing Aid Dealer 23:23, 1972
Carlson EV: Smoothing the hearing aid frequency response. J Audio Eng Soc 22:426–428,
    1974
Cox RM: Acoustic aspects of hearing aid-ear canal coupling systems. Monogr Contemp
    Audiol 1:1-44, 1979
Cox RM, Alexander GC: Acoustic versus electronic modification of hearing aid low fre-
    quency output, J Am Audiol Soc 4:190–196, 1983
Cranmer KS: Hearing aid dispensing—1986. Hearing Instruments 37:6–12, 141, 1986
Harford E, Barry J: A rehabilitative approach to the problem of unilateral hearing impair-
    ment: The contralateral routing of signals (CROS). J Speech Hear Disord 30:121–138,
    1965
Hawkins DB: Variability in clinical canal probe microphone measurements. Hearing Instru-
    ments 38:30–32, 1987
Hewitt C: New "free-field" earmold. Hearing Aid J 30:10, 32, 1977
Killion MC: Earmold plumbing for wideband hearing aids. J Acous Soc Am 59(S1): S62(A),
    1976
Killion MC: Design and Evaluation of High Fidelity Hearing Aids. Doctoral Dissertation,
    Univ Michigan Microfilms, 1979
Killion MC: Earmold options for wideband hearing aids. J Speech Hear Disord 46:10–20,
    1981
Leavitt R: Earmold: Acoustic and structural considerations, in Hodgson W, Skinner P (eds):
    Hearing Aid Assessment and Uses in Audiologic Habilitation (ed 2). Baltimore, Wil-
    liams & Wilkins, 1981, pp 73–114
Libby ER: Achieving a transparent, smooth, wideband hearing aid response. Hearing Instru-
    ments 32:9–12, 1981
Libby ER: State-of-the-art of hearing aid selection procedures. Hearing Instruments 36:30–
    38, 62, 1985
Libby ER: Real ear considerations in hearing aid selection. Hearing Instruments 38:14–16,
    1987
Lybarger SF: The Earmold as a Part of the Receiver Acoustic System. Canonsburg, PA,
    Radioear Corp, 1958
Lybarger SF: Earmolds, in Katz J (ed): Handbook in clinical Audiology (ed 2). Baltimore,
    Williams & Wilkins, 1978, pp 508–523
Lybarger SF: Controlling hearing aid performance by earmold design, in Larson VD et al.
    (eds): Auditory and Hearing Prosthetics Research. Orlando, FL, Grune & Stratton,
    1979, pp 101–132
Lybarger SF: Earmolds, in Katz J (ed): Handbook in Clinical Audiology (ed 3). Baltimore,
    Williams & Wilkins, 1985, pp 885–910
Mason WP: A study of the regular combination of acoustic elements, with application to
    acoustic filters, tapered acoustic filters, and horns. Bell Syst Tech J 6:258–294, 1927
McHugh ER, Purinsh MA: Evaluating the accuracy of earmold impression material. Hearing
    Instruments 35:12–13, 1984
National Association of Earmold Laboratories: Position paper, available from Westone Labo-
    ratories, Colorado Springs CO, 1970
National Association of Earmold Laboratories: The horn mold, available from Westone
    Laboratories, Colorado Springs, CO, 1981
Payne J: Personal communication, 1977
Pollack MC, Morgan R: Earmold technology and acoustics, in Pollack M (ed): Amplifica-
    tion for the Hearing Impaired (ed 2)., Orlando, Fl, Grune & Stratton, 1980, pp 91–142

Riess RL, Guthier JD: In-the-ear modification cookbook. Hearing Instruments 37:6–12, 141, 1986

Studebaker GA, Cox RM: Side branch and parallel vent effects in real ears and in acoustical and electrical models. J Am Audiol Soc 3:108–117, 1977

Sullivan RF: An acoustic coupling-based classification system for hearing aid fittings. Hearing Instruments 36:16–22, 1985

Joseph P. Millin

4

Practical and Philosophical Considerations

*There are few areas within the field of audiology that generate more differ-
ences of opinion than the selection of hearing aids. Over the years, a wide
diversity of procedural options for hearing aid evaluations have been proposed. None has received universal acceptance. The next four chapters of this
book relate to this very problem—how we select the appropriate amplification
system for our patients.*

*In this chapter, Joe Millin discusses some of the controversies that have
arisen and proposes solutions to many of them. This chapter is placed before
the three on hearing aid selections in order to give you a greater foundation
and insight into this complex area. Many "rules of thumb" have been used for
years without much questioning on our part. They have been handed down, so
to speak, from generation to generation. In this discussion, Joe looks at many
of these "principles" with an objective eye and points out how many of them
are no longer applicable.*

MCP

There is little doubt that technological advances in hearing aid amplification
systems in the last few years have produced substantial improvement in the sound
quality of wearable amplification. It is also true that the development of prescriptive
techniques has simplified the process of selecting hearing aids (see Berger, Chapter
7). Many audiologists feel that these changes have led to improved levels of patient
satisfaction while at the same time providing audiologists with much needed relief
from the arduous, cumbersome, and questionable comparative hearing aid selection

AMPLIFICATION FOR THE HEARING-IMPAIRED, THIRD EDITION   ISBN 0-8089-1886-9
Copyright © 1988 by Grune & Stratton, Inc.   All rights reserved.

techniques that have dominated audiologic practice for nearly 40 years (see Harford, Chapter 5).

I have no quarrel with these conclusions. As the number of required clinical decisions increased with each new technical development and comparative procedures became totally unmanageable, some kind of simplification of procedures was essential. My concern is that many audiologists seem to have come to believe that current prescriptive procedures are based on experimentally established relationships between hearing aid and listener performance and, as such, represent final answers to long-standing problems in hearing aid evaluation and selection.

One of my colleagues, a young audiologist in private practice, recently expressed just such a conviction. To her there are no problems. To determine appropriate amplification for her patients, she simply uses a commercially available, computerized, prescriptive formula and orders an aid with the specified characteristics from one of her suppliers. She then uses aided sound field measures to ensure that thresholds predicted by the prescription have been achieved. Her patients, she insists, are almost invariably enthusiastic and generally satisfied. She claims that what few complaints she has are easily solved by minor hearing aid adjustments. Asked why she selected the particular prescriptive procedure she uses, she answered that they are all pretty similar and she believes the differences among them to be of no consequence. She chose, therefore, the one that she feels is easiest to use. When asked what convinced her that the procedure she prefers will, in fact, identify appropriate amplification characteristics for her patients, she replied that the authors based the system on studies of typical preferences of successful hearing aid wearers and that they further claimed very high user satisfaction. In short, the authors simply assumed that performance options chosen by successful users would produce similar success for new users. They further assumed that user satisfaction confirms the value of the method and that they need not be concerned about objective supporting data or the possibility that some other method might produce substantially greater satisfaction.

AMPLIFIER–LISTENER RELATIONSHIPS

The obvious danger in using prescriptive formulations is the temptation to use them uncritically and to discontinue the search for lawful and predictable relationships between hearing aid electroacoustic characteristics and measurable parameters of listener performance. *The difficulties in identifying these relationships are admittedly staggering, but the fact remains that they have never been established.* The result has been that no selection strategy has achieved universal acceptance among audiologists. Until we succeed in determining valid and reliable relationships between instrumental and human performance variables, we cannot actually know how effective our current procedures are or whether some are substantially superior to others. At a time when our ability to control amplifier performance has become relatively unlimited, we cannot make optimum use of this capability because we do not have universally accepted and validated general rules by which we can effectively identify and specify the most appropriate amplifier characteristics for prospective hearing aid users. In other words, *now that we can have almost anything we want, we are unable to say with certainty exactly what we do want for our patients.*

Our failure to generate general selection rules has also exposed us to criticism from other professions, particularly otolaryngology (ACO Report 1977) and traditional dealers, who wonder how we can criticize them for lack of knowledge when we have, ourselves, no definitive procedures. As things stand, it is probable that there are nearly as many procedures for selecting hearing aids as there are audiologists, and the intrinsic worth of none of these procedures is precisely known. In his introduction to this book, Carhart, speaking of the various hearing aid selection procedures, stated the problem effectively:

> The reader can not help but emerge with the feeling that clinical audiology does not have a positive stand, but that any method for which an audiologist can present a thoughtful argument is probably as good as any dissimilar method for which another audiologist can present a comparably thoughtful argument. The implication is that the two methods are of equal merit. Such indecisiveness can not be considered the mark of maturity in the profession. Clinical research of sufficient rigor and extent must be conducted to resolve the underlying issues. Clinical audiology must assume responsibility for dealing directly and positively, and as a total profession with the issue of the relative merits of alternative methods for hearing aid selection.

The fact is that audiologists have not assumed such responsibility and only a very few are attempting to find answers to clinical problems. *So long as evaluations of hearing aid needs are performed solely on rational grounds, unsupported by convincing experimental evidence, with each audiologist using whatever system seems best, procedures used by audiologists will be no more defensible than those of any other persons, no matter how limited their training or suspect their motives.* At present we often operate more from personal conviction and unverified opinion than from any base of experimental data.

WHAT MANY AUDIOLOGISTS SEEM TO BELIEVE

To get an idea of what some of these convictions and opinions are, I have, for some months, been asking a few simple questions of audiologists from various work settings. The primary issue was, "What, if any, general rules can we state that will will help us select and fit hearing aids for our patients? That is, what can we say for certain, based on convincing research, about the relationship between hearing aid performance and listener performance?" I also posed the same questions to two "traditional" dispensers and a group of students in a graduate hearing aid seminar.

There was remarkable agreement among members of this diverse group. Their general conclusions are summarized below.

Selective Amplification Concept Endorsed

There was general agreement that a patient's hearing aid gain should vary in some proportion to differences in hearing threshold from frequency to frequency. In other words, they believed in the concept of selective amplification, although they could not precisely agree on what the relation between gain and hearing loss should be, nor could they cite any research supporting its value. Although a few of them mentioned Lybarger's (1963) observation that successful hearing aid users generally select gain equal to about half of their hearing loss at each frequency, none of the respondents felt this or any other formulation to be a complete or adequate basis for selecting hearing aids.

Low-Frequency Attenuation

Most, but not all, respondents agreed that low frequencies should be attenuated in noise, although none were willing to specify how steep the attenuation skirt should be, nor could they say how to determine at exactly what frequency this attenuation should begin. The dissenters insisted that some patients complained that attenuation of lows resulted in unacceptable sound quality whether in noise or in quiet. There was a general impression that regardless of whether they like low-frequency suppression in noise, patients prefer restoration of the low frequencies in quiet.

Output Limiting

Although there was general agreement that patient discomfort should be avoided by some kind of output limiting, no one had strong convictions about the relative value of the several forms of active compression, and several felt that symmetrical peak clipping was at least as effective as active compression. Several schemes were mentioned for establishing the level at which output should be controlled, but it was acknowledged that there is no definitive research supporting the value of any output limiting procedure (see Pollack, Chapter 2).

High-Frequency Extension

There was also a general belief that patients whose residual hearing is reasonably intact at frequencies above 4000 Hz may benefit by extension of the amplifier's upper cutoff frequency. Although new broadrange receivers, new earmolds, and a whole new methodology have been developed to extend the upper frequency limit of hearing aids (Killion 1981), there is little research attesting to its value, and none of the respondents were willing to specify how to determine exactly how much extension is necessary or desirable.

Frequency Response Smoothness

There was also a conviction that an irregular hearing aid frequency response degrades speech intelligibility and that smoothing the response by whatever means often results in significantly better listener performance. The respondents were aware of the work of Jerger and Thelin (1968), but not of Dillon (1983). Although they generally agreed on this issue and were aware of Killion's (1981) treatise on how response smoothing can be accomplished by using damping inserts, only one respondent claimed to do this regularly. Others admitted that they rarely, if ever, actually do anything to smooth frequency response, although they did claim to select instruments with smooth responses. Several of the dispensers do not even keep the necessary dampers for smoothing the hearing aid response on hand. A recent paper by Cox and Gilmore (1986), incidentally, casts some doubt on the value of this concept.

Questions pertaining to particular problem cases tended to reveal uncertainty. For example, when asked what to do for a patient who claims to hear everyone but his wife, they first facetiously suggested referral to a psychologist, but then all claimed to need more information. None could state precisely what information would be helpful or what they would do with it once provided. They generally agreed that high frequency gain would probably need to be increased, although no one could give any general statement on how to ascertain which high frequencies should be increased or by how much.

The Value of CROS

There appears to be some disillusionment with CROS and its variations, and only one of the dispensers had recommended any form of CROS fitting in the last 2 years. Part of the problem seemed to be lack of knowledge of precisely how to use the many varieties of CROS fittings that have been proposed (see Pollack, Chapter 8). Only two of the dispensers had made even limited use of them. One of these, however, had converted some users to conventional fittings if the aidable ear had significant hearing loss. In general, it was not that the CROS system was unsuccessful acoustically, but rather that many patients felt inconvenience or undesirable cosmetic factors outweighed the benefits.

A Surprise

There was one surprising observation. Two of the dispensing audiologists indicated a move away from almost exclusive use of in the ear fittings and a return to fitting behind-the-ear (BTE) aids. They felt this gave them substantially greater capability for modifying instrument response, a reduction in feedback problems and, for some users, both greater comfort and greater cosmetic hideability. I have always been somewhat amazed by the growing predominance of in-the-ear (ITE) aids. It is obvious that (BTE) aids, which permit use of "skeleton" type earmolds, are more hidable if the wearer has hair behind or over the ears.

Prescriptions a "Starting Point"

All except one respondent acknowledged using prescriptive techniques in determining hearing aid specifications for patients, but they claimed, without exception, that they considered the prescription to be "only a starting point" from which they would make appropriate alterations as needed. Asked how they decided which alterations to make, they generally avoided precise answers by stating that it depended on the user's complaints. Further probing elicited the response that the principles we have already reviewed, plus a few more, guided the alteration process.

Most agreed, for example, that reduction in high-frequency response was the general solution for complaints of tinniness or harshness, although again, just how to decide how much reduction, and at what frequencies, was not specified. A few attributed harshness to irregular frequency response. The general solution for the opposite effect, that is, a "boomy," hollow, or muffled sound, was to attenuate low frequencies.

I came away from these sessions with audiologists with some very clear impressions, not the least of which is that we know surprisingly little that is experimentally validated. All parties make general kinds of statements about how to fit aids, but none will venture to offer precise rules or strategies. Most admit to using prescriptions of one kind or another. All of these claim that the prescription is only a "starting point," but none will say how or what rules they use to modify the initial fitting. In short, there are no certainties. In fact, despite dramatic electroacoustic advancements, selection and fitting science has changed little in the last 30 years.

Gap between Technological and Clinical Developments

If you contrast these vague and indefinite selection and fitting principles with the precise procedures that have become available for measuring, specifying, and modifying hearing aid electroacoustic performance, it becomes apparent that the gap between advancements in hearing aid technology and the successful clinical application of these advancements continues to grow. *Clinical innovations continue to lag behind engineering accomplishments*, as they have for 50 years. It is surprising that manufacturers have any idea what direction product development should take, given that until very recently they have received so little input from dispensers. Nonetheless, most of the improvements or the innovations in hearing aid design come either from hearing aid manufacturers or from the radio and recording industries.

Lack of Rules Acknowledged

I am sure there are those who will challenge the idea that we have no established rules for selecting or fitting aids. Often those who are in the forefront of new developments or are recognized theorists are the first to acknowledge that we don't always know what to do with our new capabilities. Killion (1981), for example, in his landmark paper on earmold plumbing, describes how earmold modifications can extend extend high-frequency output to very high frequencies in the region of 10,000 or even 12,000 Hz, but then acknowledges that their value is as yet uncertain: "Just how many of the special earmolds described below will have enduring value is uncertain. . . . The earmold options described in this report may prove useful until the final answers are in." Staab (1985), discussing the potential advantages of digital hearing aids, states unequivocally that "A major problem today is that amplification needs of the hearing impaired are not actually known. Digital aids may be useful in studying hearing and hearing aid needs." Sandlin and Krebs (1980) say: "It is our view that technologically the status of hearing aid performance capabilities far exceed our skills to utilize them meaningfully in our evaluation processes relative to selection and fitting of electroacoustic devices." Duffy and Zelnick (1985) state that "If time and effort is to be devoted to the determination of an appropriate hearing aid for a person with a specific type of hearing impairment, the procedure utilized should be predictive of the benefits the individual will derive from the hearing aid selected, as it will be used in everyday life. Unfortunately, hearing aid selection procedures often employed today are unable to meet this objective." Harris (1976) states the problem somewhat differently: "Even if one has a good candidate and theoretically ideal prosthesis for him, there is no validated way to measure, much less to predict, what that aid does in the wearer's daily life."

Defense of Selection Methods

One should always look for the research basis of any selection procedure, regardless of its theoretical basis. When you do so you will find, for the most part, that the justification for many procedures is not experimental, but merely a claim that the system is practical, has proved effective based on experience, or has been well accepted by patients (Duffy and Zelnick 1985). There is nothing whatever wrong with such statements, as long as the reader recognizes that they are nothing more than claims, and not experimental evidence. Some formulators do, however, provide data describing the performance of people fitted by their method (Berger et al. 1980)

TRADITIONAL HEARING AID EVALUATION AND SELECTION PROCEDURES

We have not always been so unsure of ourselves. Carhart (1946a,b,c; 1950), working in the World War II military hospital program, developed procedures based on experimental methodology. Often referred to as "traditional," "conventional," or "comparative" procedures, they managed to achieve extensive, but not universal, acceptance. The primary procedure is clinical comparison on prospective hearing aid users of the performance of several hearing aids selected for trial on the basis of predetermined criteria. An aid is sought that provides (1) the greatest improvement in SRT, (2) the best word discrimination score (WDS) in quiet, (3) the widest dynamic range, and (4) the ability to maintain satisfactory speech discrimination in the highest level of noise.

The logic of the comparative procedure is so compelling that it is still used by many clinicians today. Serious challenges to its validity have been made, however, beginning with a study by Shore et al. (1960) demonstrating that "the reliability of these measures is not good enough to warrant the investment of a large amount of clinical time with them in selecting hearing aids." They further concluded "that one does not find substantial or striking differences among the results of hearing tests obtained from patients using different hearing aids or different tone settings of hearing aids."

The Diminished Clinical Use of Traditional Comparative Procedures

This study precipitated the abandonment of traditional evaluation procedures in two major clinics (Resnick and Becker 1963, Shore and Kramer 1965), and there is little doubt that it seriously undermined confidence in the traditional procedures. Another serious setback for these procedures was Resnick and Becker's conclusion, on the basis of the Shore et al. study, that comparative evaluations were unreliable and possibly invalid, and their recommendation that audiologists transfer the duty of selecting hearing aids to reputable hearing aid dispensers and concentrate instead on patient counseling.

The fact that the Shore et al. study casts doubt on their reliability was only a small part of the problem with comparative procedures. When they were developed during World War II, there were only a limited number of instrument models available (all worn on the body), and only a modest amount of modification of performance of individual aids was possible. Comparison of this limited number of options was practical, but the advent of the microminiaturized, integrated circuit dramatically increased the number of possible fitting options. Amplifiers could now be placed in eyeglass frames, in BTE enclosures, and finally in the ear canal. Further options emerged with the development of earmold modification strategies, such as venting to reduce low frequency response, and the use of earmold modifications to extend high-frequency response (Killion 1981). With the introduction of head-worn instruments, new questions emerged. Should comparisons be made on such options as binaural fitting or directional microphones? Should output be limited by clipping, linear compression, or nonlinear compression? Should some version of a CROS fitting be used?

All of these questions needed answers, in addition to the traditional problem of determining appropriate hearing aid frequency response. Obviously, if all of these options were submitted to comparison, the number of potential comparisons would be nearly unlimited. Comparative evaluation, even if it had been possible to demonstrate its validity, was no longer practical. There was now a pressing need for a means to quickly assess the value of all of these options for individual patients, and this need was, unquestionably, the major force behind the development of the many "prescriptive" selection procedures that now seem to be the dominant methods for selecting hearing aids for clinical patients.

PRESCRIPTIVE OR FORMULA FITTING

Numerous prescriptive systems for specifying appropriate hearing aid performance characteristics for clinic patients have been proposed (Lybarger 1963, Markle and Zaner 1966, Reddel and Calvert 1966, Gengel et al. 1971, Butts and Creech 1972, Kee 1972, Byrne and Tonnison 1976, Shapiro 1976, Bragg 1977, Berger et al. 1980, Skinner et al. 1982, Cox 1983, McCandless and Lyregaard 1983, Libby 1985). For many years these procedures received very limited attention, but as disillusionment with comparative procedures grew, some prescriptive procedures have gradually grown in popularity. All such formulas or prescriptive techniques are based in great part on some version of selective amplification (see Chapter 7 for an extensive review of prescriptive fitting approaches).

Selective Amplification

The concept of selective amplification has persisted ever since the development of the electronic hearing aid (see Carhart, Introduction.) Stated simply, selective amplification is the manipulation of frequency response in an attempt to optimize patient performance. There is compelling and almost irrefutable logic in the simple notion that a patient's gain requirements should be greater at frequencies where hearing loss is great than at frequencies where loss is slight. Beyond this generalization, however, we have, at best, only an approximate idea how hearing aid gain and hearing loss should be related. As Carhart points out, "Clinical audiology has not yet formulated any systematic general theory as to the role and proper applications of selective amplification" (see Introduction).

THE PERVASIVENESS OF THE SELECTIVE AMPLIFICATION CONCEPT

Selective amplification has taken many forms, but is always based on manipulation of the relationship between the patient's pure tone audiometric configuration and the frequency response of that patient's hearing aid, always with the goal of optimizing speech understanding. While there were certain major differences in experimental methodology, the usefulness of selective amplification was analyzed in both the Harvard Report (Davis et al. 1946) during the vacuum tube aid era and in the Shore et al. (1960) study with transistorized instruments. Both studies suggested that the value of the selective amplification concept could not be verified with available measures. The Harvard Report concluded:

The appropriate frequency characteristic for a hearing aid is not correctly indicated by current principles of "audiogram fitting" or "selective amplification." A uniform frequency characteristic that can be varied by a tone control between "flat" and moderate accentuation of high tones will provide the most satisfactory performance for all or nearly all cases of hearing loss. . . . For the usual hard-of-hearing patient any detailed "fitting" is wasteful of time and effort. The differentials between instruments that are indicated by most current tests are largely illusory.[*]

Despite the evidence against selective amplification, few other factors are really considered in comparative procedures. It is also the major component in prescriptive formulations.

Establishing the amount of hearing aid gain a patient will use outside the clinic, for example, is not a problem for the clinician. The patient will invariably make this decision. In my experience, instructing the patient to use higher or lower gain control adjustments is useless. In the first place, the patient will not do it, and in the second place, the level chosen by the listener is, in all likelihood, the best level for that person, given a particular amplifier (Yantis et al. 1966). Any higher level will possibly result in discomfort, while lower levels will result in reduced speech intelligibility. Furthermore, gain is a function of frequency response, since it is expressed in terms of the average of gain at selected frequencies taken from the frequency response curve. It would appear, in fact, that *the slope and smoothness of the frequency response could be critical determiners of the amount of gain the listener will choose to employ* (Jerger and Thelin 1968). In any event, the only problem with choosing gain is to assure that the overall gain of the amplifier is adequate and that at the listener's preferred setting, the instrument is not driven into saturation by input signal levels typically encountered by the patient.

FREQUENCY RESPONSE MODIFICATION IN SPECIALIZED PROCEDURES

Published descriptions of specialized fitting techniques may not identify them as forms of selective amplification, but examination of their theoretical bases make it evident that they are, in fact, attempts to optimize performance by frequency response modification. CROS fitting is one example. While initial reports (Harford and Barry 1965, Harford 1966a,b) were concerned largely with overcoming the effects of the "dead" side of the head, it soon became apparent that the open mold provided drastic reduction of low-frequency response and was useful in fitting hearing losses with the greatest deficit in high frequencies and normal or near-normal sensitivity in the lower frequency range. An added benefit, of course, is that the open mold permits "natural" (undistorted) reception of low frequencies. The

---

[*]Reprinted from Davis H, Hudgins CV, Marquis RJ, et al: The selection of hearing aids. (Harvard Report). Laryngoscope 56:58–115, 135–163, 1946.

open mold, therefore, is used as a means of manipulating hearing aid frequency response (Dodds and Harford 1968, 1970), which is what selective amplification is all about (see Chapter 8 for discussion of CROS fitting.)

Similarly, low-frequency emphasis aids for "deaf" children, whether based on an increase in the low-frequency response of conventional hearing aid amplifiers or on frequency transposition (Erber 1971, Ling 1964) are based on frequency response manipulation and thus fall into the selective amplification category. They differ from traditional practice, however, in that they amplify speech in the freqency region where the patient's sensitivity is best, based on the assumption that the high frequency region is essentially nonfunctional.

SELECTIVE AMPLIFICATION BASIS OF TYPICAL PRESCRIPTIVE
TECHNIQUES

Each of the prescriptive systems provides some method, based on selective amplification, for calculating specific hearing aid performance data by specifying mathematical operations to be performed on each patient's pure tone data to arrive at a "gain-frequency response" that is presumably appropriate for the listener. Some systems also provide a means for specifying hearing aid saturation sound pressure levels (SSPL), usually from uncomfortable loudness (UCL) data. There is a growing conviction that specification of output limitations is important, primarily for the purpose of compressing the wide variation in speech intensities within the restricted dynamic range of individual patients, although there is no universal method for determining how this should be most effectively achieved.

The prescriptive system of Berger et al. (1980) seems to have been adopted in many clinics nationwide, and it will serve well for use as an example of such formulations. This system specifies different divisors to be divided into the patient's thresholds at each audiometric test frequency. The resultant values plus a reserve of 10 dB are then sent to a manufacturer to be built into an aid for the patient or, in some cases, an aid with the specified values can be taken from the dispenser's inventory. Specific SSPL levels by frequency can also be designed into the hearing aid.

Clinician Must Choose System

Since each formula generates a different set of amplifier characterics for a given patient, the audiologist is faced with the task of deciding which system seems most likely to produce optimum communicative success for the listener. This can be a difficult decision, given that there are no experimentally established relationships between instrument performance and listener performance, and that each of the various schemes is backed by different arguments, some largely speculative, others using available hearing aid research to varying degrees.

The Berger et al. (1980) system, based in part on Lybarger's (1963) half-gain concept, makes substantial use of research on typical habits of instrument usage by "successful" hearing aid wearers. One can question, of course, whether typical behavior is necessarily optimum behavior, especially since the aid users on whom the data were based did not have unlimited opportunity to try all possible fitting options, but instead, were influenced by the particular beliefs of the dispenser or audiologist from whom they obtained their hearing aids. *No matter how well satisfied a patient may be, we have no way of knowing whether that patient might be even better satisfied with a different aid.* Despite this limitation of dependence on typical behavior, it is at present the most convincing data we have and, of the many formulas, I find that of Berger et al. (1980) to be the best reasoned. I use it routinely in our clinic, along with some additional measures that I consider important. Despite uncertainties surrounding formulas, I do not see substantial differences between fittings recommended by this formula and those arrived at by comparative procedures. This fact more than any other makes it difficult to justify the tedious comparative process. Other audiologists may disagree.

OTHER SELECTION STRATEGIES

There are other selection strategies that are not, strictly speaking, either typical comparative or prescriptive techniques, but involve features of one or the other (Cox 1985, Schachterle 1986, Zelnick 1982). The somewhat complex concept by Cox might be said to be eclectic, in the sense that it makes use of a number of other strategies, but it is also a useful flowchart to guide the dispenser in making systematic choices among various options, including some involving either comparisons or prescription. The value of these various systems is difficult to evaluate, as indeed, are all systems. The individual audiologist, having no true validating data available, must simply decide among them as reason dictates. Many choose, of course, to develop systems of their own.

One strategy that appears to have merit is described by Matkin (1984). An amplifier is selected that generates a sensation level for speech sufficient to permit optimum perception of all critical speech elements. To ensure that this has been accomplished, the patient's aided sound field audiogram is compared to the speech spectrum, which is superimposed over it. If I interpret Matkin's text correctly, this procedure involves a form of hearing aid comparison. Incidentally, he concludes that the Lybarger (1963) and the Berger et al. (1980) approaches provide insufficient gain in the higher frequencies.

Pascoe's (1975) concept of achieving an aided "uniform hearing level" for his patients has features in common with Matkin's strategy, since it would appear that good audibility for the entire speech spectrum would result from its use.

PRACTICAL AND THEORETICAL ISSUES IN PRESCRIPTIVE SELECTION AND FITTING

It is interesting that in private discussions there is substantial debate over the value of prescriptive selection techniques. Critics see formulas as arbitrary and oversimplified. They want to know why 2 is the precisely correct divisor at 500 Hz or why 2.5 wouldn't do as well. They ask how to be sure that the listeners will, during their daily pursuits, adjust the gain to the exact levels specified in the formulas. Anyone with experience with the formulas, of course, knows that listeners often do not use the predicted level.

Prescription advocates, on the other hand, argue that one must name some divisor at each frequency and so they have done so, based on the best evidence they feel is available. They do not claim the values to be sacrosanct, although they want you to make sure you have achieved them by making "objective" measures.

What the two sides are arguing, in fact, is *validity*. There is simply no convincing evidence that any system clearly identifies optimum hearing aids for listeners, although a recent study, using unusual criteria, claims that they do result in "the selection of different hearing aids for a given patient" (Humes 1986). No matter how well reasoned or convincing a formulation may be, however, its value, or that of any other method, will be known only after experimentation convincingly demonstrates that the system consistently identifies optimum or near-optimum electroacoustic conditions for individual patients. No such validating data has yet been obtained.

The efficiency and convenience of formula fitting are substantial. Only threshold and UCL data, and sometimes most comfortable loudness (MCL) data, are needed. Children without speech or adults who, for one reason or another, cannot be evaluated with speech tests can be fitted quickly without need for a second appointment or lengthy evaluation. Furthermore, the formula provides a clear goal, and success in achieving it can be objectively measured by free-field testing. I know of no data showing that other systems will produce better fittings or more satisfied hearing aid users. It is, therefore, very difficult to justify the use of programs that are more complex or take a great deal more time to execute. These are important advantages.

Some Troublesome Questions

Prescriptive fitting, on the other hand, raises many questions. One must believe, for example, that appropriate amplification for improving hearing performance, including enhancement of speech intelligibility, can be predicted solely from pure tone or other non-speech data and, further, that all persons with identical audiograms should have identical hearing aids, no matter how speech scores or other data might differ among patients. The formulas also imply that thresholds for tones, comfort levels, or tolerance levels are more important controlling features for predicting speech understanding than speech measures and that the critical objectives in fitting hearing aids are to establish optimum frequency response, adequate intensity, and normal loudness response. This could be an overpreoccupation with the purely intensive aspects of audition. *By concerning ourselves solely with loudness and intensity, we may be overlooking parameters that are more critical to successful function of the faulty auditory mechanism.*

We are just beginning to examine other potential strategies. With growing sophistication in microcircuitry, both digital and analog, we can begin to examine how speech might be recoded into unconventional units that may be better perceived by impaired ears. A discussion of some of these potential strategies can be found in ASHA (Signer 1985).

The Constantly Recurring Issue of Frequency Response

If frequency response manipulation is important, and I suspect that it is, it seems totally unlikely that a single response will serve a patient equally well in all environments. In fact, it may be that the interaction of frequency response with environment is as important as its interaction with the patient's threshold contour. It is possible—in fact, likely—that several frequency response options should be available to patients as they move from one acoustic environment to another. In fact, one of the presumed goals of digital hearing aid development is to analyze different environments and automatically select the response that is most beneficial for the patient (Staab 1985). Unfortunately, our lack of knowledge of relationships between amplifier-listener parameters could mean that, again, we will have this capability before we know how to apply it. Students, by the way, are sometimes surprised to discover that many aids dating back to the late 1940s had a switch that allowed temporary suppression of low frequencies (Millin 1984). Some aid users claimed to use this option regularly, while others tended to leave it in one position or the other. Today, many aids offer a normal- and high-frequency emphasis control (often labeled "N" and "H"), but I have seen no research whatever to determine how much use is made of this user option.

During my dispensing years, I attempted to solve listener problems by studying particular environments that gave my users difficulty. In addition to frequency response modification, solutions often required switching the aid to the opposite ear, binaural fitting, CROS-type variations (see Chapter 8), special microphone placement, and other strategies related to the effects of environmental noise, head shadow, reverberation, or weak signals. In more than a few cases, the solution was a desk-top amplifier, remote TV speaker, or other assistive listening device, rather than a hearing aid.

These experiences suggest that factors other than midrange frequency response may be of critical importance in aid selection and fitting. Formulas do not, for example, generally deal with extension of the upper frequency range (Triantos and McCandless 1974, Killion 1981) or reduction of low frequencies in noise. One virtue of the evaluation method described by Jerger and Hayes (1976) is that it permits testing of positional effects and, as such, broadens the scope of hearing aid evaluations to take cognizance of factors other than frequency response, which has been the major preoccupation of both the prescriptive and traditional procedures for 50 years. These and countless other issues must be understood before true sophistication in specifying hearing aids can be achieved.

The greatest danger in adopting any universal selection strategy at this time, when we know so little about a number of factors that may be important, is that we may retard the search for better methods. Students in particular often seek "cook-book" solutions to complex problems and tend to accept, uncritically, schemes promoted by teachers or other authority figures. At present, formulas should be regarded as useful interim strategies representing hypotheses to be tested and re-vised as research and experience dictate.

Speech Testing and Formulas

I am particularly bothered by the absence of speech tests in prescriptive proce-dures. Until such time that nonspeech stimuli can be proven to successfully predict a patient's hearing for speech, I feel compelled to use speech measures to test the adequacy of formula recommendations. I consider it mandatory to evaluate in some manner how the patient performs, using a real hearing aid worn appropriately on the head and listening to real speech, preferrably in noise.

A number of speech tests can be used for this purpose, and audiologists differ on which are most useful, but I find certain free-field comparative measures to be of particular value. An unaided soundfield WDS obtained at a relatively high level (say, 40 dB SL re: sound field SRT) appears to be a useful rough estimate of optimum ability to discriminate amplified speech with a linear amplifier, although the flat response of the audiometer may not be ideal for the patient. This score can serve as an absolute minimum performance level to be reached with a hearing aid when speech is presented at conversation level (60–65 dB SPL) with the patient instructed to set hearing aid gain for comfort. This presentation at conversational level is, it seems, critical, not only because it is a problem level, but because failure to achieve a score close to the estimate obtained above suggests that the frequency response or gain of the aid is not appropriate when the aid is adjusted as it would be in ordinary use. If a better "fit" can be found, the estimated performance score should be met and hopefully even exceeded, since an ideal hearing aid frequency response could presumably produce a WDS superior to that obtained with a flat response audiometer.

Another set of measures I like to compare are unaided and aided WDS scores obtained in the field with a conversation level input. The difference between these two scores can serve as a rough estimate of the minimum improvement that we should anticipate with an adequate fitting. Furthermore, a hearing aid with appro-priately modified frequency response could, presumably, permit the patient to achieve a score exceeding that obtained at the test level. If, however, the patient's unaided score at conversation level is relatively high, one must be more careful in fitting an aid, to assure that significant benefit is acheived.

An example can be instructive. Some years ago a colleague asked me to observe a woman who, when given a W-22 word list in the field, achieved a WDS of 48 percent. Since her loss was mild, we judged this score to be quite low. My colleague had tried several aids, all with reasonably dissimilar frequency responses. Using a conversation level input, the best score he could obtain with any aid was 28 percent. I could observe no procedural errors and I then tried more aids on the patient with the same result, that is, scores in the 20–30 percent range. Even though we could discern no tolerance difficulties, we tried a compression aid on the theory that we may somehow be overloading the ear. There was no change. We then tried binaural aids, convinced that they would result in better scores. There was still no significant change. Finally, we took her into the waiting room wearing one of the monaural fittings, and she found speech to be both objectionable and unintelligible.

There are, of course, always shortcomings in any hastily arranged clinical trial. Among other things, her trial earmolds were doubtless less than ideal, and we had only limited control of frequency response. Nonetheless, we became convinced that there was simply something about amplifiers that adversely affected her ability to discriminate speech. Even though we tentatively assumed that she was simply a poor candidate for amplification, we were aware that her communication problems were substantial, despite the mildness of her loss. We therefore arranged a clinic sponsored trial by persuading a dealer to loan us an aid for this purpose. After 7 weeks of trials, during which we made what we thought were appropriate aid modifications based on her complaints, she simply gave up in despair. Aided speech discrimination tests revealed the shortcomings of amplification for this patient and predicted her rejection of an aid during the trial period. This kind of experience convinces me of the critical importance of using speech tests in selecting hearing aids and evaluating their performance. Had we simply used a prescriptive technique, we would have glibly prescribed a set of electroacoustic characteristics for the patient, totally unaware of her reaction to amplification. I have since seen other comparable cases and I suspect that other audiologists have also.

After years of experience using speech measures to compare hearing aid effects, I am convinced that frequency response differences produce more dramatic performance differences for some listeners than for others. Only speech testing will identify such persons. A very few listeners, however, actually do more poorly aided than unaided. Alteration of frequency response generally does little to improve the performance of such persons, and they tend not to be good hearing aid candidates. The case just described is an example.

VALIDITY OF SELECTION STRATEGIES

No matter how well reasoned they may be, it must be remembered that all prescriptive procedures, as well as all comparative procedures, lack experimental validation; nor, with one possible exception (Humes 1986), have there been studies comparing the effectiveness of the various prescriptive procedures. It is true that the levels recommended by the various formulas can be verified by coupler or field measurement and that these measures have good repeatability. This "objectivity" is, in fact, often touted as a major virtue of formulas. *The fact, however, that the fitting goals can be measured reliably does not necessarily mean that the goals, themselves, are valid.* The greater issue is not whether you can obtain the levels specified by a system, but whether the levels do, in fact, represent an appropriate fitting for the patient.

Certain formulators have provided convincing evidence that the level of user satisfaction achieved by some of these formulas is relatively high, and, at present, it appears as though we have little choice but to depend on this kind of testimonial evidence. *It has not been demonstrated, however, that one formula produces better results than any other or that any formula clearly identifies optimum or near-optimum hearing aid performance characteristics.* The problems of establishing the real-world validity of these prescriptive procedures, as I will elaborate on below, are so formidable that few experimenters are willing to attempt to solve them.

THE CURRENT EMPHASIS ON MEASUREMENT STRATEGIES

I suspect all of us have seen audiologists measure a patient's aid in a test box unit and then use the obtained gain/frequency response to estimate aided thresholds for the patient, apparently blissfully unaware that the obtained results could be seriously in error because the patient's ear impedance may only remotely resemble the impedance of the test system coupler. As Pollack points out in Chapter 2, the HA1/HA-2 coupler, which is most commonly used in these test box systems, was never intended to simulate human ear impedance (Romanow 1942). Furthermore, even the superior Zwislocki type coupler (see Chapter 2) simulates, not individual patient ears, but an average (median) adult ear. Students should remember that *coupler data, no matter how accurately they may simulate hearing aid performance in average ears, cannot be used to ascertain performance in the ears of real patients, since there is no way of knowing how much the impedance of the patients' ears may deviate from average.* In addition to the substantial variability of the impedance of normal ears around the mean and factors such as the smaller ears of children, audiologists see many persons with mixed losses where the conductive component is not remediated for one reason or another. For such reasons the impedance of clinic patients varies substantially and only "real-ear" measurements of some kind will determine what SPLs will actually occur in a given patient's ear. It is this individual data that is most often needed in selection and fitting.

Real-Ear and Functional Gain

The development of two procedures for measuring aided performance has received much attention. The first is to obtain aided and unaided thresholds in sound field. The difference is the "functional gain" of the hearing aid, and if plotted (assuming a linear amplifier), also represents a frequency response. This measure is subject to all the errors related to threshold testing, but can be accurate if done carefully.

The data provided in this manner are sometimes called "use data" since they are obtained at the gain level used by the wearer and not at either a maximum or a reference test gain setting. Since these data provide aided thresholds on actual patients, they can be especially useful in hearing aid fitting and in evaluating whether the aided thresholds predicted by a particular prescriptive procedure have been achieved. The biggest disadvantage is that data are obtained only at standard, audiometric test frequencies, which is a pretty limited representation of the overall gain/frequency performance of a hearing aid. It is also a relatively time-consuming process. This "real-ear" measure provides gain data for each individual patient and does not require the use of a coupler.

The probe microphone method, also a real-ear procedure, inserts a very slim probe microphone tube alongside the earmold (or hearing aid in the case of an ITE model) and deep into the canal close to the drum. Presumably, this provides precise sound pressures produced by a hearing aid at the tympanic membrane. There is also a microphone outside the pinna. Signals are presented through a loudspeaker, and the test system makes simultaneous measures at the pinna and in the canal. When compared, these values can provide data not only on the gain of a hearing aid but also on the "insertion loss" that occurs when a mold is put into the ear canal, which, of course, obstructs the canal and alters its natural resonant properties.

One problem with both the soundfield and probe microphone methods is the presence of standing waves at the ear produced by reflections from surfaces in the test room. The ear, if it moves, passes through regions of varying sound pressure, thus yielding unstable data.

There appear to be at least three imperfect but useful solutions to this problem. The first is to fix the head with some kind of brace, so that it cannot move, although not all patients take well to this procdure. The second solution is to scatter the sound in the field by various methods so that the soundfield is relatively diffuse. While this can only be done imperfectly, it is possible to establish a region around the head that varies only slightly with head movements. Although some commercial probe systems supposedly "level the soundfield" prior to testing, these levels are achieved precisely only if there is absolutely no change in head position during consecutive signal presentations. A third possibility, with which I have had partial success experimentally, is to use a fast acting compressor to stabilize pressures at the ear.

A second problem with probe microphone measurements is, that at very high frequencies, especially at 8000 Hz and above, wavelengths are sufficiently small that pressure waves are propagated in the ear canal, presumably setting up very short standing waves (Sivian and White 1933). Slight changes in the positioning of the microphone probe tip can place it anywhere in the standing-wave pattern, thus producing data different from that at the eardrum. Attempts to establish standardized threshold data for frequencies above 8000 Hz and up to 18,000 Hz have been hampered by this problem, and thresholds reported in various studies differ from one another by as much as 55 dB (Cunningham and Goetzinger 1974, Harris and Myers 1971, Northern et al. 1972, Northern and Ratkiewicz 1985, Rudmose 1961, Zislis and Fletcher 1966). At this time it is not clear whether these differences result from calibration problems, that is, problems of establishing precise eardrum sound pressures, or whether they reflect tremendous true threshold differences among listeners at the upper frequency limit of hearing. It is probably some of each.

Depending on the degree of care taken by the clinician, both of these systems can provide valuable data up to at least 6000 Hz. There are, however, important differences in the data obtained by each method. The functional gain method provides aided behavioral threshold data, which can be used to check how well aided thresholds correspond to the thresholds predicted by a prescriptive procedure. It also provides reasonably accurate measures of the acoustic gain of an aid for individual patients under conditions of use. The limited number of frequencies tested is, however, an unfortunate shortcoming of the method, since potentially detrimental peaks and valleys in the frequency response of a hearing aid would not be seen.

Data obtained by probe tube procedures do not provide aided thresholds. These can be estimated, however, from probe data, if proper conversion data are used. Aided thresholds are most often needed when using a prescriptive procedure in which fitting success is verified by comparing the thresholds predicted by the formula with those actually achieved by the patient (e.g., Berger et al. 1980). It is also possible, and probably most convenient, to calculate and display the predicted thresholds prior to patient testing, although these predicted aided thresholds must be converted to predicted aided drum pressures. The patient test will then display the achieved drum pressures on the same graph, so that discrepancies between predicted and obtained data can be instantly compared.

One might say that these drum pressures, unlike soundfield thresholds, are not contaminated by voluntary responses, and are, therefore, more objective than aided thresholds. This is true, although one must remember that there is almost no application in which these data do not have to be, sooner or later, related to behavioral data. Depending on the data preferred by individual audiologists, the particular purposes to which the probe microphone systems can be applied, vary greatly. Their potential, in fact, appears to be almost unlimited, and they have many advantages over test boxes and functional gain meaures. Furthermore, they provide data rapidly, with relatively good accuracy and with many data points.

Measurement Goals

The systems just described offer, without question, certain important measurement advantages over the older test box systems. On the other hand, the basic value of these more reliable and probably more valid data depends on the use to which they are put. Most often they are used to ascertain how signals at the ear are altered by a hearing aid. The critical question then becomes, "Now that we are convinced that we know exactly what the patient's hearing aid is doing, what criteria do we use to decide whether the values we obtained are, in fact, appropriate for the listener?" In short, what is our goal? What do we want the hearing aid to do, and is it doing it? This is where the audiologist's selection and fitting criteria become the critical issue. Measures of hearing aid performance, no matter how accurate, are meaningless until we establish values that we are sure are appropriate for the patient. The Berger procedure recommends that aided free-field measures be obtained on the patient when the aid is returned from the manufacturer, with due attention given to problems of field testing. The resulting thresholds are then compared to those that have been predicted by subtracting the recommended gain values from the patient's unaided thresholds in the aided ear. If they differ by more than a few decibels, they recommend that the instrument be modified. While this system is "objective" in the sense that it assures that the prescribed aided values are actually obtained, we should remember that these prescribed values may or may not be optimum or near-optimum values for the patient, in terms of numerous criteria, such as speech intelligibility, sound quality, listening comfort, or user satisfaction.

THE IMPORTANCE OF THE COMPARATIVE TECHNIQUE

Despite the decline in the use of the comparative technique as a clinical tool for hearing aid selection, it is important to recognize that some form of comparative evaluation will almost certainly continue to be the primary method for examining the relation between instrument performance and patient performance. I can think of no research on this subject that did not use either some form of the Carhart comparative procedure or some form of paired comparison. With rare exceptions, research on amplifier effects involves examination of how variation in amplifier characteristics produces changes in certain criterion measures, such as word discrimination scores, thresholds, loudness level preference, relative intelligibility, relative quality, or simply instrument preference.

Assumptions Underlying Traditional Procedures

While the tutorial paper by Resnick and Becker (1963) affected clinical practice and generated controversy (Millin 1963, Jeffers and Smith 1964), its most important contribution was the formulation of the three basic assumptions that constitute the rationale for hearing aid comparison: (1) there are significant differences among hearing aids in terms of how they enable the user to understand everyday speech; (2) these differences change from one user to the next, that is, there is an interaction between people and hearing aids; and (3) these differences can be demonstrated reliably by monosyllabic word (PB 50) intelligibility scores.

These are still the underlying theoretical operating assumptions for hearing aid research. Regardless of whether they are valid, they must be embraced if amplifier comparisons are to be justified.

If the first assumption is false and one hearing aid is as effective as any other, it is obvious that there can be no possible justification for performing comparative evaluations. Neither would there seem to be any reason to use a prescriptive technique. We must believe, therefore, that hearing aid differences are meaningful. There is clearly a general conviction that this is true.

The second, more subtle assumption of an interaction between people and hearing aids requires the clinician to believe that the relative effectiveness of various hearing aids differs from patient to patient. There is considerable disagreement regarding this issue. While users of prescriptive techniques do not assume that the best hearing aid for any one patient is best for all patients, they do believe that existing interactions are predictable and thus the best instrument can be identified by application of the prescriptive formula. If research were to show that listeners with identical audiograms perform best with different hearing aids and identification of the best aid cannot be predicted from audiometric data, then, presumably, only a comparative procedure could identify the optimum aid for each patient. In order to justify comparative evaluation of aids on every patient, therefore, one must believe that precise prediction of patient amplification needs cannot, given the present state of the art, be predicted from unaided audiometric data.

There seems to be general agreement among audiologists that the third assumption is false, and that word intelligibility scores cannot unambiguously and reliably detect hearing aid effects. One way of interpreting the small differences in scores resulting from differences among hearing aids is to assume that speech discrimination tests are relatively insensitive to amplifier effects. In addition to the apparent lack of sensitivity of conventional word lists, they tend to be unreliable, and the magnitude of differences obtained when identical tests are repeated tends to be greater than effects generated by amplifier differences. Hence amplifier effects are obscured. If it is true, however, that amplifier differences have little influence on word identification, one might ask why they should should be important in discriminating conversational speech. We are back, therefore, to the first basic proposition of Resnick and Becker (1963) as to whether there are significant differences among hearing aids in terms of how they enable the user to understand everyday speech." The presumption is that typical monosyllabic word lists carry minimal information and thus are not representative of the linguistic sophistication of real interpersonal communication.

Attempts have been made, therefore, to generate tests using more "realistic" or meaningful test items in which redundancy is high and in which syntactical structure more nearly resembles genuine coversational content (Berger 1967, Jerger et al. 1966). Furthermore, by introducing meaningful materials or common grammatical and syntactical forms, some underlying linguistic sufficiency is presumably sampled by the test. The greatest problem with this concept is that the test items are almost invariably too easy. Scores tend to hover near perfect performance, and differentiation among hearing aids is actually reduced. There is the further formidable problem that the redundancy of meaningful material is dependent on the experience of the listener, and thus the effects of experience and amplifiers are confounded.

The tendency, therefore, has been to fall back on the lower redundancy of monosyllabic word lists. The theory seems to be that if the information in the stimulus is minimal, it will be difficult enough to discriminate that superior amplification systems will enable the listener to identify more items than inferior systems. It is assumed that any listener who can identify minimum information-bearing items readily will have even less difficulty with information-rich sentences. The validity of this assumption is assumed, but one must wonder how strictly this interpretation can be trusted.

Clinically, the important factor is not simply whether the reliability of a procedure is good, but whether it will differentiate between the effects of amplifiers unambiguously. Only if the effects of aids are larger than the inherent variability of the test employed to detect them will it be possible to make correct, unambiguous decisions. Present tests appear to lack the kind of precision necessary to make clear-cut decisions within a reasonable period of time, at least when making comparisons among amplifiers. Thus the search for stable, practical tests continues.

The Value of Speech Tests

I hasten to say, in spite of these factors, that it is probably a serious error to write off speech tests simply because they have a high degree of variability. It seems safe to say, despite their variability, that they often provide vital information. Just as it is much easier to "fake" an IQ test downward than upward, so, in my judgment, is it almost impossible to score 96–100 percent on the W-22 test if you have very poor speech discrimination. Nothing confirms my clinical hunches any more certainly, when I think I have found an appropriate fitting for a patient, than to see the patient produce a very high WDS. Neither does anything confirm a fitting problem more surely than a very low WDS. The sound field comparisons discussed earlier in this chapter are based on my conviction that speech data, if evaluated carefully, can be of vital importance in decision making.

Some Research Considerations

Ideally, two general conditions should be met in order to compare the effects of amplification on a listener. The first is that any independent variable, such as frequency response, should be specified very precisely. To do this properly, amplifiers with smooth, unambiguous response curves would be needed. Several slopes could then be chosen to test on the listener.

The second requisite condition, almost impossible to achieve, is that all performance variables of the trial aids other than the frequency response (the independent variable) be held constant. That is, each aid should have equivalent maximum gain, distortion, transient response, noise floor, and maximum output, to name only a few measurable parameters. The problem is that the independent variable, in this example frequency response, is not really independent of these other parameters and thus cannot literally operate as an independent variable (Chial and Hayes 1974, Bode and Kasten 1971). As frequency response is changed, some of the other properties will also change, and until changes in all but the independent variable can be rendered ineffectual, changes in patient scores may or may not be largely dependent on differences in frequency responses among aids rather than on uncontrolled differences among other factors.

VALIDITY

If, by virtue of some good fortune, a procedure should be developed that would permit reliable ranking of hearing aid performance for patients, a critical question would remain. Will the hearing aid that is found to provide the best performance for a patient in the clinical setting maintain its superiority when used by the patient outside the clinic in everyday life? Simple as this may sound, the problems of validity testing are so formidable that, to my knowldege, no serious effort to ascertain the predictive validity of any selection procedure has ever been made.

The most imposing problem is generating criteria that will adequately estimate performance in the many environments patients will typically encounter. Like our clinical measures, the reliability of such criteria must be established, after which their validity as appropriate indicators of performance must also be determined. The problem of developing reliable measures of real-world performance is even more complex than the development of clinical tests because there are many uncontrollable sources of variability in everyday environments. Unfortunately, any attempt to manipulate these variables artificially represents an intrusion into the natural events that influence listening and thus tends to contaminate the validity of the measures. In fact, it appears that the mere act of observing the listener's behavior represents such an intrusion, particularly if the listener is aware of being observed. Problems of this kind discourage investigations of test validity. Nonetheless, until we are able to validate the predictive ability of our selection strategies, we can only hope that they are maximally effective, and there is always the possibility that they are of little value.

UNTESTED AXIOMS AND HYPOTHESES

Numerous clinical rules of thumb have been accorded wide acceptance over the years, although they are in fact only assumptions. Here are a few examples. All other things being equal:

1. Fit the ear with the best speech discrimination.
2. Fit the ear with the flattest audiometric curve.
3. Fit the ear with the highest tolerance level.
4. Fit the ear with the poorest pure tone thresholds.

The list is long, and comments on only a few are necessary here. I take issue with them, not because they are necessarily unreasonable, but because they are, in fact, untested hypotheses. If their validity is ever tested, I suspect that most of them may prove to be fallacious. I have seen patients with mild hearing losses, for example, who insist that they hear better with amplification in the ear that has better pure tone thresholds, despite the fact that audiometric tests showed no significant interear differences in discrimination or tolerance. In fact, I know of one audiologist who argues that a patient with a mild loss in one ear and a moderate loss in the other will often be better off if a hearing aid will bring the mild-loss ear to a higher level of functioning than the moderate one. This audiologist states the question something like this: "Which would you rather have, one ear that functions almost perfectly and one that functions poorly, or by fitting the poorer ear, two ears that function fairly well?" The audiologist's argument is that the better ear can, in many patients, be made functionally much closer to normal than the poorer ear. The audiologist lets the patients decide, through a trial, which solution they prefer and insists that if either ear can be fitted to achieve a very low threshold and high speech discrimination without tolerance problems, the patient will invariably prefer to be fitted in that ear. Whether he is right or wrong may not be apparent, but one must conclude that the argument is logical enough to lead us to question the "fit the poorer ear" principle.

There are still physicians who tell patients that hearing aids are of no value to persons with "nerve loss," despite the fact that the overwhelming majority of hearing aids are used by persons with sensorineural hearing loss. Another often heard claim is that amplification is of no value for patients with poor discrimination for speech, when it should be obvious that any improvement over unaided hearing will be welcome by the person with severe difficulties.

Another source of concern is the clinician who advocates some pet hearing aid evaluation theory with fanatic zeal, as though it were the final answer to all selection and fitting problems. The more strongly such persons defend their theory, the less convincing is their objectivity or competency. When audiologists strongly advocate a particular evaluative system, knowing that no system enjoys scientific verification, I secretly suspect that they are very insecure in their beliefs and I am led to question both their motives and objectivity.

THE FUTURE

Digital Hearing Aids

The latest catchword is "digital." It is assumed that some form of digital processing will enable us to make dramatic improvements in amplifier capabilities. Among these possibilities are elimination of feedback, near-perfect control of frequency response, and the use of adaptive filtering, that is, adapting the electroacoustic response of hearing aids to changing environments. At present the problem is that the analog-to-digital-to-analog (A/D/A) conversion that is needed to achieve this function requires unacceptable amounts of storage and retrieval time as well as relatively bulky hardware and softwear, too much to be used in an acceptable wearable amplifier. This condition is doubtless temporary, however, and these functions have already been accomplished in "quick time" in large, nonportable amplifiers.

Dispensing and Private Practice

It is important to remind ourselves that the entrance of audiologists into the dispensing field and the resulting increase in private practice activity, as well as the broadening of our financial base, may well have saved audiology from extinction and finally provided the opportunity for the continuing relationship with clients that is necessary to provide a complete service to the hearing-impaired. Of equal importance, however, was the much needed opportunity to function independently and to escape from dependence on institutions for employment.

OPPORTUNITY FOR SELF-REALIZATION

This tendency of graduates to seek institutional employment is seriously retarding the growth of our profession (Millin 1984). Frankly, as a traditional hearing aid dealer in the 1950s, I had more income, more status, and certainly more opportunity for self-direction than did most institutionally employed audiologists, and judging from the comments of many former students now employed in institutional settings, I certainly derived more satisfaction from and my work and had more fun doing it than they do.

I heartily recommend that teachers everywhere strongly encourage audiology students to give dispensing and private practice serious consideration as employment options. In the long run this will provide the greatest satisfaction as well as the greatest financial rewards. It will also do the most to advance the profession. I am discouraged by the constant concern of students about the prospects of "finding a job" as though working for others is the only option open to them. Most physicians, optometrists, and dentists, to name a few professionals, create their own jobs. Audiologists should consider doing the same.

This is not to say that there is anything inherently wrong with institutional employment, but only that institutions tend to pay less, control more, and offer less opportunities for self-expression and hence provide less personal satisfaction than private practice. Certainly, not all audiologists should enter private practice. Many persons simply don't have the temperament for it.

Many eager, energetic, and ambitious young graduates, on the other hand, should recognize that great personal satisfaction as well as great financial rewards are likely to be found in dispensing and in private practice. For too many years, it seems to me, the speech and hearing profession has undervalued itself and has been too willing to see its practitioners in supportive rather than primary roles. Dispensing and private practice offer a welcome opportunity for self direction and greater self-realization. [For a more complete discussion, see Millin (1984).]

CONCLUSION

Hopefully, as the healthy and important emphasis on engineering developments continue, audiologists will intensify their search for underlying fitting principles that will help us to make optimum use of these developments as well as to eliminate much of the uncertainty that now characterizes our thinking. All the remarkable electronic advances will simply have limited value until we understand how to apply them. Our need for valid procedures is, in my judgment, acute.

The Paradox of Audiologic Research

A few years ago an earlier version of this chapter was being quoted by hearing aid dealers to show that audiologists were no more knowledgeable than they. This was at FDA hearings, and I was unaware that the chapter was being used in this way. I was asked by ASHA to submit testimony clarifying my position. I emphasized that just as the medical profession does not understand the common cold, so audiologists are seeking solutions to problems in amplification, and in the process we have had the courage to publicize our failures as well as their successes.

This paradox has been with us for many years. While traditional dealers confidently dispense and fit hearing aids, untroubled by selection issues, audiologists, seeking solutions to selection problems, discover more often than not that formal experiments cannot confirm their cherished concepts (Millin, 1984). Thus, for example, the "Harvard Report," early on, was unable to verify the value of selective amplification. Other attempts either failed altogether or found weak effects at best, although some reasonably convincing evidence is accumulating after some 40 years. Comparative procedures were found to be unreliable by Shore et al. (1960) and recently Cox and Gilmore (1986) have challenged the value of frequency response smoothing and have questioned the proposition that response irregularities prevent the subject from achieving adequate audibility and sensation levels for the speech spectrum.

The same fate befell attempts to experimentally confirm the value of binaural amplification, although testimonial evidence favoring it is abundant. There has been recent evidence questioning the value of low-frequency suppression, at least in one experimental noise environment (Edner 1986), although the same experiment did demonstrate relatively strong frequency response effects when the response was shaped by the listeners. As yet I have seen no data supporting the value of extension of frequency response to include higher frequencies, although neither have I seen evidence denying its value.

These issues must be resolved. There are times when I wonder whether any procedure or any scheme whatever can be vigorously defended. This is simply not a healthy position to be in. I cannot bring myself to believe that these basic questions cannot be answered, and attempts to resolve these issues are advancing at a faster rate than ever before. Whole volumes of research and commentary have emerged in recent years (Studebaker and Bess 1982, Libby 1985). Numerous individuals, many of whom have been cited herein, are also seeking answers to selection problems.

I am also unable to accept the proposition that alterations in frequency response, that is, the concept of selective amplification, does not work. It is inherently unreasonable to accept the proposition that a flat response is appropriate for all persons, regardless of differences in the amount of hearing loss across frequency. I have never talked to any audiologist who denied the value of selective amplification.

Unquestionably, our criterion measures are part of the problem, and new ones are being tried to determine whether meaningful relationships between people and hearing aids can be clarified (Cox 1983, 1986; Humes 1986, Studebaker et al. 1982). Whatever method finally emerges, we must continue to search for these relationships.

The Possible Effects of Subject Selection

I cannot help but wonder whether part of our failure to find such relationships may result from our somewhat simplistic approach to subject selection. Classifying subjects in mild, moderate, or severe sensorineural hearing loss categories or by degree of audiogram slope, as if, in some manner, this guarantees that the subjects within each group will be homogeneous in their response behavior, could be very risky. Difficult as it may be, we probably need to find ways to determine whether certain complex audiometric patterns, including, in addition to the pure tone pattern, word discrimination data, tolerance and dynamic range data, loudness patterns, and doubtless other kinds of information, the need for which is not yet recognized, may not separate out groups that are internally consistent in behavior but differ substantially from other groups. If such categories of behavior do exist, their discovery might facilitate the discovery of consistent group/amplification relationships. Despite the discouraging progress of the last 50 years, I am optimistic, in view of the accelerated research under way everywhere, that answers to most of these questions will soon be forthcoming.

REFERENCES

ACO: Report of ACO Subcommittee on Hearing Aids. Newsletter of the American Council of Otolaryngology, September, 1977
Berger KW: The KSU speech discrimination test. Kent, OH, Kent State University, 1967
Berger KW, Hagberg EN, Rane RL: Prescription of Hearing Aids: Rationale, Procedure and Results, Kent, OH, Herald Publishing House, 1980
Bode DL, Kasten RN: Hearing aid distortion and consonant identification. J Speech Hearing Res 14:323–331, 1971
Bragg BC: Toward a more objective hearing aid fitting procedure. Hearing Instruments 28:6–9, 1977
Butts FM, Creech HB: Tracing the MCL: An approach to hearing aid selection. Paper presented at the Convention of the American Speech and Hearing Association, 1972
Byrne D, Tonnison W: Selecting the gain of hearing aids for persons with sensorineural hearing impairments. Scand Audiol 5:51–59, 1976
Carhart R: Selection of hearing aids. Arch Otolaryngol 44:1–18, 1946a
Carhart R: Volume control adjustments in hearing aid selection. Laryngoscope 56:510–526, 1946b
Carhart R: Tests for the selection of hearing aids. Laryngoscope 56:780–794, 1946c
Carhart R: Hearing aid selection by university clinics. J Speech Hearing Disorders 15:106–113, 1950

Chial MR, Hayes CS: Hearing aid evaluation methods: Some underlying assumptions. J Speech Hearing Disorders 39:270–279, 1974

Cox RM, Gilmore C: Damping the hearing aid frequency response: Effects on speech clarity and preferred listening level. J Speech Hearing Res 29:357–365, 1986

Cox RM: Using ULCL measures to find frequency/gain and SSPL90. Hearing Instruments 34:17–21, 1983

Cox RM: Hearing aids and aural rehabilitation: A structured approach to hearing aid selection. Ear Hearing 6:226–239, 1985

Cunningham DR, Goetzinger CP: Extra-high frequency hearing loss and hyperlipidemia. Audiology 13:470–484, 1974

Davis H, Hudgins CV, Marquis RJ, et al: The selection of hearing aids. (Harvard Report). Laryngoscope 56:58–115, 135–163, 1946

Dillon H: Earmold modifications for wide bandwidth flat response hearing aid coupling systems for use in audiological measurements. Austral J Audiol 5:63–70, 1983

Dodds E, Harford E: Modified earpieces and CROS for high-frequency hearing losses. J Speech Hearing Res 11:204–218, 1968

Dodds E, Harford ER: Follow-up report on modified earpieces and CROS for high frequency hearing losses. J Speech Hearing Res 13:41–43, 1970

Duffy JK, Zelnick E: A critique of past and current hearing aid assessment procedures. Audecibel, Fall, 1985, pp 10–23

Edner RG: The effects of electroacoustic frequency response modifications on persons with sensorineural hearing loss. Kent, OH, Kent State University, 1986

Erber NP: Evaluation of special hearing aids for deaf children. J Speech Hearing Disorders 36:527–537, 1971

Gengel RW, Pascoe D, Shore I: A frequency response procedure for evaluating and selecting hearing aids for severely hearing impaired children. J Speech Hearing Disorders 36:341–353, 1971

Harford ER: The clinical application of CROS. Arch Otolaryngol 83:455–464, 1966a

Harford ER: Bilateral CROS. Arch Otolaryngol, 84:426–432, 1966b

Harford ER, Barry J: A rehabilitative approach to the problem of unilateral hearing impairments: The contralateral routing of signals (CROS). J Speech Hearing Disorders 30:121–138, 1965

Harris JD: Introduction, in Rubin M (ed): Hearing Aids: Current Developments and Concepts. Baltimore, University Park Press, 1976

Harris JD, Myers, CK: Tentative audiometric threshold-level standards from 8000 to 18,000 Hertz. J Acoust Soc Am 49:600–601, 1971

Humes LE: An evaluation of several rationales for selecting hearing aid gain. J Speech Hearing Res 51:272–281, 1986

Jeffers J, Smith C: On hearing aid selection, in part a reply to Resnick and Becker. ASHA 6:504–506, 1964

Jerger J, Hayes D: Hearing aid evaluation: Clinical experience with a new philosophy. Arch Otololaryngol 102:214–225, 1976

Jerger J, Malmquist C, Speaks C: Comparison of some speech intelligibility tests in the evaluation of hearing aid performance. J Speech Hearing Res 9:253–258, 1966

Jerger J, Thelin J: Effects of electroacoustic characteristics of hearing aids on speech understanding. Bull Prosthetic Res 159–197, 1968

Kee WR: Use of pure tone measurement in hearing aid fittings. Audecibel 9–15, Winter, 1972

Killion M: Earmold options for widebnd hearing aids. J Speech Hearing Disorders 46:10–20, 1981

Libby ER: State-of-the-art of hearing aid selection procedures. Hearing Instruments 36:30–38, 1985

Ling D: Implications of hearing aid amplification below 300 cps. Volta Rev 66:723–729, 1964

Ling D, Maretic H: Frequency transposition in the teaching of speech to deaf children, J Speech Hearing Res 14:37–46, 1971

Lybarger SF: Simplified fitting system for hearing aids. Radioear Spec Fitting Manual 1–8, 1963

Markle DM, Zaner A: The determination of gain requirements of hearing aids: a new method. J Auditory Res 6:371–377, 1966

Matkin ND: Wearable amplification: A litany of persisting problems, in Jerger J (ed): Pediatric Audiology. San Diego, College Hill Press, 1984, pp 125–145

McCandless GA, Lyregaard PE: Prescription of gain/output (POGO) for hearing aids. Hearing Instruments 34:16–20, 1983

Millin JP: Conventional hearing aid selection. ASHA 5:880–881, 1963

Millin JP: Hearing aid dispensing programs, in Jerger J (ed): Hearing Disorders in Adults, San Diego, College Hill Press, 1984, pp 149–171

Northern JL, Downs MP, Rudmose W, et al: Recommended high frequency audiometrics thresholds. J Acoust Soc Am 52:585–594, 1972

Northern JL, Ratkiewicz B: The quest for high frequency normative data. Seminars Hearing 6:331–339, 1985

Pascoe DP: Frequency responses of hearing aids and their effects on the speech perception of hearing-impaired subjects. Ann Otol Rhinol Laryngol 84 (Suppl 23), 1975

Reddell RC, Calvert DR: Selecting a hearing aid by interpreting audiologic data. J Auditory Res 6:445–452, 1966

Resnick DM, Becker M: Hearing aid evaluation—a new approach. ASHA 5:695–699, 1963

Romanow FF: Methods for measuring the performance of hearing aids. J Acoust Soc Am 13:294–304, 1942

Rudmose W: Data collected on the standardization of the Tracor, Incorporated, ARJ-4HF and RA-114HF extra high frequency audiometers. Austin, TX, Tracor, Inc., 1961

Sandlin RE, Krebs DF: Preface, in Libby ER (ed): Binaural Hearing and Amplification, Vol I. Tampa, Zenetron Inc., 1980

Schachterle B: Hearing aid selection: One dispenser's point of view. Seminars Hearing 7(2), 1986

Shapiro I: Hearing aid fitting by prescription. Audiology 15:163–173, 1976

Shore I, Bilger RC, Hirsh IJ: Hearing aid evaluation: reliability of repeated measurements. J Speech Hearing Disorders 25:152–170, 1960

Shore I, Kramer J: A comparison of two procedures for hearing aid evaluation. J Speech Hearing Disorders 28:159–170, 1965

Signer MB: Hearing aids: Future prospects. ASHA 27:29–32, 1985

Sivian LJ, White SD: On minimum audible sound fields. J Acoust Soc Am 4:288–321, 1933; Erratum 5:60, 1933

Skinner MW, Pasco DP, Miller JD, et al: Measurements to determine the optimal placement of speech energy whithin the listener's auditory area: A basis for selecting amplification characteristics, in Studebaker GA, Bess FH (eds): The Vanderbilt hearing-aid report. Monogr Cont Audiol 161–169, 1982

Staab W: Digital hearing aids. Hearing Instruments (November) 14–24, 1985

Studebaker GA, Bess FH (eds): The Vanderbilt hearing aid report. Monogr Cont Audiol, 1982

Studebaker GA, Bisset JD, VanOrt DM, et al: Paired comparison judgements of relative intelligibility in noise. J Acoust Soc Am 72:80–92, 1982

Triantos TJ, McCandless GA: High frequency distortion. Hearing Aid J, (June) 1974, 9–10

Yantis PA, Millin JP, Shapiro I: Speech discrimination in sensorineural hearing loss: Two experiments on the role of intensity. J Speech Hearing Res 9:178–193, 1966

Zelnick E: Selecting frequency response. Hearing Aid J 35(3), 1982

Zislis T, Fletcher JL: Relation of high frequency thresholds to age and sex. J Auditory Res 6:189–198, 1966

Earl R. Harford

5

Hearing Aid Selection for Adults

Everyone who fits or prescribes hearing aids has his or her own system for selecting what he or she thinks is the appropriate amplification system for the patient. The myriad of methods and the general lack of agreement among audiologists as to what is the best procedure for selecting and evaluating hearing aids for adults has led to confusion on the part of many of us. With the development of formula methods for selecting amplification characteristics, and the fact that no two formulas result in precisely the same gain and output requirements for the same hearing loss, the confusion and disagreements continue.

For the most part, many of the approaches that have been presented over the years appear to be defensible. Unfortunately, with the present state of the art and the available clinical tools, no one procedure can be proved to be superior to the others. In this chapter Earl Harford examines some of the classic and current approaches to hearing aid selection and evaluation. He carefully presents his preferred approach, utilizing real-ear measurements. Earl brings many years of theoretical and clinical background to this endeavor, including development of the original CROS hearing aid. The content of this chapter should stimulate a good deal of thought and discussion among the hearing health community

MCP

AMPLIFICATION FOR THE HEARING-IMPAIRED, THIRD EDITION
Copyright © 1988 by Grune & Stratton, Inc.

ISBN 0-8089-1886-9

Advances in the design and manufacture of the hearing aids and the manner in which audiology is practiced has changed the hearing aid selection process. Prior to the customized in-the-ear (ITE) and in-the-canal (ITC) hearing aid and professional dispensing, the audiologist functioned as an independent assessor of the benefits of amplification and referred the patient to a hearing aid dealer to obtain the product that the audiologist specified. Thus it was common practice for the audiologist to test a patient while wearing several different hearing aids in an effort to select one with which the patient performed well, or up to that patient's potential. The audiologist would then specify that model hearing aid and send the patient off to purchase it. This form of audiologic practice reached its peak during the 1960s when nearly all hearing aids were predesigned production models that "came off the shelf." The testing procedure that allegedly culminated in a decision to procure a certain hearing aid was called the "hearing aid selection" or "hearing aid evaluation" procedure. Now, what used to be a one-visit procedure has evolved into a multivisit ongoing process.

The traditional hearing aid selection procedure may still hold some merit in certain instances where shelf model hearing aids are prescribed and the audiologist does not maintain a dispensary. Even this rather cautious statement is debatable. Dr. Millin has some interesting discussion on this issue in Chapter 4. This situation is becoming less in evidence with the passing of time. Today, hearing aid selection is a process that emerges as a result of multivisit interaction between the dispensing audiologist and the patient. The fact of the matter is, this ongoing process of hearing aid selection is not unlike that practiced by some hearing aid dealers for more than 40 years.

This type of hearing aid selection has the advantage of total control by the person who prescribes the product. If it appears that a change in the design, type, or manufacturer of the product is indicated, it is a relatively simple maneuver by the audiologist when dispensing the product. Minor or major acoustic modifications can be made to earmolds and custom ITE hearing aids in the clinic shop without fear of alienating the relationship with a third party who sold these products to your patient. In short, because the audiologist who dispenses has total control of the product and because *most* patients want and can benefit from custom amplification, hearing aid selection has become an ongoing process rather than a one-visit procedure. In fact, I will go one step further in expressing my present opinion about the audiologist's role in amplification services for the hearing-impaired. Audiologists who are not dispensing the product they prescribe, and are not equipped and skilled in making modifications, should refer patients to someone else who is prepared to handle the entire selection process. In my opinion, *it is an injustice to patients to split them between two parties who are attempting to accomplish the same objective. Audiologists who do not dispense, fit, modify, and service hearing aids should be content to limit their role in the hearing health care field to evaluating hearing problems and referring patients to an audiologist who dispenses and provides remedial services.*

THE HEARING AID SELECTION PROCEDURE

Hearing aid selection as a clinical practice originated in the military aural rehabilitation programs during World War II. Hearing-impaired military personnel were admitted to three or four facilities across the United States as inpatients and placed on a rehabilitation regimen. Each hospital had a team of medical and non-medical specialists who examined ears, tested hearing, fit hearing aids, provided lip reading instruction, and offered auditory training. They maintained a library of body-worn hearing aids, which were the only type available at that time. Experiences during this era indicated, but did not prove that (1) a given hearing-impaired patient is likely to obtain more benefit from one hearing aid and less help from another, (2) a hearing aid that is very effective for one patient is not necessarily equally effective for all patients, and (3) differences in patient performance from one hearing aid to another can be measured by some type of reliable test. These three assumptions are not discussed here. Joseph Millin has handled this well in the previous chapter. Suffice it to say that these three observations may have had merit in 1945, but the past 40 years have seen many changes. Thus the original rationale for embarking on some type of testing schedule aimed at selecting appropriate amplification for a patient has lost much of its value. We know and accept the first two assumptions as correct. Today, we have national and international standards for measuring and reporting the performance characteristics of wearable hearing aids. We are easily able to measure and categorize appropriate electroacoustic and acoustic characteristics for a cross section of the clinical population. Hearing aid test boxes are nearly as common as audiometers in clinical settings. There is little excuse for prescribing amplification for one type of loss that is, in fact, designed and intended for a very different type of loss. Little differences seem to make little difference to the user.

The major problem centers around the third assumption from the 1940s; that is, we are able to use some type of psychophysical measurement to distinguish between an appropriate and inappropriate hearing aid while being worn by a patient. Again, Dr. Millin treats this assumption very well in Chapter 4.

Just within the past few years there have been five major developments that contributed heavily to the virtual demise of the routine traditional hearing aid selection procedures that involve psychophysical tests. First, *custom-made ITE (and canal) hearing aids now constitute the majority that are dispensed.* Eyeglass hearing aids are nearly extinct, and the behind-the-ear (BTE) hearing aid is destined to a similar future, albeit not as complete. Second, *audiologists in greater numbers are finally recognizing the value of binaural hearing aids.* Consequently, there will be fewer unhappy hearing aid users. Third, *it is common practice for audiologists to dispense hearing aids.* Hearing aid dispensing and fitting alone offer accelerated training and knowledge of wearable amplification that scarcely any graduate degree program could provide only 5 years ago. Fourth, *real-ear probe measurements are gaining popularity in the hearing aid selection process.* Fifth, *components such as miniature transducers and chips, as well as manufacturing technology, are result-ing in a more stable, dependable, quality product.* Most manufacturers obtain their components from the same source. There are few, if any, secrets in the manufacturing industry. Consequently, hearing aids are more similar today across manufacturers than at any time in history.

What Shore, et al. (1960) told us many years ago is more valid today than ever. That is, *audiologists should spend less time and energy selecting amplification for their patient and more time assisting them in learning how to obtain maximum benefit from their hearing aids.* If everyone could accept this advice and practice comfortably, this chapter could be brought to a close rather swiftly, sparing the reader any further pain, and suggesting that Derek Sander's chapter be the next one to consult. Unfortunately our topic is not quite that simple. There remains quite a lot to be said about selecting appropriate amplification for the hearing-impaired, albeit we are no longer as systematic as in times past (thank heavens!). My comment is not intended to imply less rigor. Instead, it implies that I do not advocate the lengthy search for a superior hearing aid through the use of inferential clinical tests, (PB word lists, etc.).

Differences of opinion have always existed regarding the best way to select amplification for a hearing-impaired person. Audiologists tended to adopt a procedure that seemed to work effectively for them and with which they were comfortable. Audiologists were trained from the beginning that they should have documentation for their clinical decisions. Thus, if they could place a test score in a patient's file, regardless of its validity, this should minimize the guilt of prescribing a hearing aid based on clinical judgment and experience!

Unquestionably, there is need for a clinical procedure that is quick, uncomplicated, and objective and that correlates with everyday communicative performance. It is quite likely that a practice that employs a single clinical procedure is unrealistic and impractical. Patients vary in their needs for amplification and ability to use hearing aids. It is more realistic to think in terms of a variety of techniques so that appropriate amplification can be selected for individual patients. This principle may become more popular as more audiologists become directly involved in hearing aid dispensing.

Regardless of the specific procedures used to select hearing aids, the fundamental initial objectives of the audiologist can be summarized as follows: *(1) assess the patient's need for amplification, 2) estimate how well the patient can be expected to function with an amplifying system, and 3) determine the characteristics needed for optimal amplification.* At the conclusion of this stage of the process, the patient is likely to be advised according to one of the following possibilities:

1. Retain the present amplification as is because it is functioning well and providing optimal benefit.
2. Retain the present amplification, but with some specific modification.
3. Procure new amplification according to specific or general characteristics.

4. Abstain from the use of amplification at the present time, but return for periodic evaluation.

CANDIDACY FOR AMPLIFICATION

In the earlier days of wearable amplification, there seemed to be two distinct groups of hearing-impaired persons: those who could use hearing aids and those who could not, based on the nature of their hearing loss. Today, this dichotomy has virtually disappeared. Advances in hearing aid technology over the past 30 years offer much greater flexibility for providing effective amplification for a wide variety of hearing problems, ranging from mild to profound hearing losses. *I consider anyone who manifests some degree of communicative difficulty due to a hearing loss as a candidate for amplification.* It is not a question of who can and who cannot use amplification. Instead, it is a question of how much benefit can be expected from amplification. Although the audiometric profile is important, *it is by no means the sole or primary factor in determining candidacy for amplification.* There are at least two other factors that should be considered when judging candidacy for amplification: *lifestyle* and *motivation.* These factors impact on the degree of the person's hearing loss and ultimately reflect the consequences of the actual auditory deficit on quality of life. Stated differently, it is rare when a loss is so mild that it cannot be successfully fit with amplification, *provided the person's communicative ability is affected by the loss.* A mild hearing loss can affect communication in a variety of ways, depending on the person's lifestyle and own standards for daily performance. For example, I have a Swedish colleague who has a mild hearing loss and has hearing aids, and when I recently asked him if he uses his aids, he said, "only while I am visiting the U.S. or another foreign country. I do not need them when I am communicating in Swedish." In brief, *the more demands one has on one's hearing and the more motivated one is to hear better, the better the prognosis for successful hearing aid use, regardless of the audiometric characteristics of the hearing loss.* A case in point is shown is Figure 5-1.

On the other hand, there are patients who manifest an obvious communicative problem in the majority of daily listening situations who deny a handicapping hearing loss. A case in point is a resort owner who recently visited our clinic at the insistence of his wife and grown sons. His audiogram is displayed in Figure 5-2. To date, no one has been able to convince him that his hearing loss warrants corrective amplification, even though he has a 50-dB bilateral hearing loss and used binaural ITE hearing aids for a week before returning them to the dispenser.

During the pioneering days of the wearable hearing aid, a significant number of people using amplification had a conductive hearing loss due to otosclerosis. Surgery for this malady was in its infancy. Such individuals were very good hearing aid users, while those with sensorineural hearing impairment ordinarily reacted negatively to the crude amplifying devices of this early era. Consequently, from that

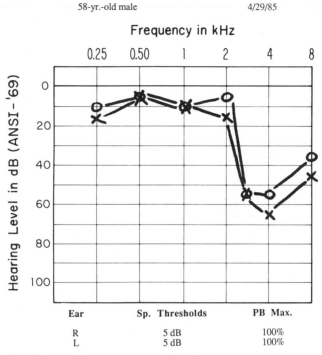

Ear	Sp. Thresholds	PB Max.
R	5 dB	100%
L	5 dB	100%

Fig. 5-1. Audiogram and speech audiometric scores of a 58-year-old male administrator who uses binaural ITE hearing aids full time.

time until the present, certain myths have emerged about the candidacy for a hearing aid. Unfortunately, these misconceptions continue to prevail, particularly among some members of the medical profession who apparently fail to remain current with developments in aural rehabilitation. Listed below are some common *false notions* about candidacy for a hearing aid:

1. Persons with a sensorineural hearing loss cannot be helped by a hearing aid.
2. Those with a unilateral hearing loss do not need an aid, nor can they be helped by one.
3. Those with a severe or profound hearing loss cannot be helped by wearable amplification.
4. Persons with a severe speech discrimination loss cannot be helped by hearing aids.
5. Those with a marked high frequency loss cannot use hearing aids effectively.
6. Persons with a mild hearing loss cannot benefit from hearing aids.
7. Those with a tolerance problem cannot use aids effectively.

8. Persons with assymmetrical hearing loss should not be fit with binaural amplification.

Sensorineural Loss

To some, it may seem surprising to note that there are still those who believe that patients with sensorineural hearing loss cannot benefit from amplification. Unfortunately, such is not the case. In an article entitled "The hidden handicap of deafness," Dr. Samuel Rosen (Shambaugh and Rosen 1975), a prominent Otologist, was asked, "When can a hearing aid help?" He responded to this question by saying "Of course, if it's a sensorineural loss, no hearing aid will help." Clearly, this statement is totally false, yet it appears in a publication that finds its way to many physicians' offices and is read by patients and physicians throughout the country. Such a statement could do irreparable harm to countless numbers of hearing-impaired persons. This false notion was placed first on my list because it continues to warrant persistent public and professional attention. Some hearing aid manufacturers capitalize on this misconception by advertising that "now there is a hearing aid for 'nerve deafness'!" On the other hand, it is refreshing to read the brief report

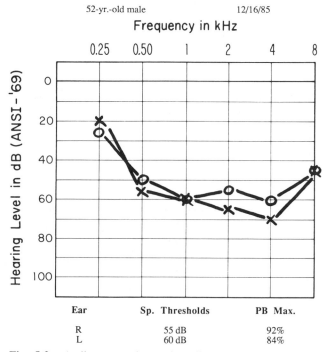

Fig. 5-2. Audiogram and speech audiometric scores of a 52-year-old resort owner who denies a hearing handicap and refuses to use hearing aids, even canal aids.

by Jerome Goldstein, M.D. (1986). It is aimed at the primary-care physician, and one section attempts to dispel the myth that persons with "nerve deafness" cannot be helped by hearing aids.

Unilateral Hearing Loss

Prior to the mid-1960s, persons with normal or near-normal hearing in one ear and an unaidable hearing loss in the opposite ear could not be helped by a hearing aid. Four factors constitute an unaidable ear when the opposite ear is normal or near normal: (1) a profound loss of sensitivity so that sounds amplified by a hearing aid cannot be heard with any degree of usefulness, (2) a severe speech discrimination (recognition) loss, (3) an ear in which it is medically inadvisable to place an earmold, and (4) a marked tolerance problem for amplified sounds.

As a result of the development of CROS (contralateral routing of signals) (Harford and Barry 1965), many persons with unilateral hearing loss are now using amplification. Although CROS amplification is often effective for some persons with this type of loss, others seem to adjust well to a unilateral hearing impairment and prefer not to use amplification. This same statement can be made about persons with a bilateral hearing impairment. The important point is that a form of amplification is, indeed, available for persons with a unilateral hearing loss. The reader should consult Chapter 8 for a detailed discussion on CROS amplification.

Not all persons with a unilateral hearing loss need to resort to a CROS hearing aid. Some can use an aid directly in the impaired ear. This type of fitting for a person with impaired hearing in one ear is superior to CROS because it offers binaural hearing with one hearing aid (BHOA) (Harford and Musket 1964). Obviously, for this approach to be successful, the patient's impaired ear must be aidable and amplification must be acoustically comfortable.

Severe Hearing Loss

Patients with severe or profound bilateral hearing loss, in either residual hearing, recognition for speech, or both, should not be ruled out as potential hearing aid candidates. It is worth keeping in mind that any improvement in ability to communicate will be welcomed by the patient who hears and/or understands minimally because of impaired hearing. These persons can be desperate, and denial of amplification could be a great injustice to many of them. The ability to detect warning sounds as well as other environmental noises can justify amplification for the profoundly impaired. Care should be taken to incorporate a standardized lipreading test into the hearing aid selection procedure for certain patients. Dodds and Harford (1968) emphasize the value of utilizing a lip-reading test in conjunction with auditory cues from a hearing aid. Indeed, many patients who appear to derive virtually no benefit from hearing aids on auditory tests, and who are poor visual communicators without amplification, may perform exceptionally well when combining visual cues with amplification. The decision to contraindicate hearing aid use for a person with a severe hearing problem should not be based solely on the results of auditory tests.

High-Frequency Loss

In the past, if a person had a hearing loss beginning above 1500 Hz, amplification was, more often than not, contraindicated. This was because hearing aid and earmold technology had not yet developed to the point where low- and midfrequency amplification could be appropriately reduced while amplifying the high frequencies.

This is no longer the case. With the development of open earmolds, tube fittings (see Chapter 3) and feedback reduction circuits (see Chapter 2), most people with a high-frequency precipitous loss can be successfully fit with amplification. We now are less often confronted with the problems of low frequency over amplification, which can result in the "barrel" effect and poor speech intelligibility in the presence of background noise when fitting persons with this type of loss.

Mild Hearing Loss

Advances in the electroacoustic characteristics of hearing aids, earmold acoustics, and ITE instruments have led to wearable amplification for persons with mild hearing loss. Also, there are now nonelectronic acoustic resonators on the market for mild losses. It is too early to judge their merits and effectiveness. Pollack presents a discussion of these devices in Chapter 8.

Just as important as technical developments, clinicians in greater numbers now recognize that *even minimal hearing loss can cause significant communicative problems for certain individuals.* Perhaps this awareness is an indication that some clinicians are joining the ranks of those with mild-high frequency hearing impairment and, as a consequence, are gaining firsthand experience with this type of problem. Whatever the reason, it is true that many persons with mild hearing loss are now benefiting from amplification in many daily situations. These situations include theater productions, auditorium presentations, conferences, meeting rooms, classrooms, and similar situations. Certainly, persons with mild hearing loss are candidates for at least part-time hearing aid use. Only the potential user is able to determine whether amplification for this degree of loss is worth the expense, inconvenience and effort. The audiometric characteristics on two such persons are illustrated in Figures 5-3 and 5-4.

Tolerance Problems

One of the most difficult cases to fit successfully is the patient with a severe tolerance problem. Even though there have been some refinements in output limiting in the past decade, patients with a narrow dynamic range are often tenuous candidates for hearing aids. Yet, some persons in this category are using aids, at

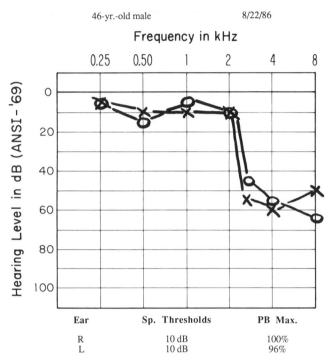

Fig. 5-3. Audiogram and speech audiometric scores of a 46-year-old male salesman who uses binaural ITE hearing aids the majority of the time.

least with partial success. Thus the patient who manifests a narrow dynamic range (often described as a recruitment problem) may be helped by hearing aids, but there are many persons in this category who refuse amplification mainly because of extreme acoustic discomfort, especially in groups and noisy places.

Clinical Approach to the Determination of Candidacy

Perhaps the most expedient way to establish a person's candidacy for a hearing aid is to inquire directly about, or observe, difficulty in hearing. Although it is not essential in all cases, *a good prerequisite to candidacy for a hearing aid is the patient's acceptance of a hearing loss and level of motivation to improve communicative efficiency.* These two factors are interwoven. In brief, there are two easily defined criteria to establish candidacy for hearing aid use that can be put in the form of questions: Do you have trouble hearing or understanding in some situations? Do you want to improve your hearing? If the answer to both of these questions is in the affirmative, and the patient has had competent medical consultation, that patient automatically becomes a candidate for a hearing aid. Although this approach gets right to the point in the majority of cases, it is by no means foolproof. Certainly,

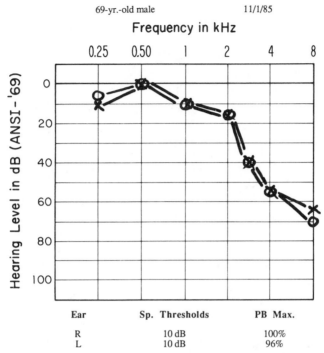

69-yr.-old male   11/1/85

Frequency in kHz

Fig. 5-4. Audiogram and speech audiometric scores of a 69-year-old male minister who uses binaural ITE hearing aids the majority of the time.

Ear	Sp. Thresholds	PB Max.
R	10 dB	100%
L	10 dB	96%

audiometric data can be useful in some cases for determining candidacy for a hearing aid. In the majority of cases, however, the audiometric data serve as confirmation of clinical observation and case history information.

Recent advances in technology and application of hearing aids offers such flexibility that we are now able to provide benefit for nearly all types of hearing loss. It is essential to add to this statement an important factor that can influence a person's candidacy for amplification; that is, the environment in which the patient spends a major portion of the time, both at work and elsewhere. Many patients complain that their greatest communicative problem is in noisy places. As a rule, hearing aids are not as effective in noisy environments as they are in quiet. With the newer input compression circuits, variable filtering, so-called signal processing circuits, and other electroacoustic manipulations, people with sensorineural losses are able to function considerably better in noisy environments than was the case only a couple of years ago. If, however, a patient is led to expect dramatic help from hearing aids in noisy situations, the prognosis for satisfaction from amplification must be guarded. *Realistic expectations from miniature amplifying systems is of paramount importance.* Many times we hear the patient report that a hearing aid helps the least where it is needed the most. Thus it is essential that the clinician carefully appraise the patient's lifestyle and communicative problems and counsel the patient realistically during the hearing aid selection process.

After medical and/or surgical treatment has been completed or deemed unnecessary, or it is determined that amplification would not aggravate ongoing medical treatment, and the patient expresses some degree of motivation to investigate hearing aid use, the patient becomes a candidate for a hearing aid. Thus the nonmedical remediation process begins. Obviously, the first step in this process is to learn more about the patient.

The objective of our service is to provide our patients with convenient, comfortable, manageable, beneficial, and acceptable amplification. A cross section of the hearing-impaired adult population is composed of two-thirds over the age of 60 years, about equally divided between men and women. When I was a student of the late Raymond Carhart at Northwestern University, I was taught that all patients should first be considered "problem users" until proved otherwise. This was in the days when we knew almost nothing about amplification (compared to our level of knowledge today) for the hearing-impaired and even less about how to select hearing aids. Today, I approach the clinical population with the reverse philosophy, specifically, that *every patient should be considered a routine candidate for hearing aids, unless proven otherwise.* This seems to be a more accurate appraisal of the reality of our clinical population. In brief, the adult hearing-impaired population falls into two groups: (1) those who are easily fit with hearing aids and adjust readily to them and (2) those who are difficult to fit and/or have problems using them to their benefit. The former group is many times larger than the latter. There is a separate group of patients who need to be included: veteran hearing aid users, and these, too, are either routine or problem users.

If we accept the fact that most hearing-impaired patients are predictably good users of modern hearing aids, we should conclude that all patients who seek help from amplification need *not* be managed the same way. It is inefficient and unnecessary to subject a routine patient to the same rigorous time-consuming, expensive clinical process that is often necessary for a problem user. Thus flexibility is an important characteristic for the effective audiologist engaged in amplification services for the hearing-impaired. We must exercise common sense with each patient and not be so rigid that we "overkill" an otherwise routine candidate for hearing aids. This is probably one of the most difficult transitions the student of audiology must make when leaving the university and entering private practice. *Unfortunately, many students do not have a realistic practicum exposure during their formative years and enter the professional world with unrealistic expectations.* The fact is that most patients are not in the mood to spend an inordinate period of time while their hearing health care provider tries to figure out how to help them. Most patients come to the audiologist with a hearing problem and want to know, within a reasonable period of time, what can be done to correct it. The audiologist's responsibility is to find a feasible solution to the problem as efficiently as possible. Naturally, if the audiologist determines that the patient is likely to have considerable difficulty handling amplification, this information should be conveyed to the patient as soon as possible in order to prepare him or her for a more extensive clinical venture.

AUDIOLOGIC EVALUATION

We assume that the cause of the patient's hearing loss has been investigated by a physician. Any medical and/or surgical remediation to treat the loss is either ruled out, completed or, if still active, will not influence the use of amplification. Even though the patient may have consulted a physician, the audiologist should be on the alert for any sign of an active pathology or conductive component during the evaluation and as long as he may continue to manage the patient with amplification. The audiologist may see a patient prior to the physician. The audiologist must use professional judgment as to the need for a current medical consultation.

Case History

Some clinicians prefer to obtain a history from a patient at the outset of the first visit. Others do a hearing evaluation first and then the history. We use an abbreviated intake history that the patient completes when checking in for an appointment (Appendix A). We review this form before starting with the patient and sometimes do the hearing tests and complete the history after the testing. Other times, we complete the history first, and then do the testing, which is probably the most popular approach. In any case, remember that flexibility is a keynote to a viable, effective clinical practice. The important thing to remember is that we are audiologists engaged in the non-medical remediation of hearing impairment. This is not to say that we should not explore some medical matters. The audiologist may well be the first hearing health care professional to serve a particular patient. Thus it could be important for purposes of screening to ask about tinnitus, history of otitis media, vertigo, aural fullness and pressure, fluctuations in hearing, ear pain or discomfort, and other physical complaints that could signify the need for an otologic consultation. The main point is that we should be spending our time on a more social-oriented history to learn about the communication problems of our patient.

Suffice it to say that there are vast differences in the lifestyles of people and, as a consequence, the demands placed on their ability to communicate. Some people depend on their communicative process to earn a living, while others do not. The objective of a good history is to obtain as clear and complete a profile as necessary in order to understand the lifestyle and communicative needs and problems of the patient. Sometimes there are specific yet less obvious communicative problems that need to be illuminated at the outset. Consider, for example, the bus driver with a right unilateral hearing loss and the funeral director with a mild bilateral high-frequency loss. This point could be expanded to include a long list of special communicative situations that represent a major problem for the person who is experiencing it. The effective clinician is one who studies people in their daily activities and develops a sense of awareness and understanding for the various consequences that can accrue as a result of a specific type of hearing deficit.

A partial list of points that warrant investigation, categorized into the past, present, and future are listed in Table 5-1.

The last item in Table 5-1 is very important because it expresses the patient's expectations and sets the stage for the balance of the visit. Other factors include

Table 5-1
Pertinent Information from a Patient's Case History

Past
    Duration of hearing loss
    Nature of onset (sudden vs insidious)
    Mode of progression (unchanged or gradually worse)
    Stability of the loss (fluctuating or constant)
    Understanding of the cause of the hearing loss
    Understanding of medical and/or surgical help for the loss
    Patient's perception of hearing aids
    Prior efforts to improve hearing
    Prior experiences with hearing aids
    Prior training in communicative skills
    Alterations in lifestyle resulting from the hearing loss

Present
    Station in life (family constellation, work, social, recreation, etc.)
    Self-appraisal of hearing loss
    General health of patient, including any visual or manual dexterity problems
    Difficult and easy listening situations
    Impression or awareness of others of patient's hearing loss
    Effect on patient's work and/or social activities

Future (what the patient anticipates in the foreseeable future)
    Occupational and/or vocational changes
    Retirement
    Educational pursuits
    Extended and/or frequent travel
    Increased or decreased social and/or work demands
    What the patient wants to learn from today's visit to the audiologist

what the patient's biases or feelings are about using a hearing aid. Is the patient especially vain about appearance or using a "badge of handicap" (a hearing aid)? Does the patient wish to investigate a particular type or brand of hearing aid because of an advertisement, friend, or some other reason?

These points represent an example of some of the factors that the clinician should consider when entering into the decision-making process that we shall see unfold as we proceed. We cannot expect patients to volunteer all the information we need to help us make logical decisions about the type of amplification we prescribe. We need to be aware of the infinite number of variables that impinge on this process and anticipate as many of them as possible at the outset to avoid going off in the wrong direction.

Hearing Handicap Assessment Scales

Various scales and profile questionnaires have been advocated for assessing or appraising the extent of handicap imposed by a hearing impairment. These can be referred to as hearing handicap assessment scales or profiles. One of the first to promote this concept was Davis (1948), with what he called the *Social Adequacy Index*. This concept led to a more refined scale proposed by High et al. (1964) several years later. Probably the most vigorous effort in this area has been the extensive work of Alpiner and his associates (1978), who developed the Denver Scale of Communication Function. Some other research on the subject of assessing the handicap imposed by a hearing loss on an individual has been reported by Noble and Atherly (1970), Giolas (1970), Rupp et al. (1977), Giolas et al. (1979), Ventry and Weinstein (1982), and Schow and Nerbonne (1982). The reader should also refer to Dr. Sanders' chapter in this text.

The use of some type of scale may have merit but is a time-consuming process. Of course, people vary considerably in their communicative needs. Audiometric results alone are inadequate for judging the need for amplification in many individuals. An honest self-appraisal may help a patient reach a more realistic level of understanding. A questionnaire can be sent by mail to potential patients, and a preview of the result might serve as a guide for the allocation of staff time and extent of a scheduled evaluation. It may be risky to rely too heavily on this technique, however, because some people are poor judges of their own communicative problems. In any event, listen carefully to your patients and remember what they say. Even though they may be poor correspondents, there is something to be learned from everyone, and it may help you serve that particular patient and others more effectively.

Basic Audiologic Assessment

The significance of a good history was stressed in the previous section. The patient has described any communicative problems. Consequently, the audiologic evaluation should yield test results that verify the patient's complaint(s). Every patient who comes to the audiologist for hearing help can be placed in one of four basic audiologic categories corresponding to the primary communicative complaint and/or unaided test results: (1) impaired sensitivity with good speech discrimination (Fig. 5.5A), (2) impaired sensitivity and speech discrimination (Fig. 5-5B), (3) impaired discrimination with good sensitivity (Fig. 5-5C), and (4) no measurable hearing loss (in the soundfield) (Fig. 5-5D).

Once the clinician has obtained a descriptive profile of the patient's lifestyle, communicative needs and problems, and a comprehensive evaluation of that patient's hearing, it is time to explain the test results and make decisions about the type of amplification to be pursued.

PRESELECTION OF AMPLIFICATION

I label this step in the selection process as the "preselection" because we must allow for future changes in early decisions. The preselected amplification often

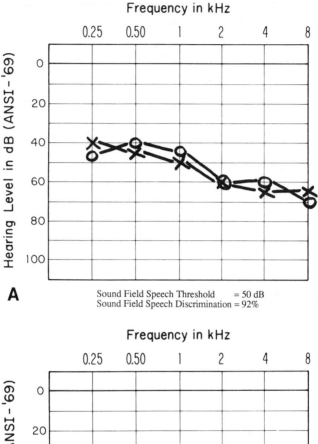

Frequency in kHz

A

Sound Field Speech Threshold   = 50 dB
Sound Field Speech Discrimination = 92%

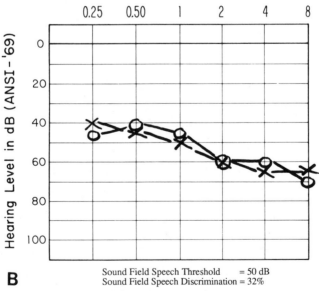

Frequency in kHz

B

Sound Field Speech Threshold   = 50 dB
Sound Field Speech Discrimination = 32%

Fig. 5-5. Four audiometric profiles that represent the majority of the hearing-impaired population: (A) a bilateral loss of auditory sensitivity for speech, but with good recognition (discrimination) ability for amplified speech; (B) a loss in sensitivity for conversa-

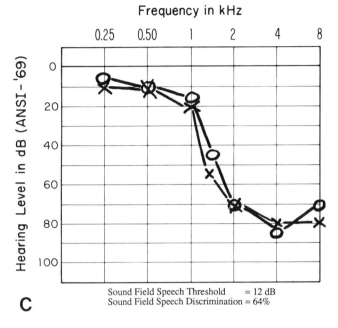

Frequency in kHz

Sound Field Speech Threshold   = 12 dB
Sound Field Speech Discrimination = 64%

C

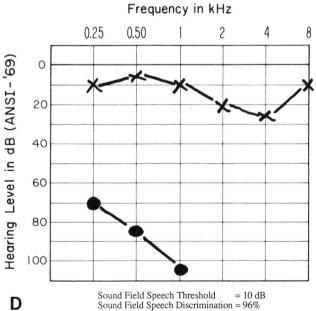

Frequency in kHz

Sound Field Speech Threshold   = 10 dB
Sound Field Speech Discrimination = 96%

D

tional speech as well as amplified speech intelligibility. (C) normal sensitivity for conversational speech but impaired intelligibility; (D) normal sensitivity and intelligibility for speech on soundfield tests in the clinic, but still complaining of a perplexing communicative problem.

becomes the final hearing aids for routine adult patients when prescribed by the experienced audiologist. Even so, initial specifications are subject to change as the patient begins to use the new amplification and reports back on daily experiences. When the audiologist reaches this stage of the remediation process, much information is available to apply to preselection decisions, such as audiologic profile, lifestyle, patient preferences, approximate level of motivation, physical limitations, and special auditory limitations. In addition, logical electroacoustic and acoustic features need to be determined when selecting amplification for trial listening. The audiologist should have criteria for the electroacoustic characteristics that seem to be most appropriate for a specific patient. These criteria may be based on the audiologist's or someone else's formula. The reader will find a detailed discussion on this topic in Chapter 7.

Three major pitfalls should be avoided when preselecting appropriate amplification: (1) monaural instead of binaural, (2) BTE instead of ITE (or canal), and (3) overamplification. Each of these three problem areas is addressed in the following paragraphs.

Monaural versus Binaural

First, I believe that binaural hearing and amplification is superior to monaural hearing and amplification. For more on this subject, refer to Chapter 8. I do not feel compelled to defend this position in this context, but one would not need to go far to find some audiologists who will take exception to my position. At the same time, these persons will advocate binaural amplification for children because of its superiority. *If binaural amplification is important for children, why is it not important for adults?* My approach is to always give binaural amplification first priority and then try to justify why I would prescribe a single hearing aid for a patient with a bilateral hearing loss. I am unaware of any dependable clinical tests that will help me identify who will and who will not benefit from binaural amplification. Test results from monaural versus binaural hearing can be like statistics; that is, you can make the result come out the way you want. Therefore, I have total control in dispensing of the product; I start my patients with binaural amplification and, during the process of initial use, give them the opportunity to decide whether one aid is as good as two aids. If so, the patient returns one aid. Over the past 6 years, only 5 percent of our patients have chosen to return one aid and use monaural amplification. This result is based on a total number of more than 1000 patients.

There are some obvious reasons for prescribing one hearing aid for a patient: (1) nonaidable ear,* assuming that the opposite ear is aidable, (2) normal or nearnormal hearing in one ear and aidable hearing in the opposite ear, and (3) a person who is sedentary or a virtual recluse. As stated earlier, the audiologist should not allow

---

*A non-aidable ear in this context is defined as an ear that manifests one or a combination of the following: a profound or complete loss of auditory sensitivity, severe tolerance problem, severe speech discrimination loss or atresia, stenosis, chronic otitis media, or external otitis.

cost to influence professional judgment. This is a very personal matter that should be the patient's responsibility.

The audiologist runs the risk of "short changing" the patient by second guessing that the patient cannot or should not spend money for something. Of course, the audiologist can and should discuss "trade-offs" or compromises relative to costs. This can be risky, however, because of the unknowns at this stage of the ongoing selection process. Perhaps that is one of the reasons we encourage our patients to start with binaural amplification and allow them to come to an ultimate conclusion over a period of several weeks.

It seems that a common misconception prevails relative to the fitting of binaural amplification. More specifically, binaural hearing aids should be used when there is a considerable communicative problem and the hearing loss is the same in both ears. This is a far too limiting criterion. Figure 5-6 illustrates examples that contradict this false notion. Each of these three patients have been using binaural amplification full-time for more than 2 years, having started with monaural amplification for several years prior to that. None is willing to give up the hearing aid in the poorer ear.

In-the-Ear (or Canal) versus Behind-the-Ear

There are advantages and disadvantages to ITEs and BTEs at this point in time, and some important facts should be stressed about each type. First, there have been considerable improvements in the design, construction, and quality control of ITEs in the past few years. Manufacturers now provide a variety of circuits, allowing for application to a broader segment of the hearing-impaired population. In fact, most acoustic modifications that apply to earmolds can now be used in ITE instruments. The small canal aids are not as flexible as the larger ITE instruments. Second, the research and clinical application of in situ measurements allow the audiologist to evaluate more precisely the function of the ITE aid. Third, the location of the microphone and its juxtaposition to the output of the amplified signal in the ear canal has favorable acoustic advantages. Finally, there is *very strong* consumer preference for ITE and ITC hearing aids because of their aesthetics, comfort, and convenience. Nevertheless, *the competent audiologist will not allow consumer preference to preclude good clinical judgment if a BTE aid is likely to provide more benefit than and ITE or ITC aid.* Table 5-2 lists the advantages and disadvantages of each style of instrument.

The main objective of the preselection process is to match amplification to the needs of the patient. This match includes comfort and convenience, as well as type, electroacoustic, and acoustic considerations. The size and shape of the patient's auricles and ear canals must be studied. There are some people who have stiff or small auricles that cannot accommodate even a small postauricular aid comfortably. An ITE aid is a practical solution. Conversely, there are those with shallow conchas and tiny ear canals who are best fit with BTE aids.

In general, older persons find ITE aids more convenient to insert and remove,

46-yr.-old male   6/6/85

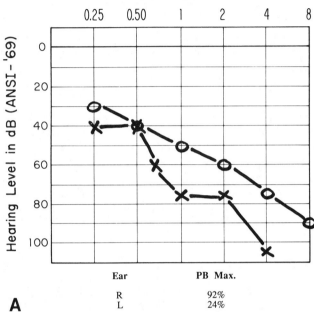

Ear	PB Max.
R	92%
L	24%

A

60-yr.-old male   11/30/83

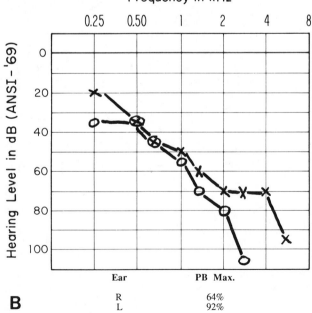

Ear	PB Max.
R	64%
L	92%

B

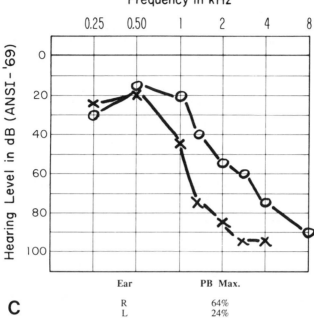

Frequency in kHz

C

Ear	PB Max.
R	64%
L	24%

Fig. 5-6. Audiogram and speech recognition scores for three male patients (A–C) using binaural amplification full time. Each used monaural and BICROS hearing aids prior to binaural amplification. Each patient reports that binaural amplification is infinitely superior to monaural (better ear) or BICROS, in spite of significantly poorer speech discrimination in one ear.

Table 5-2

Advantages and Disadvantages of BTE and ITE Fittings

Type of Aid	Advantages	Disadvantages
ITE/ITC	Probable acoustic quality Convenient to manage Comfortable Strong consumer preference	More fragile Less predictable performance Wax in output channel Susceptible to feedback problems Presents loaner problems unless patient has own earmold
BTE	More variety of electroacoustic adjustments More predictable performance Better quality control More durable Easier to service in clinic Easier to vent and modify earmold	More cumbersome Competes with eyeglasses for space in some cases More conspicuous for some users Less acceptable to consumers

as well as easier management of the volume control. Changing the battery can be a problem with either an ITE or BTE. Canal aids can be a problem for older patients. Even though they are relatively easy to insert, they can be difficult to remove and it may be difficult to operate the volume control. Also, changing the tiny size 312 battery in a canal aid can be a problem compared to the 13 battery in the conventional ITE. The new A-10 battery is even smaller than the 312. It has been my experience that the majority of older patients prefer ITE aids and are able to manipulate them more easily than postauricular aids.

Overamplification

The terms *overfit* and *underfit* have been used in the hearing aid field since its inception. The interpretation is evident; overfitting is providing the patient with more amplification than necessary to the extent that it causes discomfort or, at least, unnecessary annoyance. Patients who are underfit do not have enough "use" or "full-on" gain to satisfy their listening needs, so as to render the amplification inadequate. When selecting hearing aids for a new user, however, it is better to err in the direction of an underfit than overfit. Unfortunately, there has been a long-standing tendency for audiologists to overfit their patients. One reason may be because audiology clinics are usually quiet environments, but this may be an oversimplification. It is wise to use output limiters and vent the aid or earmold as much as possible. The limiter can be adjusted at a later time to allow more output, and vents can be partially or completely closed. Keep in mind the binaural summation principle. A patient requires less gain from each of two hearing aids than from one aid in order to have the same degree of loudness perception.

It seems popular today to practice the one-half gain rule, for example, 30-dB gain for a 60-dB hearing level. We have found that new hearing aid users with a pure sensorineural loss who are fit binaurally will use gain that is about one-third their hearing level. When ordering hearing aids, however, we specify 3–5 dB more than our predicted amount of use gain so as to have ample reserve. Also, it is important to stay below the discomfort level with appropriate output limitations. Output trim adjusters and compression circuits are helpful with this criterion.

There are many factors to consider when processing the preselection of amplification for a patient. Most of these I have addressed in this section. Table 5-3 summarizes these points.

Listening Experience

By this time, the audiologist should have studied the patient's hearing loss and reached certain decisions about the type of amplification, electroacoustic characteristics, and acoustic modifications that are most appropriate for that patient. It is helpful to fit the patient with an approximation of these parameters, if possible. A large variety of stock earmolds and several pair of general-purpose BTE hearing aids allow the option of fitting a range of hearing loss, either binaural, monaural,

Table 5-3
Factors in Preselection of Amplification

Type of aid(s)
    Body
    Postauricular
    ITE
    ITC
Mode of Amplification
    Monaural direct to right or left ear
    Binaural
    Monaural indirect (CROS)
    Monaural indirect and monaural direct (BICROS)
Gain
    One-half or one-third of the degree of hearing loss
Output limiting
    Do not exceed uncomfortable loudness level
Frequency Response
    Avoid too much low-frequency gain
Directional versus nondirectional microphone
    For postauricular aids only
Coupling
    Open canal or tube fitting
    Closed canal
    Variable vents

CROS, or BICROS. The purpose of this demonstration is twofold. First, it provides the opportunity to study the patient's reaction to amplification that approximates the prescription. Second, it gives patients an opportunity to experience the use of amplification and further develop their realistic expectations. We practice this technique even with veteran hearing aid users. These patients are usually good reporters and can guide us in refining our prescription.

During or following this listening demonstration, the patient and accompanying spouse, friend, or family member(s) are counseled relative to subsequent steps in the process of obtaining amplification. It is important to tailor this discussion to known facts, being careful to avoid speculations about hearing aid limitations and advantages that may never develop for this particular patient. It is best not to generalize too much about advantages and limitations of amplification at this time until more is known about how the patient is adjusting to the new hearing aids. That opportunity will come soon enough; and that is the time to deal with this important subject.

The listening experience may reveal, for the first time, clues that the patient is going to have significant problems benefiting from amplification and/or physically managing the hearing aids. If this is the case, it is wise to initiate strategies immediately that may resolve or reduce such problems. For example, in the case of custom hearing aids, it is helpful to initially order options, such as trimmers, compression circuit, feedback reduction, venting, and other features, rather than disrupt use later by returning the aids to the manufacturer.

Table 5-4 contains examples of some typical physical problems with possible solutions. Another physical problem that can virtually preclude effective hearing aid use is a collapsed or nearly closed ear canal. This condition can cause feedback before comfort and/or annoying and embarrassing involuntary feedback. Usually the only feasible solution to this problem is meatoplasty, that is, surgically removing the cartilaginous portion of the concha that closed the orifice of the external auditory meatus.

INTERPRETATION AND STRATEGIES

This is the time when it makes good sense to involve another member(s) of the family when explaining the results of the audiologic evaluation and preselection in lay terms. By use of some simple visual aids, most people can be taught quickly to interpret the results of their basic hearing tests. In most cases, they can be helped to understand why they are having the kind of communicative problems they reported during the history-taking session. It is wise to educate your patients to better understand the nature of their hearing loss before discussing a feasible solution.

Most patients expect to receive a prognosis for hearing aid use. They should be told what degree of improvement they should expect from the rehabilitative approach you recommend. Stated somewhat differently, this is the time when the audiologist must face the challenge of answering a basic question: "Based on my experience and knowledge and the nature of this patient's hearing loss, lifestyle, and level of motivation, what can I expect as an outcome?" This is the time to start educating the patient, and others close to that patient, about realistic expectations.

Table 5-4
Typical Physical Problems and Possible Solutions

Physical Problem	Complete or Partial Solution
Auricles	
Small	ITE or ITC
Soft	
Close to head	
Canals	
"Stiff," "bony"	BTE with soft mold
Fingers, hands, and arms	
Arthritis	ITE with extended volume control,
Missing	nail notches, extended handle
Poor dexterity	

Experience seems to be the prime factor that will improve the audiologists' accuracy in prognosticating the outcome of their efforts.

The next logical step is to establish strategies for reaching the objectives and goals set forth in the prognosis. For example, "Mr. Carlson, I see no reason why you cannot use amplification effectively in your daily activities and do quite well. You can use any type of amplification that is available. The choice is yours to make. Also, you are likely to hear best if you use a hearing aid in both ears, rather than one. Now, let's talk about the pros and cons of each type of hearing aid." It is not necessary to spend a lot of time involving the patient in the decision-making process. It can be very effective, however, to allow the patient to participate in this part of the process, unless the patient characteristically cannot make decisions easily and indicates a desire for you to issue directives. There are these kinds of patients, and you need to recognize them and be prepared to be very direct.

It may be helpful to keep in mind that you are not in a position to sit in judgment of certain kinds of decisions, such as what is too expensive for the patient to handle. Obviously, if a patient categorically admits to having $X to spend on amplification, this must become a factor, but it should not preclude telling that patient what, in your best professional judgment, will offer optimal benefit for the hearing problem. Then, it is the patient's decision to settle for less, not yours. A patient comes to you for help. Your responsibility is to prescribe amplification that allows the patient to obtain optimum acoustic compensation comfortably and conveniently. This should be the standard reference point. The patient should be helped to understand what is compromised by settling for anything less than what is prescribed.

This issue arises occasionally when binaural hearing aids are prescribed. The patient may admit to wanting only one aid, like a neighbor uses. In cases where there is little or no difference between ears, I urge the patient to choose the ear to be aided. *The patient has already decided to compromise optimum benefit, and I want him to start taking some responsibility for the consequences.* Let us continue with the scenario. Let us say the patient chooses the left ear because the right ear is used for the telephone. A hearing aid is ultimately fitted and the patient returns for follow-up visits only to report that he or she really is not very pleased with the aid. The patient admits to enjoying television more now but still cannot hear his or her spouse and other passengers while driving the car. The ongoing process, of course, is to explain why the patient has trouble in the car and should decide whether it is important enough to the patient and the patient's spouse to try an aid in the right ear, also. Thus *the process continues until the patient reconciles any compromises or follows my original prescription.* An important concept to bear in mind is that there are those individuals who will not follow your recommendations end up unhappy with the fitting and then complain to anyone who will listen about how terrible you are. There is little that you can do about this situation other than to counsel as thoroughly as possible and try to be sure that your patients understand that they are making decisions that may be contrary to their overall best interests.

PRESCRIPTION

For 30 years I referred to this step in the process as the "selection" or "recommendation" but now I prefer to use the term "prescription," believing that it most accurately describes this process. I find the term *recommendation* carries a weak connotation. The term *selection* has a similar message. Appendix B illustrates the prescription form we have used for the past few years and found to be most effective. This form becomes a permanent part of the patient's file. It is used by our dispensing office personnel to prepare the purchase agreement and the manufacturer's order form. It can also be used to obtain purchase authorization from third-party payers.

The patient has had an opportunity to use preselected amplification and, the audiologist has had an opportunity to evaluate the patients reactions to it. The results have been discussed, and presumably the patient has decided to proceed with the selection process. The next step is to take good ear impressions. The fit of the earmold or the custom hearing aid is an extremely important ingredient in the acceptance and fit of amplification. Also, the fit can have a direct influence on the performance of the hearing aid. The reader should become familiar with this process, as presented in Chapter 3.

THE FITTING

The fitting is the beginning of the most crucial stage in the hearing aid selection process, which occurs anywhere from a few days to several weeks following the initial visit. This is when the patient is introduced to the new amplification. The audiologist must ensure that the hearing aids fit comfortably and provide the type of amplification that was prescribed. It is wise to be certain that the hearing aids shipped to you by the manufacturer meet your expectations and are functioning flawlessly. If you fail to check the aids carefully and one or both fail to function properly at the time of the fitting, you could be in for an embarrassing situation.

The typical patient arrives at the fitting appointment rather apprehensive. This is particularly true for the new hearing aid user. If for no other reason, the patient is anxious because this is a new experience, but there is usually more involved. The patient has had the time since the last appointment to ponder the decision to use amplification and is wondering whether the hearing aids will be beneficial. Possibly this patient has heard still more negative tales about hearing aids since the last visit. This heightens the patient's anxiety even more than simply the newness of the situation and the unknown experiences that lie ahead. Perhaps even more importantly, the patient is coming face to face with the reality of having a hearing handicap and is about to become the owner of a badge that announces this fact to all that can see it.

Some patients seem totally unaffected by this situation, which is all well and good. Even so, the audiologist should be aware of those who are not quite so secure.

These patients warrant special understanding to help them relax and participate in this stage of the process. The reader is well advised to study Chapter 10 because many of the points covered by Dr. Sanders apply directly to the hearing aid fitting.

Do the Hearing Aids Fit Properly?

This must be the first step. Regardless of the type of hearing aids being fit, they must be comfortable. This is where a good-quality dental-lab type grinder-buffer is an invaluable tool for the audiologist. Such a tool can be obtained through hearing aid accessory suppliers. Even with the most perfect ear impressions, sometimes it is necessary to alter the contours of an earmold or custom hearing aid so it will fit more comfortably.

How Do the Hearing Aids Sound?

I refer to this stage of the fitting and verification process as the *subjective adjustment*. On exceedingly rare occasions, I prescribe hearing aids without trimmers, that is, at least frequency and output adjusters. I specify a frequency trimmer even for a precipitous high-frequency hearing loss with normal hearing in the mid and low frequencies. Most low-frequency reduction potentiometers (tone control) will reduce circuit noise by as much as 3 dB. This can be a desirable result for patients with sensitive hearing for low frequencies who may otherwise complain of hearing circuit noise in quiet environments. I adjust the trimmer, starting with the setting I feel is most appropriate for the patient and adjusting toward the opposite setting. While making this change I seek the reactions of the patient. As I introduce more low-frequency gain, for example, it is not uncommon for patients to report that sounds are louder, noises harsher, and that their own voices are more objectionable. Sometimes, however, a patient will prefer more low-frequency amplification than I would predict, saying that sounds are less metallic and more natural.

I prefer to have the patient regularly use one-half to two-thirds rotation of the gain (volume) control. Just barely "on" suggests too much gain, and "full-on" indicates inadequate gain. Ideally, I want them to be able to increase the gain, without feedback, in certain listening situations. Therefore, I check carefully for feedback at full-on gain. Naturally, when fitting hearing aids with vents, one may encounter feedback before full-on gain. This is acceptable, provided the patient reports good speech intelligibility before feedback. I prefer to achieve ample gain with the output trimmer set to less than maximum. This condition allows some reserve in the event that the patient's hearing levels should somewhat deteriorate over the life of the hearing aids. Sometimes we have to reduce the size of the venting at this stage. Also, the audiologist must be certain the ear canal is completely free of wax, which is a common cause of feedback.

Once the hearing aids have been adjusted for optimal acoustic comfort and the patient reports they feel comfortable, it is time to verify their performance while being worn.

VERIFICATION OF PERFORMANCE

The next logical step in the fitting process is to obtain measurements that will document the performance of the amplification while it is being worn by the patient. Various techniques have been used or proposed for this purpose over the past 40–50 years. Gerald Studebaker (1980) offers a summary of these techniques. Only the most popular procedures will be described here.

A hearing aid test box with its accompanying printout capability is an indispensable instrument in a clinical hearing aid selection setting. It is common knowledge that the performance of a hearing aid is likely to change when it is inserted into the ear of a human being. In fact, it is difficult to deny that the user and the hearing aid function as a totality. Therefore, test box measurements, including KEMAR or other manikins, should be used for their intended purpose, that is, to measure and monitor the performance of a hearing aid according to manufacturer's specifications under standardized laboratory conditions. A test box or manikin should not be used to verify the response of a hearing aid as it is worn.

When it comes to measuring the performance of a hearing aid while it is being worn, there are two categories of techniques. One may be called an *indirect, behavioral, inferential, or psychophysical technique* that actually measures the patient's performance without and with amplification. The other category may be referred to as a *real-ear or in situ* technique. This second category is a physical measurement of acoustic stimuli in the patient's ear canal. The patient plays a passive role by offering the ear canal for the site of the measurement. Stated differently, the patient's performance is not being tested. Instead, the hearing aid system per se is being measured at the location of the output of the amplified signal. Specifically, the ear canal.

Indirect methods using speech are an outgrowth of Carhart's (1946) methodology established in military aural rehabilitation centers during World War II. This procedure involves unaided and aided measures of speech thresholds, tolerance levels, and speech discrimination performance in quiet and in the presence of competing signals. Carhart advocated the concept that the user and the hearing aid function as a totality. He contended that there is a measurable interaction between the patient and the electroacoustic characteristics of the hearing aid, and that factors such as the acoustic coupling can affect the user's performance. There have been some modifications to Carhart's original procedure over the past 40 or more years.

Speech Audiometry

The use of speech tests to measure the so-called benefits of wearable amplification have been challenged and criticized for more than 25 years, starting with the classic article by Shore et al. (1960). Test-retest reliability of "standardized" speech materials notwithstanding, there are other variables. Since the patient typically responds orally to test stimuli, the examiner is being tested simultaneously. Thus written or some type of visual responses are recommended to control this variable.

Recorded stimuli should be used routinely to eliminate differences among the clinicians' delivery of test material. Further, performance on auditory speech discrimination tests does not necessarily correspond to changes in the electroacoustic characteristics of a hearing aid, unless these changes are greatly exaggerated (Harris et al. 1961, Jerger et al. 1966 a,b). Conversely, if aided performance does not measure up to expectations on a speech audiometric test, the audiologist cannot necessarily identify the reason for the limited performance. Stated differently, speech stimuli do not identify the cause of inferior performance with a hearing aid.

When we carefully scrutinize published reports on the subject of hearing aid selection, monitoring, and verification procedures, we must reach the inescapable conclusion that *not a single procedure using speech stimuli has ever been established as a valid and reliable clinical method for consistently verifying the performance of a hearing aid while it is being worn.* Probably a major reason for this void is the difficulty in developing a clinical test that yields a good correlation between test performance and a person's daily communicative efficiency with amplification. *Auditory speech discrimination, as measured in the clinic using available standardized test materials, does not measure or predict with any degree of accuracy, how the patient will function in everyday life situations.* The reason is obvious. There are many variables that influence a person's communicative ability, including the acoustic environment, the patient's ability to use visual clues, temporal and prosodic clues, alertness and emotional states of the patient, communicative demands on the patient, command of language, and the oral delivery of other speakers, as well as other factors. These variables are difficult, if not impossible to measure.

Functional Gain

An alternate to the use of speech materials for the verification of hearing aid performance is functional gain measurements, that is, the difference between unaided and aided thresholds for warble tones or narrowbands of noise, in a sound-field. Initially, audiologists resorted to functional gain when fitting children with hearing aids and other patients with limited language or unintelligible speech. As more clinicians recognize the weakness of speech tests and the lengthy procedure involved, they turn to functional gain as a way of obtaining some documentation on the performance of a hearing aid. The promotion of formulas for interfacing of electroacoustic parameters to hearing loss has stimulated interest in functional gain measurements. Many audiologists are now selecting and verifying hearing aids for their patients almost entirely on electroacoustic characteristics that conform to a specified formula of their choice. They may adapt one carte blanche from the literature, or develop a formula of their own. The reader is urged to consult Chapter 7 in this book for an in-depth discussion of formulas. My discussion on this subject pertains to clinical methods that provide for a verification of specific electroacoustic parameters based on a formula of choice. Functional gain measurements allow for verification of formula. In fact, most formulas assume the use of a functional gain measurement.

Functional gain has the advantage of fairly limited patient participation, but the patient must still respond to an acoustic stimulus. Functional gain measurements can be used to determine whether the gain and maximum output of a hearing aid conform to predetermined values, based on a formula. In fact, predetermined values need not be established. That is, a formula need not enter the picture at all. The audiologist may simply wish to know the gain and maximum output of the hearing aid at discrete frequencies. If so, functional gain, using warble tones or narrow-bands of noise, has the potential to provide this information.

Functional gain measures have certain disadvantages. Only discrete frequencies are selected to "sample" gain. Clinicians typically assume a straight line from one data point to the next, such as seen on an audiogram. The output of a hearing aid can spike or dip dramatically within a relatively narrow frequency range. You will see these spikes and dips later in this chapter, when in situ measurements are illustrated. Another weakness of functional gain is the fact that the patient must be relied on to obtain data. That is, functional gain, like speech audiometry, is an indirect, behavioral measurement that is subject to psychophysical variables.

A third weakness, and one that cannot be discarded lightly, is the time involved in obtaining the measurements. Recall that at the outset of this chapter, I stressed the importance of moving along, being careful not to bore or fatigue the patient. One may argue that it does not require much time to obtain functional gain measures at six or seven frequencies. But remember, we could be involved in binaural amplification and we may need to make one or more adjustments to both hearing aids that requires a functional gain retest each time a change is made. Stated differently, minutes add up to hours.

Still another weakness of functional measurements is the calibration of the stimuli. Continuous pure tones generate standing waves that are likely to "break up" or vary in level from moment to moment in the same location or from place to place in the same room. In brief, continuous pure tones are not appropriate for functional gain measures. Warble tones are more stable over time and location, but they, too, can vary unpredictably in a typical clinical audiology sound room. Narrowbands of noise are more stable than warble tones but do not identify the peaks and valleys so often seen in the frequency response of hearing aids. Also, one must exercise much caution in measuring the soundfield stimulus and transferring these data to earphone measures, especially when assessing the maximum output levels of a hearing aid. Harford et al. (1983) address this issue to some extent.

In Situ Measurements

An in situ measure is a real ear technique that provides direct quantitative data about the electroacoustic characteristics of the amplified sound delivered to the patient's ear canal. It is gaining rapidly in popularity and will probably become the method of choice for verifying the performance of a hearing aid in the clinical setting. It is a simple, quick procedure that requires only the passive cooperation of the patient. In Chapter 2, Pollack describes, in detail, in situ measures as a clinical technique.

I have been using in situ methods routinely for verifying hearing aid performance since 1979 (Harford 1980a,b: 1981: 1984) and I find ear canal measurements useful for the following purposes:

1. Gain/frequency response
2. Real-ear SSPL$_{90}$ (re: SSPL$_{90}$)
3. Second harmonic distortion
4. Reserve gain (use vs full-on or under feedback)
5. Quality or morphology of the frequency response
6. Effect of electroacoustic adjustments
7. Effect of acoustic modifications
8. Binaural matching
9. Comparison of one hearing aid to another
10. Directional microphone effect
11. Comparison of CROS and BICROS
12. Evaluating assistive listening devices
13. Evaluating auditory training instruments

Figures 5-7 and 5-8 illustrate the application of real-ear measures for verifying the effect of tone adjustments while wearing a hearing aid.

CARE AND USE OF THE HEARING AID

The final step during this stage of the hearing aid selection process is to ensure that the patient is able to handle the instruments and understands basic care and maintenance. All manufacturers supply an owner's instruction booklet with each new hearing aid, but it is wise to reinforce these basic points. The audiologist should ensure that the patient can insert the earmold or custom hearing aid and is able to manipulate the volume control and other switches. During this final phase of the fitting and verification, it is wise to counsel the patient, spouse, and/or others relative to realistic expectations. A positive approach is much better than one loaded with reservations and precautions. It is important, however, to impose certain limitations so that the patient does not overuse the hearing aids too early in the adjustment period. It is worthwhile to consult Chapter 10 for more information.

FOLLOW-UP VISITS

It is essential that patients return for *at least* one postfitting and verification visit in order to ascertain whether the new amplification is, indeed, appropriate and beneficial. *If patients do not return, you cannot assume that you have been successful!* It seems reasonable to have the patients return 2 weeks after their fittings. Of course, they should be advised to return sooner if for any reason they are unable to use their new hearing aids. Sometimes a pressure point or contact ulcer will develop that requires sanding and buffing of the earmold or custom hearing aid.

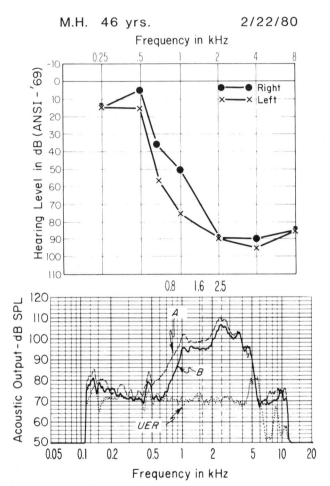

Fig. 5-7. Audiogram (A) and results of insertion gain (B) procedure for the right ear of a 46-year-old patient. Curves A and B in insertion gain graph illustrate differences in the frequency response adjustment on his hearing aid. Curve A represents the "N" tone setting and curve B, the "H" tone setting. This measurement provides the gain/frequency response for this particular hearing aid while it is being worn with two different tone adjustments. Reproduced from Harford ER: The use of a miniature microphone in the ear canal for the verification of hearing aid performance. Ear Hearing 1:329–337, © by Williams & Wilkins, 1980. With permission.

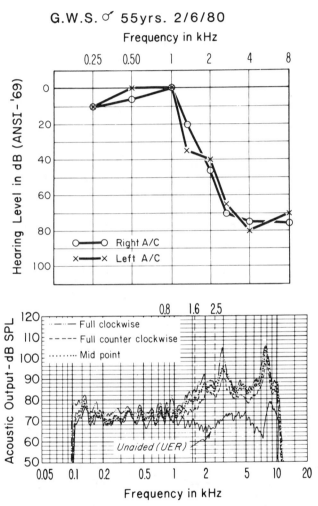

Fig. 5-8. Audiogram (A) and insertion gain (B) measurements for a patient for whom a custom ITE aid was prescribed. Insertion gain measures show changes in acoustic output and the smoothness of the frequency response when adjusting trimpot on the hearing aid. Reproduced from Harford ER: A new clinical technique for verification of hearing aid response. Arch Otolaryngology 107: 461–468, 1981. With permission.

When the patient returns, it is important to obtain information concerning the following:

1. The amount of use. On a scale of 0–100 percent, how much of the time has the patient used the aids?
2. Are the hearing aids physically comfortable?
3. Describe experiences where the aids were beneficial.
4. Describe uncomfortable experiences.
5. What else does the patient wish to report?
6. Does the patient's spouse, friend, or other family member have observations to report or questions to ask?

Based on these reports, some modifications may be necessary, such as more or less venting, trimmer adjustments, shortening the canal portion of the earmold or custom hearing aid, or others. The main point to keep in mind at this stage of the selection process is to determine whether the patient is "on a typical course of adjustment" or is experiencing problems that are out of proportion to usual expectations. This is a fundamental principle to understand. The audiologist must come to recognize a typical complaint or expressed problem for a particular type of hearing loss and convey to the patient the message that there is no need for much concern. The audiologist must emphasize that this is, indeed, typical and that matters will improve with time. It is at this point in the hearing aid selection where the naive or inexperienced audiologist could lose a patient's confidence or, at the least, create problems that otherwise are unnecessary. I stress again the importance of a positive attitude.

It is equally important to recognize, accept, and deal with a patient's report that expresses a problem that warrants direct action, such as a recasing of a custom-made aid, new earmold, change of circuit or hearing aid, a major modification in design of mold or aid, or other change.

Each time a modification is made, the audiologist has the option to verify the effect of the change on the physical characteristics of the output of the hearing aid (in situ measures) or on the patient's performance (psychophysical measures). Real-ear, in situ measures have the supreme advantage of speed, detail, and reliability. Thus each time a change is made, it should take only a matter of seconds to verify the effect of the change.

Of course, it is always gratifying to hear a patient applaud the benefits of the amplification you prescribed, fit, and verified, but this is not always the case. Hopefully, with more experience, your batting average will improve. If the patient is satisfied, what else can you do? I suggest that you wish your patients well, remind them of your interest in their hearing health care, and advise them to return voluntarily or by invitation in a year or prior to the expiration of their warranty. Then, if the hearing aids need maintenance, this can be accomplished at minimum or no cost. This encourages a patient to return with a year-end report that further verifies the success of your hearing aid selection.

Our program includes a 1–1½-hour hearing aid orientation and information session during the first visit following the fitting. This session is designed for both the patient and his spouse, friend, or other family members. These small group sessions are limited to five or six new and problem hearing aid users. The group is "led" by an audiologist who has had several years' experience with these sessions. The audiologist uses slides, recordings and other audio-visual aids, as well as a fun quiz to teach and reinforce some basic areas of popular concern.

CONCLUSION

Generally speaking, hearing aid selection and fitting techniques have not progressed at the same rate as technological developments in hearing aids. To emphasize this point, hearing aid design and technology allowed for practical binaural amplification 35 years ago. To this day, the prescription and use of binaural amplification is still not the method of choice by many audiologists (Mueller 1986). Hearing aids continue to get smaller and more technical. The new A-10 battery and microprocessors will carry us into still another generation of sophisticated miniaturized amplifiers. It behooves the audiologist to stay abreast of current developments and exercise ingenuity in the practical application of these advances for the benefit of the hearing-impaired. It would be to the advantage of everyone if audiologists and manufacturers worked more closely in product development and application.

Regardless of the pessimism expressed above, audiologists have made some progress with hearing aids, but the late Raymond Carhart's words at the outset of this text warrant careful thought, although it has been more than a dozen years since he wrote them. I invite the reader to return to the last three or four pages of the Introduction (before Chapter 1 in this volume) and study Carhart's thoughts once again. Time is passing and technology is advancing. Any audiologist who intends to maintain a leading role in hearing aid rehabilitation would do well to follow the advice of Carhart.

REFERENCES

Alpiner JG: Evaluation of communication function, In Alpiner JG (ed): Handbook of Adult Rehabilitative Audiology. Baltimore, Williams & Wilkins, 1978, pp. 30–66

Carhart R: Tests for the selection of hearing aids. Laryngoscope 56:780–794, 1946

Davis H: The articulation area and the social adequacy index for hearing. Laryngoscope 58:761–778, 1948

Dodds E, Harford ER: Application of a lipreading test in a hearing aid evaluation. Speech Hearing Disorders 33:167–173, 1968

Giolas TG: The measurement of hearing handicap. Maico Audiological Library Series 8:6, 1970

Giolas TG, Owens E, Lamb SH, et al: Hearing performance inventory. J Speech Hearing Disorders 44:169–195, 1979

Goldstein J: Hearing loss and the primary care MD—an overview. Hearing J 39:23–24, 1986

Harford ER: The use of a miniature microphone in the ear canal for the verification of hearing aid performance. Ear Hearing 1:329–337, 1980a

Harford ER: A microphone in the ear canal to measure hearing aid performance. Hearing Instruments 31:14–15, 32, 1980b

Harford ER: A new clinical technique for verification of hearing aid response. Arch Otolaryngology 107:461–468, 1981

Harford ER: The use of real-ear measurements for fitting wearable amplification. Hearing J 37:20–25, 1984

Harford ER, Barry J: A rehabilitative approach to the problem of unilateral hearing loss: The contralateral routing of signals (CROS). J Speech Hearing Disorders 30:121–138, 1965

Harford ER, Leijon A, Liden G, et al: Audiometric earphone discomfort level and hearing aid SSPL$_{90}$ as measured in the human ear canal. Ear Hearing 4:185–189, 1983

Harford ER, Musket, C: Binaural hearing with one hearing aid. J Speech Hearing Disorders 29:133–146, 1964

Harris JD, Haines HL, Kelsey PA, et al: The relation between speech intelligibility and the electroacoustic characteristics of low fidelity circuitry. J Auditory Res 5:357–381, 1961

High WS, Fairbanks G, Glorig A: Scale of self-assessment of hearing handicap. J Speech Hearing Disorders 29: 215–230, 1964

Jerger J, Malmquist C, Speaks C: Comparison of some speech intelligibility tests in the evaluation of hearing aid performance. Speech Hearing Res 9:253–258, 1966a

Jerger J, Speaks C, Malmquist C: Hearing aid performance and hearing aid selection. J Speech Hearing Res 9:136–149, 1966b

Mueller HG: Binaural amplification: Attitudinal factors. Hearing J 39:7–10, 1986

Noble WG, Atherley GRC: The hearing measure scale: A questionnaire for the assessment of auditory disability. J Auditory Res 10:229–250, 1970

Rupp RR, Higgins J, Maurer JF: A feasibility scale for predicting hearing aid use (FSPHAU) for older individuals. J Acad Rehab Audiol 10:81–104, 1977

Schow RL, Nerbonne MA: Communication screening profile: Use with elderly clients. Ear Hearing 3:135–147, 1982

Shambaugh G, Rosen S: The hidden handicap of deafness. Med World News 16:53–60, 1975

Shore I, Bilger RC, Hirsh I. Hearing aid evaluation: Reliability of repeated measurements. J Speech Hearing Disorders 25:152–170, 1960

Studebaker G: Fifty years of hearing aid research: An evaluation of progress. Ear Hearing 1:57–62, 1980

Ventry IM, Weinstein BE: The hearing handicap inventory for the elderly: A new tool. Ear Hearing 3:128–134, 1982

Appendix A

Intake History

Name _____ Age _____ Today's Date _____

What is your occupation? _____

Who referred you to the Audiology Clinic? _____

What concerns you the most? Hearing loss _____ Dizziness _____ Ear noises _____
                        Other (specify) _____

1. If you think or know you have a hearing problem, please answer the following: otherwise, go to question 2.

   a. Do you have a problem hearing in the following situations?
      While listening to another person at a distance of 6 feet? Yes _____ No _____
      In groups and noisy places? Yes _____ No _____
      While using the telephone? Yes _____ No _____ If yes, which ear do you prefer?
      Right _____ Left _____ No preference _____
      At work? Yes _____ No _____
      At home? Yes _____ No _____
      In social and recreational situations? Yes _____ No _____

   b. From which ear do you hear better? Right _____ Left _____
      Both about the same _____

   c. What do you think caused your hearing loss? _____

   d. Did your hearing loss come on suddenly _____? Gradually _____?

   e. When did you first notice the loss? _____

   f. Has it gotten worse over time? Yes _____ No _____

   g. Does it fluctuate from time to time? Yes _____ No _____

   h. Does anyone in your family have a hearing problem? Yes _____ No _____
      If yes, who? _____

2. Have you ever had ear surgery? Yes _____ No _____

3. Do you presently have "tubes" in your ears? Yes _____ No _____ Don't know _____

4. Do you take any medicines regularly? Yes _____ No _____

5. Are you bothered by noises in your ears or head? Yes _____ No _____
   If yes, Right _____ Left _____ Both _____ Head_____

6. Are you ever dizzy? Yes _____ No _____ If yes, please describe: _____
   _____

7. Have you *ever* been exposed to loud noises for any length of time? Yes _____ No _____
   If yes, for how long? _____

8. Have you ever used a hearing aid in the past? Yes _____ No _____

9. If you are using a hearing aid now, please answer the following. If you are *not* using an aid, go to question 10.

   a. Which ear is aided? Right _____ Left _____ Both_____

   b. How long have you used an aid? _____

   c. How long have you had your present aid? _____

   d. Are you satisfied with the aid? Yes _____ No _____

10. What do you want to learn from your visit today? _____
    _____

Appendix B

Hearing Care Specialists

Creekside Professional Building
6600 Excelsior Blvd. Suite 150
St. Louis Park, MN 55426

Hearing and Prescription

Name _____ UH# _____ Date _____

BTE/Standard Products	ITE
Manuf. _____ Model _____	Manuf. _____ Model _____
Ear choice: L ___ R ___ Binaural ___	Ear choice: L ___ R ___ Binaural ___
Battery: _____ Air/Mercury	Battery: _____ Air/Mercury

Options:
___ Telecoil   ___ Boot
___ Hook _____ ___ Cord type _____
___ Receiver   ___ Cord length
___ Other _____ ___ Color _____

Adjustments:
Tone ___ Output ___ Gain ___ AGC ___

Remarks: _____
_____

Earmold: L ___ R ___ Binaural ___

Style: Material:
___ #1 (w/snap ring) ___ Lucite
___ #2 (phantom)   ___ Other _____
___ #2HF
___ #3 (full shell)   Attachments:
___ Other _____   ___ Glue tube
___ Sound separator ___ Other _____
___ Select-A-Vent   Tube Size: _____

Loss   Ear texture:
___ Mild   ___ Soft
___ Moderate   ___ Medium
___ Severe   ___ Firm
___ Profound

Options:
___ Gain potential   ___ IROS A/B
___ Frequency pot.   ___ Select-A-Vent
___ Output limiter   ___ Sound separator
___ Telecoil   ___ Removal notches
___ Macro vent   ___ Built-up VC
___ Short canal   ___ Other _____

Cord length _____ Color _____

Specifications:

	L	R	
MCL			dB HL
UCL			dB HL
Gain			dB
SSPL			dB
Slope			

	L	R	
$SSPL_{90}$ not to exceed			dB SPL

Remarks: _____
_____

Medical Release: _____
Audiologist: _____

This prescription is valid for a maximum period of 6 months from above date, or less if there is a significant change in hearing. After 6 months, further evaluation would be required prior to obtaining a hearing aid.

Richard C. Seewald
Mark Ross

6

Amplification for Young Hearing-Impaired Children

For most hearing-impaired children, the early and appropriate selection and use of amplification is the single most important habilitative tool available to us. These words set the tone for this chapter by Richard Seewald and Mark Ross—a realistic, holistic approach to the problem. One of the most frustrating aspects of selecting a hearing aid for a young child is the inability to quantify the accuracy of our decision. Although real-ear measurements take us further, we are still not where we would like to be. With this in mind, Richard and Mark present special considerations for dealing with these situations. Beyond this, they describe, in humanistic terms, suggestions for parent counseling as the key to the successful use of amplification by a child.

MCP

The major problem of most hearing-impaired children is that they have trouble hearing! Before one rejects this remark as facetious or trite, let us look closely into its implications. Certainly the congenitally hearing-impaired child's deviations in communication skills development and their resulting effect on all facets of the child's life are a direct consequence of the hearing impairment. Although there are a variety of opinions regarding the specifics of the relationship between the degree, type, and configuration of the hearing loss and the consequent problems, no one could logically argue that a strong relationship does not exist. On what habilitative measures, however, do the professions involved with the young hearing-impaired child focus most of their time and energy? In what areas do the articles in profes-

AMPLIFICATION FOR THE HEARING-IMPAIRED, THIRD EDITION
Copyright © 1988 by Grune & Stratton, Inc.

sional journals and papers read at professional meetings show the greatest concentration? To answer the question negatively, these papers concentrate not on measures designed to reduce the problem at the source, namely, the hearing loss itself, but rather on efforts that are essentially remedial and focus on correcting abnormal developmental patterns.

The underlying premise of this chapter is that *for most hearing-impaired children, the early and appropriate selection and use of amplification is the single most important habilitative tool available to us.* Audition is the normal route through which speech and language develop. The overwhelming majority of hearing-impaired children have a great deal of residual hearing (Boothroyd 1972, Elliot 1967, Goodman 1949, Hine 1973, Huizing 1959, Montgomery 1967), which, when properly exploited through amplification, can still serve as the primary channel for communication purposes (Fry 1978). By focusing on audition in an enriched natural language environment, the child's own potential capacity for speech and language development is used as our most significant ally in all habilitative endeavors. We have expanded on this point elsewhere in more detail (Ross et al. 1982, Ross and Giolas 1978). Once optimum audition through amplification is accomplished, enriched speech and language experiences, special tutoring, and innovative media can be effectively applied to the remaining deficits and needs. The first step, however, must be focused on the quality and quantity of auditory input provided to the child so that the natural development of speech and language can be maximized.

It is not easy to ensure this first step when the selection of appropriate amplification is being considered. With adults, we see a diverse variety of methods of selection and evaluation of hearing aids, all of which remain subject to questions and ultimate validation. We can be informed and aware of the appropriateness of our selection, however, by the feedback we get from verbal adults who are able to express their preferences and concerns. For young children, we have amassed a similar proliferation of selection and evaluation procedures, but are without clear feedback regarding the validity of our recommendations. *Thus, with children, our selection may remain inappropriate or inadequate during the early stages merely because we cannot obtain immediate constructive feedback from them.* We have not yet developed generally accepted procedures for assessing the effectiveness of the final product, namely, appropriately selected amplification.

Our current approach for selecting and evaluating the effectiveness of amplification is defined in four distinct yet interrelated steps. For the purpose of introduction, these steps will be briefly mentioned, although all will be described in greater detail in the ensuing pages.

The first and most basic step is quantifying the child's residual hearing. We need to know as much as possible about the child's hearing as quickly as possible, but what we don't know should not stop us from proceeding with amplification. We must always be aware, as should the child's parents and teachers, that we will need to make modifications and perhaps even major changes as we learn more about a child and that child's auditory status.

The second step is to define and provide the electroacoustic dimensions that will optimize auditory learning for the child. At this step we must draw extensively on our knowledge of speech and environmental acoustics, psychoacoustics, speech perception, and psycholinguistics and combine that knowledge with what we do know of the child's unique residual hearing characteristics. The end result of this process is a specific set of electroacoustic dimensions and selection of a system capable of providing these dimensions.

Our third step is concerned with evaluating the adequacy and success of the selection process. In other words, in the interaction between a child's residual hearing and that child's electroacoustic system are we able to observe and measure the predicted growth in auditory behavior and in speech and language development. Although audiometric validation is an important component in this process, substantiation of the adequacy of our selection will not come from the audiometric assessment alone. At this stage we are looking for continued documentation from unsolicited and elicited reports from parents and others involved in the habilitation program; from documented growth in auditory skills and speech and language performance; and from behavioral manifestations on the part of the child in the clinic, at home, in the classroom, and in other real-life situations.

Our fourth and final step is the process of modifying and monitoring the electroacoustic system as more data accumulate regarding the child and that child's performance. Implicit in this fourth step are two assumptions. First, the selection of amplification for young children is an ongoing process that extends beyond one or two clinic visits, and beyond the typical confines of a "clinic," into the more important realities of a child's daily living. We look at the selection and evaluation of amplification as an integral part of the total habilitation program. Second, all initial electroacoustic recommendations are tentative, subject to appropriate modifications as information about the child's hearing and auditory development begins to accumulate, and our own knowledge in the areas of audition, linguistics, and electroacoustics increases and becomes more refined.

Throughout the process of selecting and evaluating amplification for the young child, we are continually aware that it is only one component, although an important one, in a total habilitative process. Early emphasis on amplification cannot take place in an habilitative vacuum. The successful use of amplification is apt to reflect the audiologist's ability to communicate the necessity for amplification to the parents and their active participation in this aspect of the child's program, which, in turn, depends on their understanding and their acceptance of their hearing-impaired child. This is not a stage that can be taken for granted, and it cannot be relegated to occasional casual contacts between parents and the audiologist.

"Parent counseling" does not occur magically because the audiologist sometimes talks to the child's parents or because this is what is labeled as the intention. The services of a skilled, sensitive clinician who can assist the parents in working through their feelings of anxiety and guilt that frequently accompany the discovery of their child's problems is a prerequisite for an optimally successful habilitative effort (Luterman 1979, 1984; Moses and Van Hecke-Wulatin 1981). A purely technical approach to habilitation, no matter how skilled, is apt to founder on the parent's misapprehensions and misunderstandings. Parents are essential partners in a joint habilitative effort. They have more invested and have the greatest impact on their children, particularly the younger ones, and their level of participation is often the major factor in determining the ultimate success or failure of the habilitation program. Thus, if we are to be successful in our intervention with amplification, the technical aspects of this process must be systematically integrated with a significant commitment to provide support and information sharing with parents. Additionally, we must be willing to extend our thinking and perceptions to areas outside of the clinical setting. The practice of placing a hearing aid on a child and hoping for the best does not pay the best dividends. The "perfect" amplification system for a child will be useless if it is not working or worn consistently once the child steps out of the clinic or if the optimal use of audition is not encouraged and expected in the home and educational environments.

We reemphasize that, although this chapter is devoted primarily to the procedures and technical aspects of selecting and evaluating amplification for young hearing-impaired children, it should nevertheless be understood that, *for the best results, these techniques must be embedded within a complete habilitative matrix.*

PRESELECTION CONSIDERATIONS

Assessment and Diagnosis

The comprehensive assessment and diagnosis of a young hearing-impaired child is an obvious preliminary to intervention with amplification. Does the child have a hearing impairment at all? If so, what is the type and etiology of the impairment? What is the nature of the hearing loss in terms of both severity and configuration? Do additional problems exist that can affect the child's learning and general development? What are the available resources both within and outside the child's family to support the purchase and appropriate use of amplification? These are not easy questions to answer, particularly when infants are the subject of concern. Yet, they are examples of questions that require systematic consideration for each child, through a well-integrated, cooperative team effort.

Typically we do not have complete information before proceeding with amplification. Our initial recommendations for the young child most often reflect some degree of uncertainty regarding the child and the nature and degree of impairment. In most cases, the assessment process will need to continue simultaneously with the amplification program, since ultimately the success of our habilitative efforts depends greatly on understanding the unique nature of the situation. We have often observed, for example, a real lack of commitment to amplification on the part of the parents, until their questions regarding etiology have been thoroughly explored. The process of assessment and diagnosis, then, does not end with the initial hearing aid recommendation. Naturally, as more information accumulates and insight develops regarding the child and the impairment, the amplification and general habilitative program should be modified accordingly.

The advent and widespread use of physiological measures of hearing, particularly auditory brainstem response (ABR) measures (Jacobson 1985; Worthington and Peters, 1984) and the immittance battery (Orchik and MacKimmie 1984, Popelka, 1981), as well as the results from some nonauditory diagnostic procedures such as computerized tomographic (CT) scans, are beginning to reduce the uncertainty regarding the auditory status in young children. In working toward the amplification selection process, our current preference, with regard to auditory assessment, is to utilize behavioral response procedures, particularly visual reinforcement audiometry (VRA), as early as possible. Research findings, as well as our own clinical experiences, suggest that reliable, frequency-specific, hearing sensitivity data can be obtained with children as young as seven months of age (Wilson and Thompson 1984).

We should not underestimate the value of information that can be obtained with behavioral assessment techniques. In the hands of a skilled clinician who is experienced in observing and interpreting response behavior, the results provide not only information regarding the child's peripheral hearing sensitivity but also insight into the child's ability to attend, process, and respond to acoustic signals in an age-appropriate manner (Boothroyd 1982, Northern and Downs 1984, Wilson and Thompson 1984). After one or two sessions, it is possible with the majority of children to formulate reasonable estimates regarding the degree and configuration of the hearing loss, any sensitivity differences between ears, and the type of impairment. In considering the assessment findings it is necessary to ask the questions, "Is the child's manner of responding and general auditory behavior consistent with that child's developmental age and peripheral hearing status?" If not, we must be continually alert to the possibility of complicating factors in addition to hearing loss.

Finally, the immittance test battery is an integral and routine part of the assessment protocol. It not only provides detailed information relative to the absence or presence of conductive dysfunction but can lend additional confirmation related to the presence of sensorineural hearing loss in difficult-to-test children (Green and Margolis 1983).

Regardless of the assessment techniques employed, rarely is an accurate diagnostic picture completed before the ages of 2–3 years, or well into the optimal readiness period for speech and language acquisition. Therefore, the audiologist is usually in a position in which amplification must be recommended on the basis of incomplete information or risk losing some very valuable time while precise diagnostic and auditory profiles are established. A number of studies have reported that the time between an initial diagnosis of hearing impairment and the actual fitting with amplification can be as long as one year (Worthington et al. 1985). While there are presumably a number of reasons for this, the audiologist's reluctance to recommend amplification until complete audiometric data have been obtained should not be among them.

At times we encounter the child who is not responding to high intensity auditory signals and appears to be "too deaf" to benefit from amplification. Since it is only a minority of hearing-impaired children whose hearing is so poor that they respond by vibrotactile perception primarily, and since even this limited information can provide some assistance in communication (Erber 1972, Ross et al. 1973), *it makes therapeutic sense to require amplification for all hearing-impaired children at the earliest possible age.*

A necessary qualification must be added here. Hearing aids should not be fitted to any child without prior otologic examination, clearance, and/or treatment. Such practice will not only ensure good comprehensive medical care of the hearing-impaired child but may also contribute to that child's initial adaptation to and use of amplification. In our own practice we have frequently seen prescribed medication relieve negative middle-ear pressure and middle-ear effusion, which previously contributed to annoyance with the earmold and/or an excessive amount of feedback.

Physical Characteristics and Electroacoustic Performance

HEARING AID DESIGN FEATURES AND PERFORMANCE

Before entering into the hearing aid selection process with any child, the audiologist will need to preselect a limited number of instruments for consideration on the basis of specific physical and electroacoustic criteria. The physical characteristics of hearing aids are especially relevant to consider for young children. Many of these children are highly active, human tornadoes who frequently derive great pleasure from literally covering themselves with sand, water, oatmeal, or any other available substance. Knowing this, we need to be especially concerned with the performance record of any instrument we might recommend. For example, we should know whether the hearing aid has stable operating characteristics even when submitted to unusual conditions, a respectable maintenance record, and physical characteristics that are sufficiently sturdy and durable.

The physical dimensions of the hearing aid should be appropriate to a child-size user. We continue to see examples of ear-level hearing aids with bottom facing microphones hidden in a coat or sweater collar, or a button-type receiver that is almost as large as the child's pinna tending to pull the earmold out of the ear. Another important consideration is that the controls of the hearing aid should be clearly labeled so that parents and other adults who work with the child may have reference points when monitoring the child's amplification. Other specific characteristics that will affect the performance or manageability of the hearing aid include weight and susceptibility of its components to moisture.

Additional design features the audiologist will need to consider during this preselection phase are related to the microphone type: directional or omnidirectional and compatibility with other systems the child may use within the habilitative program. It must be extremely discouraging for parents to learn that the hearing aids purchased during the prior year must be replaced because of incompatibility with either personal frequency-modulated (FM) or loop systems in use within the child's preschool classroom. During this time of developing technologies in amplification it is unlikely that the audiologist can anticipate every system interface requirement a given child may need. It would be prudent, however, for the audiologist to keep informed about the types of educational systems being used within the child's geographic location and to recommend instruments with powerful telecoils and direct audio-input options as often as possible.

In terms of electroacoustic characteristics, the key word in preselection is *flexibility*. Since the initial information concerning the child's residual hearing may be limited and since the electroacoustics of the hearing aid will, in all likelihood, be modified as more information is obtained, an aid whose electroacoustic dimensions can be easily modified to meet the child's requirements is essential. A number of hearing aids can be eliminated from further consideration on the basis of their electroacoustic performance characteristics alone. These characteristics include high internal noise and harmonic distortion levels, nonlinear volume control taper characteristics, and short battery life.

In moving from this preselection phase into the process of selecting electro-acoustic dimensions for a specific child, certain preliminary decisions need to be made regarding the earmold, the type of hearing aid to be used, that is, ear level or body type, and whether a monaural or binaural fitting will be applied within the initial stages. These decisions must be made carefully through the integration of the audiologist's clinical experience and knowledge with the available assessment findings for the individual child. Whatever preliminary decisions are made regarding an amplification system, they must account for each child's unique situation and reflect a strong and clear rationale. We say this because it is not only necessary for the audiologist to understand why a particular initial approach was chosen, but at the same time it is imperative for the parents to understand and support the specific plan of action.

HEARING AID TYPE

For the greatest majority of young hearing-impaired children, we prefer the use of postauricular hearing aids. Most manufacturers are now producing instruments that offer the electroacoustic flexibility, power, frequency range, and practical features that were once attributed only to body-worn hearing aids. Our preference is based primarily on the fact that postauricular instruments offer the advantages of microphone location in a more "normal" position, around the pinna area (Kuhn 1980), and normal separation of the microphones for binaural perception. Additionally, these instruments virtually eliminate many of the common problems associated with body-worn hearing aids, including clothing noise, broken cords, and reduction in high frequency transmission due to the sound absorption properties of the body (Erber 1973).

Despite our preference for ear-level amplification, we agree wholeheartedly with the concerns regarding feedback management and control expressed recently by Matkin (1984). There is no question that the simple reduction in distance between the hearing aid microphone and acoustic output from the receiver associated with ear level instruments increases the likelihood of feedback. Because of the rapid growth of the external ear in early childhood, control of the feedback problem requires that (1) the audiologist become knowledgeable about current earmold impression and design techniques that help to reduce the problem (Castleton 1985, Madell and Gendel 1984) and (2) parents carefully monitor the function of the amplification system on a regular basis so that when feedback occurs, it can be dealt with appropriately.

Our concern here is clearly illustrated in a field study reported by Matkin (1984) in which 8 out of 11 young children with severe to profound hearing loss were found to be receiving only limited benefit from their postauricular instruments because the parents had reduced the gain to avoid feedback. If, for whatever reason, the feedback problem cannot be dealt with effectively, or if an appropriate degree of amplification and/or frequency response cannot be provided with ear-level instruments, the option of body-worn amplification should receive serious consideration. For example, profoundly hearing-impaired children may benefit from the enhancement of the lower-frequency regions with body-worn instruments as a result of the body baffle effect (Erber 1973). Valuable auditory learning time can be lost, sometimes months, in an effort to fit the child cosmetically rather than selecting a type appropriate for that individual child. Above all, we must remain clearly focused on the ultimate goal of this process, which is to provide the young child with the appropriate quantity and quality of amplification on a consistent basis regardless of the means by which this is accomplished.

EARMOLD COUPLING CONSIDERATIONS

The preselection stage also includes specific recommendations for a particular type of earmold. In recent years we have developed an increased awareness and understanding of the acoustical properties and subsequent effects produced by earmold coupling systems (see Chapter 3). We can no longer view the earmold simply as a means for directing amplified sound to the ear canal or as a custom anchor to hold the hearing aid in place. *Rather, the earmold coupling system must be viewed as an integral part of the total electroacoustic system since it will exert its own unique influence on the amplified signal delivered to the individual.* It is primarily for this reason that young hearing-impaired children should enter the amplification selection and evaluation process with their own custom-made earmolds.

It can be assumed that the evaluation process will indicate the need for some "fine-tuning" modifications through the application of venting, filtering, and/or use of the acoustic horn. The audiologist should be able to develop a reasonable starting place with the residual hearing data in hand. For young children, we routinely recommend earmolds fabricated from soft materials such as polyvinylchloride or silicone. In addition to the safety-related benefits, we generally encounter less difficulty with feedback when using earmolds made from soft materials. With regard to earmold design, we begin with a full-shell type fitted with thick-walled tubing. For children with severe to profound degrees of hearing loss, we have found an additional buildup of material in the tragus portion to be an effective means of feedback control.

MONAURAL VERSUS BINAURAL SYSTEM SELECTION

The final preselection consideration is related to whether monaural or binaural amplification will be applied initially. Since the issue of binaural amplification continues to be somewhat controversial in our field, it will be considered as a special topic with the final section of this chapter. At this point, however, we will briefly describe our current approach to this within the framework of the preselection process.

At our facilities, binaural hearing aids are recommended initially for the majority of children we see. In addition to the generally positive auditory effects (Hawkins and Yacullo 1984, Ross 1977a), a binaural fitting is the arrangement of choice in the initial stages for two reasons. First, most young children are eventually found to have bilateral, fairly symmetrical hearing losses with between-ear sensitivity differences rarely exceeding more than 10 or 15 dB at specific frequencies. Moreover, the hearing aid evaluation procedure to be described within the next section allows the clinician to quantify any aided performance differences that may exist between the two ears. With a moderate degree of assurance, the audiologist should therefore, be able to shape the electroacoustic characteristics so that reasonably symmetrical aided performance can be achieved. Second, in our experience, parents tend to be much more receptive to the concept of binaural amplification when the child is first being fitted with hearing aids. Two-ear amplification makes sense to them at this time, and the greatest majority readily accept and support the recommendation. It is when binaural recommendations are made after a more or less successful adjustment to a monaural fitting that parental—and, occasionally, a child's—resistance, to a second hearing aid is experienced. There is, of course, always the possibility that the specific instrument selected is inappropriate for one ear, especially when we are relying on soundfield measurements, which can reflect the sensitivity dimensions of the "better" ear, at least within a portion of the audiometric frequency range, and therefore underestimate the degree of hearing loss in the second or "poorer" ear. In cases where the benefits of the second hearing aid are questionable, a clinic loaner instrument should be used until individual ear information becomes available. This loaner option should be included in any audiologic program for young children.

In summary, we have now considered the relevant aspects of the assessment and diagnosis findings and, in turn, developed a preliminary plan with regard to the physical means by which amplification will be provided initially. Thus the stage is set for entering into the process of selecting specific electroacoustic dimensions for the child. Before proceeding further, we would like to reemphasize, through a brief example, the importance of sharing with the parents the rationale for recommendations we make regarding the means by which amplification will be provided. One of us (R. Seewald) recently participated in a parent group in which only one of the children being represented was using body-worn amplification. The issue of ear-level versus body-worn amplification emerged as a topic of discussion and a number of the parents clearly described their understanding of the relative benefits of ear-level hearing aids. The mother of the child with the body-type aid reluctantly admitted that she had no idea why her child was not using ear-level amplification and eventually expressed real feelings of guilt that she was not providing the best for her child. It is clear from this example that the parents must understand why a particular approach is recommended if we are to expect them to support and feel comfortable with the specific plan we design. If parents are left with feelings of uncertainty or apprehension, we may lose our most important source of support in achieving a successful program of amplification.

ELECTROACOUSTIC SELECTION AND EVALUATION PROCEDURES

Rationale

The primary goal of the amplification selection and evaluation process is to provide the child with the maximum auditory information in a manner consistent with that child's residual hearing. Specifically, we are concerned with delivering as many of the acoustic dimensions of speech in as many situations as possible without approaching or exceeding the level at which the reception of speech becomes uncomfortable. When possible, we are further interested in reducing the influence, or competition, of irrelevant sounds that could potentially interfere with the child's perception of spoken language.

In attempting to accomplish this general goal we need to recognize and incorporate the acoustics of speech as a basis for our selection considerations (Boothroyd 1978, Levitt 1978, Ling 1978). What parameters of frequency, intensity, and duration contained in speech provide the salient auditory cues for speech perception in the normal child, and how can they be provided optimally to a child with hearing loss? To address these issues, we need to draw extensively from the areas of acoustic phonetics, psychoacoustics, electroacoustics, and psycholinguistics. Although we most certainly have more to learn regarding the interrelationship among all relevant factors, our current knowledge base, in conjunction with existing and developing technologies, brings us closer to attaining our general goal on a more consistent basis than at any prior time. It is simply not necessary for the audiologist to stand with a child's audiometric data in dB hearing level in one hand, the manufacturer's specification in dB sound pressure level (SPL) in the other hand, and utter a silent prayer!

With young children in particular, a speech-spectrum-based theoretical approach to the selection of electroacoustic characteristics appears to be the most useful for our purpose (Byrne 1981, 1982; Erber 1973; Gengel et al. 1971; Schwartz and Larson 1977b). The theoretical approach to electroacoustic selection, as described by Byrne (1981, 1982), bases selection on known or hypothesized relationships among the amplification characteristics of hearing aids, the acoustic dimensions of the speech signal, and the measurable auditory characteristics of the child. The end result of this selection approach is a specific set of electroacoustic characteristics, including frequency response and saturation sound pressure level (SSPL) functions that are predicted as being appropriate for the individual child. With this approach, the electroacoustic characteristics that we specify depend on all available audiometric information and knowledge of the most salient perceptual cues present in the acoustic speech signal. We are not overly concerned with the brand name of the hearing aids we ultimately recommend, but with the electroacoustic dimensions they embody. This is an important distinction to make. *We are not comparing brand X to brand Y, but are selecting electroacoustic system X because in our view it best meets the auditory learning requirements of the child.* It is not the name monogrammed on a hearing aid that interests us, but whether its performance is likely to provide the most relevant acoustic information to the child.

In the general approach we are currently using (Seewald et al. 1985), we make a clear differentiation between the electroacoustic selection stage and the evaluation stage of the process (Byrne 1981). This is not to suggest that selection and evaluation are unrelated activities in the overall process. On the contrary, one of the major advantages of a theoretical electroacoustic selection approach is that it provides specific criteria on which evaluation can be based. *We take the view that it is not possible to evaluate the success of our fittings with amplification without first deciding what it is that we want.* Thus we first determine the electroacoustic characteristics most appropriate for a given child as based on our theoretical model (selection) and then assess the degree to which we have approximated those requirements by obtaining real-ear measurements of performance with the selected system (evaluation). Where evaluation indicates differences between the desired and the actual performance, appropriate modifications are made to the electroacoustic system with which we are working. Thus, although electroacoustic selection and evaluation are viewed as distinctly different stages, both are necessary and interrelated aspects of this critically important process.

Instrumentation and Calibration

In developing our current approach we have attempted to design the procedures around instrumentation systems that are presently available in most clinical settings. With the exception of a microcomputer, all that is required is the instrumentation capability for performing frequency-specific soundfield audiometric measurements of hearing aid electroacoustic performance. We recognize that all clinicians who work with young children do not have access to a microcomputer system. Thus, in addition to our computer-assisted approach, we will consider alternate selection and evaluation strategies that do not require the availability of a microcomputer system.

A selection and evaluation approach presupposes that we have some means of ensuring that we are actually delivering the desired electroacoustic parameters. One basic requirement is clearly an electroacoustic measurement system. In using standard analysis devices we need to remain cognizant of the fact that the real-ear performance of a hearing aid can differ markedly and is unpredictable from its performance as defined in a standard 2-cc coupler (Hawkins and Haskell 1982;

Wetzell and Harford 1983). If this limitation is acknowledged, standard electro-acoustic measurements, in conjunction with functional gain measures, can nevertheless play a useful role in the evaluation stage of the process (Skinner et al. 1982b).

One promising alternative to the standard electroacoustic measurement system, particularly for amplification fittings with young children, comes with the recent emergence of commercially available computerized probe tube microphone systems (Berlin 1985, Jablin 1984, Libby 1985, Nielson and Rasmussen 1984). In addition to elimination of the known problems associated with standard 2-cc and real-ear performance differences, a major advantage of insertion gain and in situ response measurements of hearing aid performance with young children is the fact that, as purely physical measurements, they require only passive cooperation and avoid a variety of difficulties associated with more conventional psychoacoustic measures (Hawkins et al. 1985, Libby 1985).

Before we can comfortably recommend general application of probe tube microphone measurements with young children to the exclusion of other more conventional approaches, there are still a number of methodologic issues that remain unresolved and/or only partially understood (Hawkins and Mueller 1986), and the need exists for more systematic research regarding the application of the new technology with young hearing-impaired children (Leister and Claus-Parodi 1986). It is primarily for these reasons that we will focus our attention on procedures that require simply the availability of a standard electroacoustic analysis device. We are, however, in cooperation with others (Stelmachowicz et al. 1985), developing a modification of our general approach and computer program that incorporates the use of probe tube microphone system measurements. We believe that this will ultimately provide us with a greater degree of precision within the evaluation stage of the overall process.

In general, the standard electroacoustic analysis instrumentation is used to shape and confirm the preliminary estimates of gain and output that the selection model (to be discussed) predicts as appropriate for a given child. These coupler-based measurements are then compared to the functional gain values obtained during the evaluation stage to determine the extent to which our preliminary estimates vary from the desired real-ear performance. Where differences are found to exist, the electroacoustic system (hearing aid and earmold coupling) are modified accordingly, using the results of the standard electroacoustic analysis as the basis for resolving the differences observed. Such an approach is clearly preferred to the time-honored methods of (1) setting the gain control by increasing gain until feedback occurs, then reducing gain slightly until audible feedback is eliminated, or (2) arbitrarily setting the gain to the one-half or three-quarters "on" position.

In addition to its use within the initial selection and evaluation process, the electroacoustic analyzer serves a critically important function in the long-term management of amplification with young children. The use of this system provides us with verification that a particular instrument is performing as the manufacturer specified when it was initially fitted, and further, that the electroacoustic characteristics have remained stable over time. As practicing clinicians, we have learned that it can never be assumed that the electroacoustic system we first delivered to the child is at all the same 3, 6, or 12 months later. Our experiences with highly active young children have led us to routinely monitor the electroacoustic characteristics on at least a monthly basis whenever possible. We also strongly recommend that a complete electroacoustic analysis be performed prior to all aided behavioral assessments with children. Much time can be saved and frustration avoided by identifying performance difficulties with the hearing aid before subjecting a child to an evaluation session with a defective instrument!

The selection and evaluation approach we are currently using requires the appropriate instrumentation and test environment for performing frequency-specific soundfield audiometric measurements. Because selection of electroacoustic characteristics is based on the responses obtained in the soundfield, it is a necessary prerequisite that the test stimuli be calibrated and that the test environment and measurement conditions be carefully controlled. A comprehensive discussion of soundfield measurement-related issues has been recently provided by Walker et al. (1984). We view this as essential reading for clinicians who are concerned with obtaining valid and reliable soundfield audiometric data. In general, we are currently using frequency-modulated (warble) tones with SPL reference values which conform to those recommended by Morgan et al. (1979). These SPL reference levels for soundfield measurements (45° azimuth) have been demonstrated to coincide well with ANSI 1969 standard reference levels for pure tone stimuli presented via earphones.

SPL Reference Level

Our goal of providing the child with the most appropriate electroacoustic dimensions can be illustrated and observed by plotting all relevant data on a single graph with the same reference level. In our judgment, an SPL reference scale lends itself best to this purpose. The response characteristics of hearing aids, the acoustics of speech, and environmental noise measurements are all commonly plotted on an SPL reference scale. Through utilization of the same scale for plotting audiometric data, all relevant dimensions under consideration become more directly comparable. By way of illustration, Figure 6-1 presents a child's unaided soundfield thresholds plotted on a conventional audiogram in decibels HTL. Figure 6-2 presents the same audiometric thresholds, converted to decibels SPL, along with the 0-dB reference values (Morgan et al. 1979). With this SPL graph we can have a visual representation of the appropriateness of the electroacoustic selection, as will be demonstrated below.

Finally, it is necessary that any amplification selection and evaluation approach specifically designed for young children be realistic in terms of routine clinical practice. As our approach has evolved (see the first two editions of this book), we became concerned with the extensive number of calculations required. Clearly, any procedure that necessitates 30–45 minutes of manual computation cannot be consid-

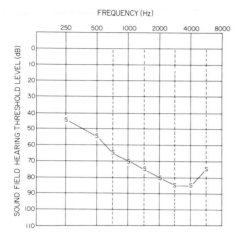

Fig. 6-1. Example of unaided soundfield thresholds plotted on a conventional audiogram in decibels HTL.

ered as feasible in terms of routine clinical practice! Our need for efficiency and accuracy in this process has led to the use of a small computer. With the use of a microcomputer, all data entry, computation, and printing of results require less than 3 minutes. In addition, we have virtually eliminated the possibility of making simple computational errors.

One additional benefit we have realized in using a computer-assisted approach is that at the end of both the selection and evaluation stages we have a clear hard copy of all relevant data entered and all results generated for the individual child. For the purposes of efficient and accurate recordkeeping, we see this as a most useful by-product of the approach we are now using.

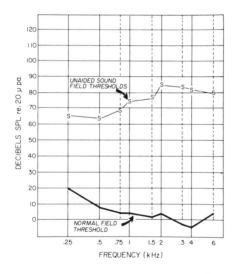

Fig. 6-2. The unaided soundfield thresholds from Figure 6-1 plotted in decibels SPL.

The Speech Spectrum

Since we are concerned here primarily with the young child's auditory perception of speech, we must consider acoustic dimensions of the speech signal in the process of selecting and evaluating amplification systems. With adults we are most often able to evaluate the success of our fittings, in terms of speech perception, through the use of appropriately designed measures of speech recognition and comprehension. Such is not the case with young children, for whom we typically have to predict speech perceptual abilities, at least in the early stages, based on our understanding of the interactions among auditory thresholds, amplification characteristics, and the complex dimensions of the acoustic speech signal.

With the primary focus on the amplification of speech signals, the clinician must be familiar with its frequency, intensity, and temporal characteristics. Furthermore, the clinician must develop or choose some working definition of the speech signal for the purposes of electroacoustic selection and for developing reasonable predictions regarding the child's potential for using residual hearing in speech perception.

One way in which the acoustic nature of speech has been studied is in terms of its long-term average spectral characteristics (Benson and Hirsh 1953, Byrne 1977, Dunn and White 1940, Pearsons et al. 1976). The long-term average speech spectrum has been shown to vary as a function of talker age and gender differences, distance, and environmental and vocal effort factors (Levitt 1982, Pearsons et al. 1976, Turner and Holte 1985). Nonetheless, some generalizations regarding the speech spectrum are possible for the purpose of electroacoustic selection and evaluation.

The overall average intensity of speech at a distance of 1 m from the talker is approximately 60–70 dB SPL, depending on the research cited. The average intensity characteristics vary as a function of frequency with the levels within the 4000–6000-Hz range approximately 20–25 dB less than the average level within the 500-Hz frequency region. Variations in intensity occur within each frequency region as well. Within each octave or third-octave band the intensity fluctuates by approximately 30 dB over time. Actually, the total intensity range associated with conversational speech has been shown to approach 50 dB when normal rhythmic variations are taken into account. This is important to keep in mind since often a single value is used to indicate the intensity of speech without recognizing that the specific value simply represents an average figure across and within frequency regions. For our purposes, however, realizing that we will be using fixed average values in the selection and evaluation process, the long-term average speech spectrum can be defined by the values presented in Table 6-1 (see also Fig. 6-3).

In general, we are attempting to amplify this average speech spectrum to provide the child with as much as possible of the raw acoustic material in speech for optimal auditory learning. As we examine the intensity contour of the average speech spectrum, it becomes clear that the selection of acoustic gain or output that reflects one average value is of little usefulness in the selection of an optimal

Table 6-1
One-Third Octave Band Levels (in dB SPL) Defining the Long-Term
Average Speech Spectrum

Frequency (Hz)								
250	500	750	1000	1500	2000	3000	4000	6000
60	66.5	62*	55	57*	57*	51*	49	47

*Interpolated.

electroacoustic system for a given child. For example, consider the child whose soundfield thresholds are displayed in Figure 6-4. The relationship between the average speech spectrum and the unaided thresholds are shown to vary quite significantly as a function of frequency. It is apparent that this child would require different degrees of real-ear gain within each frequency region if the average speech spectrum is to become audible across the complete frequency range. Thus the speech spectrum based approach to selection is most effectively utilized when the dimensions of gain and output are selected as a function of frequency region, and not by some arbitrarily defined average value of either of these electroacoustic characteristics.

At present, there is no generally accepted working definition of the long-term average speech spectrum for electroacoustic selection purposes. For example, of six speech-spectrum-based selection approaches we reviewed (Berger 1976, Byrne 1978, Cox 1983, Gengel et al. 1971, Pascoe 1978, Shapiro 1976), none chose to use the same values in defining the long-term average speech spectrum. The choice of a particular working definition is not trivial since, as Byrne (1977) has reminded us, the way in which the speech spectrum is defined is reflected directly in the specific electroacoustic characteristics selected as most appropriate. For example,

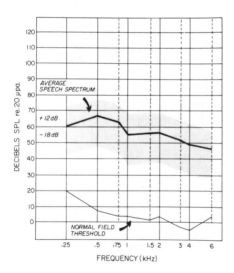

Fig. 6-3. The long-term average speech spectrum used for electroacoustic selection purposes. Note the associated 30-dB range with 12 dB above and 18 dB below the mean values across frequency.

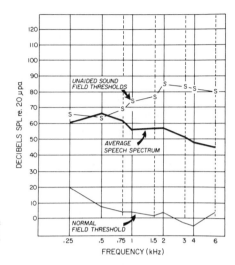

Fig. 6-4. Relationship between the average speech spectrum and the unaided soundfield thresholds for a hearing-impaired child.

the greater the level of speech, as represented by the long-term average values, the lower will be the estimated gain requirements for a given individual.

We need to recognize that, regardless of how it is operationally defined, any long-term average speech spectrum can be viewed as only a rough estimate of what the child will actually encounter in daily experiences. As noted earlier, we can assume a fair degree of variability in the acoustic nature of speech actually reaching the child that results from talker and situational differences (Pearsons et al. 1976). Nevertheless, for the electroacoustic selection process, we must choose some approximation of the speech signal that would be specifically relevant in terms of the acoustical environment and the unique auditory needs of the young hearing-impaired child. Along these lines, two issues in particular deserve consideration.

In choosing a specific set of values to represent average speech input, we must consider the relationship between distance and the resulting levels of speech reaching the microphone of the child's hearing aid. Turner and Holte (1985) measured the levels of speech produced by 5 female talkers at distances of 20 cm and 1 m and found that the sound pressure levels within each of 6 third-octave bands were 14–21 dB greater at the nearer 20-cm position. These findings have particular relevance for hearing-impaired children as we consider some of the more important language input and interactive times such as feeding, story time, and some typical parent–child play activities. Thus, as we consider the communicative environment of young hearing-impaired children, particularly the parent–child interaction, we often find that the child is in relatively close proximity to the source of speech, which is more often than not the mother. In many key learning situations, then, young hearing-impaired children are receiving speech at levels exceeding those defined by average values obtained at the standard distance of 1 m.

The second issue is the critical role that auditory self-monitoring plays for children who are in the process of learning oral language (Fry 1978). Some of our own measurements have shown the average levels of children's speech to be 80–90-dB SPL when measured at their own ears. Thus, in choosing a speech spectrum for electroacoustic selection purposes, we cannot be concerned only with approximating the average speech of others but must be equally concerned with the spectrum characteristics associated with the child's own speech productions.

In view of these considerations we have, at present, chosen to incorporate the long-term average speech spectrum described by Cox (1983) into our selection and evaluation procedures (see Table 6-1). With an overall level of 70-dB SPL, the one-third octave band values represented by this spectrum are among the highest reported in the literature.

Selection of Frequency/Gain Characteristics

BACKGROUND AND RATIONALE

We have observed elsewhere that, "after many years of research with hearing aids and literally thousands of publications, the conclusion seems to be that the more sound available to a person, the better that person hears" (Ross 1982). While there are both exceptions and qualifications to this, in general, an electroacoustic system capable of delivering an amplified speech signal that is sufficiently audible across the widest possible frequency range will allow for the optimal use of residual hearing in speech perception. We are not suggesting that the simple provision of an audible speech signal is sufficient for perception; it is, however, a necessary precondition. A child's perceptual experience will naturally be affected by the child's prior exposure to and knowledge of the auditory linguistic code (Fry 1978) as well as perceptual distortions resulting from the hearing impairment (Boothroyd 1978). For there to be any reasonable chance that the speech signal will be comprehended, however, we must first be able to guarantee that it can be detected. Thus *audibility of the speech signal can be viewed as the most basic prerequisite to auditory linguistic growth and performance.*

It is with this general notion of providing the child with an audible speech signal that we approach the task of selecting the dimensions of gain and frequency response. Regarding the concept of sufficient audibility for speech perception, the findings of Erber and Witt (1977) provide some useful direction in establishing appropriate goals for electroacoustic selection purposes. In that study, the influence of sensation level (SL) on speech perception was examined by presenting severely and profoundly hearing-impaired children with a word recognition task at SLs ranging from near detection to near discomfort. For children within the severe hearing loss range [70–95-dB hearing threshold level (HTL)], word recognition scores were found to rise rapidly as the overall acoustic level of the unshaped speech signal increased above threshold. Specifically, the 10 severely hearing-impaired children achieved their maximum recognition scores at SLs between 24 and 36 dB (mean = 30.6 dB). In contrast, the word recognition scores (2–27 percent correct) for the profoundly deaf children showed little change as a function of SL.

In addition to word recognition, Erber and Witt (1977) also obtained performance-intensity functions for the percentage of words categorized correctly according to stress pattern (monosyllable, trochee, or spondee). Thus, even if the stimulus items could not be recognized, the child's ability to use audition in perceiving word patterns was described as a function of the SL of speech. Although, as noted above, SL produced very little change in word recognition performance for the profoundly deaf children, the word categorization scores clearly improved as a function of increased SL. Overall, the highest categorization scores for the 10 children were obtained at SLs of 12–30 dB (mean = 21.6 dB SL). Even for children with minimal amounts of residual hearing, therefore, the provision of speech signals sufficiently above threshold was of documented usefulness in the auditory perception of speech.

From this we can conclude that, regardless of the degree of hearing loss (assuming the presence of some residual hearing), the speech signal must be delivered at levels sufficiently above threshold within all frequency regions where residual hearing is present. Furthermore, it appears that, because of the inherent limitations associated with increasing degrees of hearing loss, optimal SLs for speech perception will be generally lower as the severity of hearing loss increases.

Although all details of the relationship may not be clear, we can safely assume that the pattern or shape of the amplified speech spectrum reaching the hearing-impaired listener bears some relationship to speech intelligibility. Furthermore, it seems reasonable to assume that the pattern that has been shown to improve speech recognition abilities for hearing-impaired adults would be the same with hearing-impaired children. The difference, of course, is that with adults, appropriate modifications in signal processing increases their *recognition* ability, while with young hearing-impaired children, the same signal must be used in the *development* of auditory perception and speech production skills. Since speech recognition ability cannot be assessed directly with very young children, the preceding assumptions are not only logical but necessary if we are to approach the selection of electroacoustic characteristics for young children in an intelligent and systematic manner.

In light of some convincing theoretical and clinical evidence, there has been a recent surge of emphasis in hearing aid design on extending the high-frequency range of hearing aids. We know that much of the energy of voiceless phonemes, particularly /s/, /sh/, /f/, the unvoiced /th/, and /ch/, fall above 4000 Hz (Levitt 1978). The child's reception of high-frequency sounds has both phonemic and morphemic implications. The /s/ and /t/ phonemes, for example, are also plural and past tense markers, respectively. *An electroacoustic system that filters potentially valuable acoustic information does not make sense.* In this instance, one cannot extrapolate from adults to children. An adult who knows language can function quite well with the elimination of a certain degree of the redundancy in the speech signal. Not so with a congenitally hearing-impaired child, who is attempting to learn speech and language through an impaired auditory system and a low-fidelity amplification device. Hence the additional acoustic information provided by the high frequencies is likely not to be redundant at all, but rather provides the cues necessary for developing certain speech and language skills.

The results of a number of research studies with adults have supported an extension of the upper range of hearing aids (Lippmann et al. 1981, Pascoe 1975, Pascoe et al. 1973, Schwartz et al. 1979, Skinner 1980, Skinner et al. 1982a, Triantos and McCandless 1974). For example, Triantos and McCandless (1974) compared the speech recognition ability in quiet and noise of both normal hearing and hearing-impaired adults under conditions of high-frequency cutoff, one at 3800 Hz and one at 5200 Hz. Both groups of subjects demonstrated improved recognition scores of approximately 15 percent with the extended high-frequency response when the measurements were conducted in noise. No differences were found within quiet conditions. In terms of personal preference, the subjects selected the higher-frequency cutoff over the lower. Given the present technical capability of engineering hearing aids and earmold coupling systems to provide upper-frequency responses to 6000 Hz or higher, there appears to be no good reason to deprive any hearing-impaired individual, and particularly a child, of this potentially valuable acoustic information.

There is considerable debate regarding the optimal frequency response for the region below 1000 Hz (Braida et al. 1979, Leijon et al. 1984, Punch et al. 1980). It continues to be our practice, with young children, *to deemphasize but not eliminate* the amount of amplification within the low-frequency region, and particularly the output relative to the higher frequencies when the child demonstrates usable residual hearing within the high-frequency region. We base this spectrum shaping principle on studies that have shown that at high SPLs the presence of a low-frequency first formant can interfere with perception of the higher frequency second formant transitions (Danaher et al. 1978). These transitions are known to be important cues to consonant perception. By eliminating the first formant, which is generally more intense than the second, these studies have shown improved frequency discrimination of the second formant transition for the majority of hearing-impaired subjects. Along similar lines, Sweetow (1977) found superior speech recognition scores for hearing-impaired subjects in a condition where low-frequency amplification was reduced. The practice of delivering relatively high SPL low-frequency amplification to children with residual hearing extending beyond 2000 Hz is not supported by available evidence. At the same time, however, some recent research findings suggest that we may have overreacted in our attempts to avoid an upward spread of masking by low frequency energy. Punch and Beck (1986) found that an increase in the low-frequency response was related to positive subjective judgments in perceived speech quality in both quiet and noise. Insofar as syllabic recognition was concerned, they found that an increase in the low-frequency response improved scores in quiet and did not detrimentally affect recognition ability in noise conditions.

Olsen (1971) related various electroacoustic characteristics to the intelligibility of speech processed through several different hearing aids. Of all dimensions considered, he found that frequency bandwidth was the one most predictive of speech intelligibility, with wider bandwidths associated with the highest performance scores. This important relationship between bandwidth and intelligibility was more recently confirmed in an excellent study by Skinner et al. (1982a). Specifically, speech intelligibility was measured as a function of bandwidth by presenting nine different combinations of three low-frequency and three high-frequency cutoffs (266, 375, and 530 Hz; 3000, 4242, and 6000 Hz) to two highly trained listeners with moderately severe sensorineural hearing losses. The major finding was that elimination of either low- or high-frequency speech energy from the widest band-width delivered (266–6000 Hz) resulted in a reduction in word recognition ability for the two listeners.

One equally important aspect of this study was that each of the nine bandwidth combinations was presented at three different overall levels relative to the subject's most common loudness (MCL) (−7, +3, +13 dB). Performance scores were not found to be significantly different from each other when the overall speech levels were delivered at either +3 or +13 dB above MCL. When the overall level was below MCL (−7 dB) and close to threshold, however, particularly within the mid- to high-frequency range, the word recognition scores were found to be significantly lower. Thus, in support of the generalizations we made earlier, Skinner et al. (1982b) demonstrated that the greater the amount of speech energy available in terms of both bandwidth and overall level above threshold, the greater the intelligibility of the spoken message. These findings have clear implications for the selection of the frequency/gain dimensions we utilize with the young hearing-impaired child.

Given these findings, there would appear to be a definite advantage in selecting these electroacoustic characteristics based on the suprathreshold measures of auditory perception whenever possible (Cox and Bisset 1982). Some excellent selection strategies currently exist that utilize suprathreshold measures (Cox 1983, 1985; Skinner et al. 1982b). Unfortunately, with the young child, we are not in the position of being able to measure suprathreshold dimensions (such as the MCL) and therefore must base our selection of the frequency/gain characteristics on sensitivity threshold information alone (Murry and Byrne 1984).

FORMULA STRATEGIES

There are a number of threshold-based approaches to selecting frequency/gain characteristics that can be useful with young children, at least in developing a first approximation of the real-ear gain requirements (Berger 1976, Byrne and Tonnisson 1976, McCandless and Lyregaard 1983). Each of these selection approaches uses some variation of the so-called half-gain rule that proposes using an amount of gain in each frequency region approximately equal to one-half of the hearing loss within that frequency region. For example, if the hearing threshold level of an individual were 70 dB at 1000 Hz, then the first estimate of required functional gain would be 35 dB. Generally slightly less gain is prescribed by these methods within the 250- and 500-Hz frequency regions.

The selection approach proposed by Byrne and Tonnisson (1976), which was initially developed for use with children (Byrne and Fifield 1974), provides the clinician with coupler-measured gain equivalent to required real-ear gain values as a function of hearing level and frequency region for both ear-level and body-worn instruments. These coupler-measured values can be used to select and shape the appropriate frequency/gain characteristics in the standard 2-cc coupler prior to fitting the instrument for evaluation purposes. Additionally, target aided threshold values for evaluating the provision of appropriate frequency/gain characteristics are provided in tabular format for the octave and interoctave frequencies of 250–4000 Hz. Revised versions of this approach have been developed and reported by Byrne (1978), Murry and Byrne (1984), Cox (1985), and Byrne and Dillion (1986). For a comprehensive discussion of formula fitting strategies, refer to Chapter 7.

PROCEDURES

The general approach we have chosen to take in selecting the frequency/gain characteristics for young children is best described as a speech spectrum based procedure (Erber 1973, Gengel et al. 1971, Ross 1975, Schwartz and Larson 1977b). The goal is to select frequency/gain dimensions that place the long-term average speech spectrum at levels sufficiently above threshold to be useful across the broadest possible frequency range. To accomplish this goal, we have developed some frequency-specific estimates of the sensation levels at which amplified speech should be delivered to the child. With these estimates, we are attempting to deliver as much of the speech spectrum as possible at levels sufficiently above threshold to be useful in speech perception, yet simultaneously recognizing the limitations imposed by the reduced area associated with increasing degrees of sensorineural hearing loss (Kamm et al. 1978, Levitt 1982).

Our frequency-specific desired sensation levels of amplified speech, which have been modified from our earlier version (Seewald et al. 1985), are presented in Figure 6-5. On the basis of these curves, we determine the level above threshold that the average speech spectrum should be delivered as a function of HTL for each frequency region at which thresholds have been obtained. For a child with a threshold level of 70 dB at 1000 Hz, for example, a desired sensation level for amplified speech of approximately 15 dB is selected for that frequency region. Likewise, if

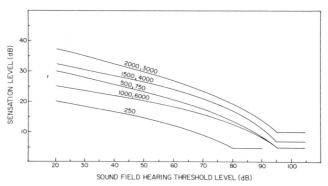

Fig. 6-5. Desired sensation levels of amplified speech as a function of hearing threshold level and frequency region.

the same child has a threshold of 80 dB at 6000 Hz, a desired sensation level of approximately 12 dB would be selected for that frequency region. The relative weighting of these desired sensation levels as a function of frequency generally approximate Pascoe's (1978) "perceived speech spectrum" with the exception of slight reduction in desired levels within the lower-frequency regions. The sensation level emphasis between 1500 and 3000 Hz has been chosen in an attempt to restore the natural amplification associated with the normal field-to-eardrum transfer function (Shaw 1980), which is typically eliminated by the presence of an occluding earmold.

The manner in which we approach the selection of frequency/gain characteristics is illustrated in Figure 6-6. First, on the basis of our desired sensation level estimates, we determine the level above threshold at which the amplified speech spectrum should be delivered within each frequency region. For the soundfield thresholds shown in Figure 6-6, the desired sensation levels for amplified speech are as follows:

250	500	750	1000	1500	2000	3000	4000	6000
16	22	19	15	18	19	16	14	13 dB SL

Second, to accomplish this goal electroacoustically, we simply calculate the difference, in decibels between the unamplified long-term average speech spectrum values and the SPLs at which the amplified speech spectrum is to be delivered. The result of these calculations, as shown in Figure 6-6, is the amount of real-ear gain required, as a function of frequency, which will allow us to deliver speech at the desired levels. In this way we have specified the desired frequency/gain characteristics for the individual child.

Having specified the amount of desired real-ear gain as a function of fre-

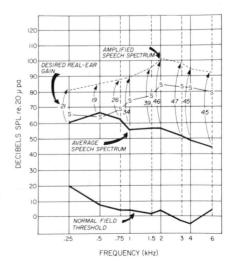

Fig. 6-6. Illustration of the frequency/gain selection process. The gain values required to place the speech spectrum at the desired sensation levels as a function of frequency are indicated.

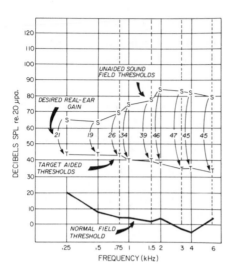

Fig. 6-7. Illustration of how the target aided soundfield thresholds are determined. As shown, the target aided thresholds are the result of the unaided soundfield thresholds minus the desired real-ear gain within each frequency region.

quency, we are now able to project what the child's aided hearing sensitivity should be. In other words, if the child is provided with the specific frequency/gain characteristics as determined above, these characteristics should be reflected, in terms of functional gain, by observing the difference between the child's aided and unaided minimal response levels. The projected or target aided thresholds, along with other relevant dimensions, are presented in Figure 6-7. These target aided thresholds will be used during the evaluation stage of the process to validate the provision of the appropriate real-ear frequency/gain characteristics.

The computer-assisted version of this approach to selecting frequency/gain characteristics requires that certain information be stored within the computer's memory and that other information be entered by the clinician. We acknowledge that most clinical audiologists obtain audiometric data in decibels HTL. Rather than ignore conventional practice, our computer program has been written such that all audiometric data are entered in decibels HTL and all hearing aid electroacoustic data are entered in decibels SPL as defined in a 2-cc coupler. This requires that the decibels HTL/decibels SPL conversion factors referred to in an earlier section (Morgan et al. 1979) be stored within the computer's memory. Other required information that is stored includes the idealized speech spectrum values presented in Table 6-1 and the nonlinear equations derived for the curves shown in Figure 6-5 used in selecting the desired sensation levels for amplified speech.

With this information stored in the computer's memory, the clinician simply needs to enter the threshold values, in decibels HTL, for the frequency regions at which reliable measurements were obtained. A series of calculations is then performed by the computer and the following information is produced in hard-copy form as a function of frequency: (1) unaided thresholds in decibels HTL and SPL, (2) desired sensation levels for amplified speech, (3) desired real-ear gain, (4) desired real-ear and coupler SSPL (to be discussed below), and (5) target aided

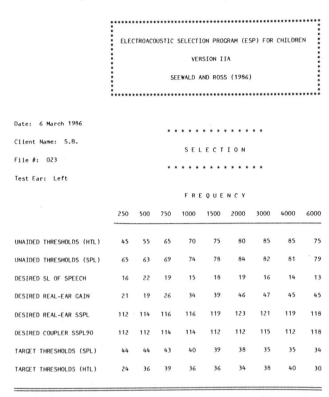

Fig. 6-8. Sample of the computer-generated output from the selection stage.

threshold values in decibels HTL and SPL. A sample of the printed output generated from the frequency/gain selection stage for the case example under consideration is shown in Figure 6-8.

Along the lines of Byrne and Tonnisson (1976) and Cox (1985), we have developed a series of tables from the selection stage of our approach for those who do not have access to a microcomputer. Appendix A provides the clinician with the desired real-ear gain values, in decibels, for nine octave and interoctave frequency regions as a function of unaided soundfield threshold (decibels HTL) for frequency-modulated tones. With frequency-specific threshold data in hand and by consulting the table in Appendix A, the clinician can determine the frequency/gain requirements that our model selects as appropriate for the individual child. Later in the process, these values will be used to determine the extent to which we have provided the desired frequency/gain characteristics to the child. Specifically, these desired real-ear gain values will be compared with the actual real-ear hearing aid performance as measured by means of either aided versus unaided soundfield threshold comparisons (functional gain) or a probe tube microphone system (insertion gain).

Selecting Output Characteristics

BACKGROUND AND RATIONALE

In our experience, *maximum output is the most important electroacoustic parameter to consider in fitting a hearing aid to young children.* It is, in our judgment, the major reason (shared with ill-fitting earmolds) for their rejection of amplification when it occurs. Constant or even occasional sounds that are uncomfortably loud or painful will elicit fear and rejection in the child not accustomed to amplified sound. For this reason, it is critical that we approach the selection of maximum output with extreme care. We need to remain cognizant of the fact that the real-ear performance of a hearing aid can differ markedly and is unpredictable from its performance characteristics as defined in a standard 2-cc coupler (Harford et al. 1983, Hawkins and Haskell 1982, Larson et al. 1977). We want to emphasize this point, because with young children in particular who have relatively small ear canals, there is every reason to expect that the 2-cc coupler will generally underestimate the amount of sound pressure a given hearing aid produces in a real-ear canal (Jirsa and Norris 1978). As with the frequency/gain characteristics, we need to somehow account for these coupler–real-ear discrepancies in specifying the maximum power output.

At present we have only limited data concerning the magnitude of the 2-cc coupler–real-ear SPL differences that may be expected for maximum power output. Two recent studies comparing hearing aid performance in a standard 2-cc coupler with real-ear measures, using commercially available probe microphone systems, suggest that for the majority of individuals, the 2-cc coupler levels can be expected to underestimate hearing aid output in the real ear (Harford et al. 1983, Nelson-Barlow et al. 1985). The coupler–real-ear comparisons obtained by Nelson-Barlow et al. revealed a mean deviation between the two measures of 10.3 dB [standard deviation (SD) = 9.1].

We have noted elsewhere (Seewald et al. 1985), as have others (Byrne 1981), that the selection of an appropriate real-ear SSPL can be viewed in terms of a compromise. On one hand, we do not want to deliver sound levels that exceed a child's discomfort level and may be potentially damaging; on the other hand, we must ensure audibility of the amplified speech signal. It is of no benefit to the child to provide "safe" output levels if the amplified speech levels are not—or are only minimally—audible. While the dangers of overamplification are real (Hawkins 1982, Rintleman and Bess 1977), it is estimated by Macrae (1985) that the effects of overamplification will occur in approximately 4 out of 1000 children with severe to profound hearing loss. Furthermore, it has been observed (Humes and Bess 1981) that the greater the magnitude of one's hearing loss, the less likely are permanent threshold shifts resulting from overamplification. Since, however, we do want to preclude *any* such effects from occurring, a cautious, but not overly timid attitude, should be adopted.

The relatively independent dimensions of output and gain must be considered simultaneously in selecting the appropriate electroacoustic characteristics. An instrument with a relatively low SSPL, with relatively high gain, will often saturate; that is, the input signal plus gain will exceed the output limitations of the hearing aid. The unfortunate result is an increase in distortion and a consequent reduction in the intelligibility of the amplified speech signal. There are times when one would desire to limit the output levels, because of behaviorally observed tolerance problems, but still maintain a relatively high level of gain. In these instances, some form of compression amplification would be an appropriate step to take (see Chapter 2).

PROCEDURES

Currently, we have no valid method for directly assessing the loudness discomfort levels (LDL) as a function of frequency with very young children. The usefulness of auditory threshold as a predictor of LDL has been assessed with the hope that threshold measures could be used in estimating hearing aid output requirements (Kamm et al. 1978, McCandless 1976). Although Kamm et al. found some relationship between degree of hearing loss and LDL in adult subjects, they concluded that individual variability was too large to permit the kind of predictive accuracy required in the electroacoustic selection process.

For our selection procedure, we have chosen to base specification of the desired real-ear SSPL on our earlier projections of the amplified speech levels. For each frequency region, we determine the desired real-ear SSPL according to the linear function presented in Figure 6-9.

It can be recalled that the projected amplified speech levels (speech spectrum plus real-ear gain), shown along the abscissa in Figure 6-9, are generated within the selection stage (see Fig. 6-8). The ordinate of Figure 6-9 represents the amount of acoustic space, in decibels that we have chosen to place between the projected

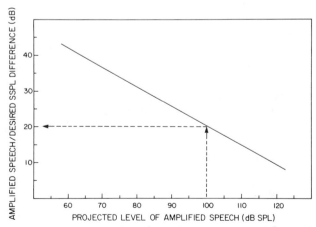

Fig. 6-9. The linear function for the relationship between the projected level of amplified speech and the difference, in decibels between the projected amplified speech level and desired maximum real-ear SPL.

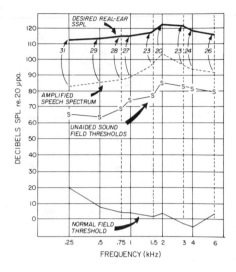

Fig. 6-10. Illustration of the SSPL selection process. As shown, selection of the desired maximum real-ear SPLs based on the projected levels of the amplified speech spectrum within each frequency region. The specific amount of acoustic space between the amplified speech spectrum and the desired maximum SPLs, within each frequency region, are determined by the linear function presented in Figure 6-9.

amplified speech levels and the level at which saturation occurs. It can be observed that the difference between the amplified speech level and desired SSPL decreases with increasing levels of amplified speech. This relationship accounts for the progressively decreasing dynamic range of auditory space associated with increasingly greater degrees of hearing loss (Levitt 1982).

To illustrate, if we project the amplified speech level to be 100-dB SPL for a given frequency region, we observe in Figure 6-9 that the desired acoustic space between this level of amplified speech and the desired maximum real-ear level is approximately 20 dB (shown by dashed line). Thus the projected amplified speech level (100-dB SPL) plus the 20 dB of "head room" results in a desired real-ear SSPL of approximately 120 dB. That is, the $SSPL_{90}$ in a coupler should result in no greater than 120-dB SPL in the real ear.

The frequency specific approach we employ in selecting real-ear saturation levels is illustrated graphically in Figure 6-10 with the differences, in decibels, between the amplified speech levels and the desired SSPLs shown as a function of frequency. For those clinicians who do not have access to a microcomputer, Appendix B can be consulted to determine the desired real-ear SSPL characteristics that our model selects as appropriate for the individual child. Since these levels have been developed in real-ear terms, they are the appropriate values to be used by clinicians who have the capability of obtaining insertion measurements of hearing aid output.

For individuals who do not have probe microphone systems available to them, the provision of appropriate real-ear saturation levels is a more difficult problem to resolve. As noted earlier, we need to account for 2-cc coupler–real-ear discrepancies in specifying the maximum power output (Byrne 1981). We had originally developed an a priori approach to this that attempted to account for real-ear–coupler differences on an individual-by-individual basis (Seewald et al. 1985). Briefly, the

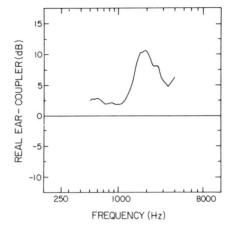

Fig. 6-11. Mean insertion to HA-2 coupler differences, in decibels, as a function of frequency reported by Nelson-Barlow et al. (1985) for 15 hearing-impaired children. All positive values indicate the extent to which the mean SPLs in the real-ear exceeded 2-coupler-defined levels.

differences between the functional and coupler frequency responses were applied to the desired real-ear output to obtain the desired coupler SSPL$_{90}$. Since this approach presently lacks research and clinical support, however, we have abandoned it for the time being.

A study by Nelson-Barlow et al. (1985) reported the mean real-ear–HA-2 coupler differences, as a function of frequency, for 15 hearing-impaired children aged 3–15 years. Their findings are illustrated in Figure 6-11 with the real-ear–coupler differences plotted as a function of frequency. In this figure, a positive number indicates that the HA-2 coupler underestimated the real-ear SPL with a negative number indication that the coupler overestimated in SPL in the real ear. It can be observed that, on average, the SPL measured within the HA-2 coupler underestimated the real-ear SPL by as much as 10 dB, with the differences varying as a function of frequency.

These findings have obvious implications for the selection of appropriate frequency/SSPL characteristics with children. For example, it is conceivable for a hearing aid with an HA-2 coupler defined maximum output of 130-dB SPL to actually deliver SPLs as high as 140–145 dB within the child's ear canal! The unfortunate consequence of this will be, at best, the available gain will be reduced in an attempt to eliminate the predictable difficulties with feedback. At worst, through overamplification, we risk long-term damage to the child's already limited residual hearing (Rintleman and Bess 1977), not to mention complete rejection of amplification on the part of the child.

Although we most certainly recognize the limitations associated with applying average correction factors in selection electroacoustic dimensions (Preves 1984), we have, at present, chosen to apply the mean HA-2 coupler–real-ear differences as a function of frequency, reported by Nelson Barlow et al. (1985) in specifying the desired HA-2 coupler SSPL$_{90}$ values. The application of this approach to our case example is illustrated in Table 6-2. By subtracting the average amount by which Nelson-Barlow et al. (1985) found the HA-2 coupler to underestimate the real-ear

Table 6-2
How the Desired Real-Ear Maximum SPL Values (in dB) Are Converted to HA-2
Coupler-Defined SSPL$_{90}$ as a Function of Frequency

	Frequency (kHz)								
	0.25	*0.5*	*0.75*	*1*	*1.5*	*2*	*3*	*4*	*6*
Desired real-ear maximum SPL	112	114	116	116	119	123	121	114	118
Mean real-ear/HA-2 coupler differences*	—	2	2	2	7	11	6	2	—
Desired HA-2 coupler SSPL$_{90}$	112	112	114	114	112	112	115	112	118

*Data from Nelson-Barlow NL, Auslander MC, Rines D et al: Probe-microphone measures in hearing-impaired children and adults. Paper presented at Convention of the American Speech-Language-Hearing Association, Washington, DC, 1985.

SPL, we have developed the desired HA-2 coupler defined SSPL$_{90}$ response for our case example.

Appendix C presents the desired coupler SSPL$_{90}$ values in tabular format for nine octave and interoctave frequency regions as a function of soundfield threshold (dB HTL) for frequency-modulated tones. It is appropriate for clinicians to consult this table in those situations where more direct probe tube microphone measurements are not possible. As can be observed in Figure 6-8, our computer program generates both real-ear and HA-2 coupler-defined values for the frequency/SSPL characteristic.

Evaluating Performance

BACKGROUND AND RATIONALE

The basic premise throughout the whole of our approach to the selection of hearing aids for children is that all electroacoustic recommendations are tentative. When working with young children, we assume that we will not possess complete information relative to their hearing status and, furthermore, that this status may change over time. Unfortunate, but common, is the child with a progressive hearing loss. We have frequently encountered instances where progression is barely detectable except when viewed over a long period of time, as well as where the progression occurs in dramatic threshold shifts. Modifications must be made in the electroacoustic parameters to reflect these changes in auditory status. In fact, the same hearing aid worn by any child year after year without modification or replacement is strongly suspect. In all probability, it is no longer an "optimal" electroacoustic system for that child.

The methods of evaluating the continued appropriateness of the system and identifying and providing the required modifications are not elaborate or theoretical.

Simply stated, they involve long-term, consistent, and persistent monitoring, evaluation, and systematic application of remedial measures.

In our amplification program we utilize several major evaluative situations. The first and most familiar to most audiology programs is the clinical evaluation. Whenever possible, we attempt to see young children in the clinical setting at least monthly and more frequently when a problem is reported or suspected. Here we rely on the various measurement techniques discussed in this chapter, including electroacoustic measurements of hearing aid performance at "use" settings, electroacoustic immittance measurements, and soundfield aided and unaided measurements to provide us with updated results.

Additional data are accumulated from some nonaudiometric assessment tools in an attempt to document growth in speech-language, auditory, social-emotional, and cognitive development. Furthermore, we rely most heavily on observation of the child through reporting of that child's behavior in various situations by parents, teachers, speech–language pathologists, and other managing adults. Related to this, one evaluative approach we have found to be most helpful, particularly within the early stages, is to request that the parents keep a daily log of the child's adjustment to and performance with amplification. This approach often provides very useful information by which the audiologist can determine the need for any modifications in the electroacoustic dimensions, and the physical arrangement of the hearing aid or earmold coupling system. Simultaneously it has the advantage of encouraging more active participation by the parents in the child's habilitative program.

Finally, the professionals primarily responsible for amplification programs, the audiologists, need to expand their observational skills and activities to other situations. It is most useful when they leave the sound-treated environments that have become their reality and become more involved in observing the children's performance in their reality of the home or classroom—both of which are extensions of our traditional "clinic."

With regard to the in-clinic evaluation of hearing aid performance, it is important for the audiologist to become familiar with all available options, since it can be assumed that no single method will meet all evaluative requirements in all situations. For this reason, we do not expect that there will ever be one single preferred way for evaluating performance with young children. Among the various approaches to this problem reported in the literature, those that are currently most popular or would seem to offer the greatest potential usefulness include: aided behavioral speech-spectrum-based procedures (Byrne and Fifield 1974, Erber 1973, Gengel et al. 1971, Matkin 1984, Ross 1975, Schwartz and Larson 1977b); acoustic reflex measurements (Hall 1985, Rines et al. 1984, Tonisson 1975); auditory evoked brainstem response measures (Hall 1985, Hecox 1983, Kileny 1982, Mohoney 1985); and real-ear, probe microphone measures (Harford 1980, Libby 1985, Nielsen and Rasmussen 1984).

As we consider integrating any of these approaches into routine clinical practice, we must remain focused simultaneously on what is perhaps a more basic and equally important consideration: *what do we want the amplification to do for the child.* As we noted earlier, it is not possible to evaluate the success of our fittings with young children without first addressing this issue. It is clear to us that a great deal more research is required with regard to both the selection and evaluation aspects of this most challenging clinical problem.

At present, we use aided soundfield threshold measures as our primary method for evaluating the provision of appropriate real-ear electroacoustic dimensions. These measurements can be obtained regardless of the particular response mode employed (e.g., visual reinforcement audiometry, conditioned play audiometry). Because we have already obtained unaided soundfield thresholds during the selection stage, we can use the aided–unaided comparison as a means for assessing the functional or real-ear frequency/gain characteristics of the selected instrument. Generally, where differences are observed between the obtained and the desired characteristics, appropriate modifications can be made to bring electroacoustic performance in line with the child's needs. We will elaborate on this point later within this section.

As with any measurement procedure, there are a number of potential pitfalls and limitations associated with aided soundfield measurements about which clinicians must become knowledgeable. Killion and Monser (1980) have identified several such problems that can affect the validity of our soundfield aided measurements, including the ambient noise level, internal hearing aid noise, standing waves in the test environment, or insufficiently steep filter slopes with narrowband noise stimuli. On the basis of a recent study, Rines et al. (1984) concluded that aided–unaided comparisons provide accurate estimates of functional gain for individuals with hearing losses greater than 35-dB HTL. For individuals with frequency regions of normal or near normal hearing, however, aided threshold measurements were found to underestimate functional gain because the aided thresholds approached intensities at which internal hearing aid noise and/or ambient room noise effectively masked aided signal perception. To circumvent this measurement problem, they suggested the use of aided–unaided acoustic reflex threshold estimates of functional gain.

As suggested earlier, we view selection and evaluation as distinctly different yet interrelated aspects of a more general process. In the transition between selection and evaluation, a specific hearing aid and earmold coupling system are chosen that, at least in theory, will provide the best approximation of the frequency/gain and frequency/SSPL dimensions as specified by the selection model we use. This amplification system will be used within the evaluation stage to assess the degree to which it meets the desired real-ear electroacoustic requirements. Where evaluation indicates differences between desired and real-ear performance, appropriate modifications are made to the system or when necessary, a different system is chosen for evaluation.

PROCEDURES

The choice and electroacoustic shaping of the amplification system to be used during evaluation are performed according to the guidelines and procedures as modified from Cox (1985) and outlined in the following 10 steps:

1. Only instruments that meet the preselection requirements, as described earlier, are considered for evaluation.
2. A specific instrument is chosen that has the electroacoustic capability and flexibility for providing the specified electroacoustic characteristics.
3. An earmold coupling system is chosen that, according to our best estimates, will provide the appropriate acoustic shaping characteristics.
4. The volume control and output controls are adjusted to their "full-on" positions.
5. The hearing aid is attached to the electroacoustic measuring device by means of an HA-2 coupler, and a frequency/$SSPL_{90}$ curve is recorded.
6. The results of this analysis are compared with the desired coupler SSPL values, and the output control is adjusted until the output levels approximate or fall below the specified values within all frequency regions.
7. With an input of 60 dB at 2000 Hz, the volume control is adjusted until the desired amount of gain is achieved (Fig. 6-8).
8. With an input of 60 dB at 500 Hz, the tone control setting is adjusted until the desired amount of gain is achieved at this frequency (Fig. 6-8). With the hearing aid controls set, a frequency/gain curve is generated with an input of 60-dB SPL.
9. The volume control is adjusted to the "full-on" position and a second frequency/gain curve is recorded on the same graph. The two frequency/gain curves are compared to make certain that at least 10 dB of reserve gain is available at all frequencies.
10. With an input of 60 dB at 2000 Hz, the volume control is readjusted until the desired amount of gain is again achieved in the coupler. The volume control is taped firmly in this position.

With the amplification system chosen and adjusted in this way, we are now prepared to fit the system to the child and perform the evaluation. Although we can expect to observe differences between the coupler-defined characteristics and what the child actually receives, in real-ear terms (Hawkins and Schum 1984), we have now documented the coupler-defined performance, which we can use at a later point to bring electroacoustic performance in line with the child's requirements.

For the greatest majority of young children we work with, our amplification evaluation is based on aided soundfield threshold measurements. Specifically, aided measurements are obtained under precisely the same conditions as those under which the unaided soundfield thresholds were assessed, with the exception that the amplification system under consideration is now in place on the child. For these behavioral measurements, the hearing aid's volume, tone, and output controls are in the same position as they were for the electroacoustic analysis. We then measure soundfield thresholds within all frequency regions for which reliable unaided thresholds were obtained.

The aided soundfield test results for our case example are presented on a conventional audiogram in Figure 6-12. The same audiometric data, converted to decibels SPL, are shown in Figure 6-13. To assess the adequacy of the amplification

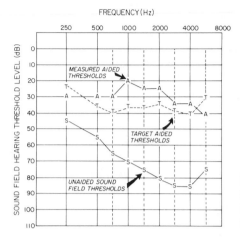

Fig. 6-12. Illustration of the actual aided and the unaided thresholds, in decibels HTL, for the case example shown in relation to the target aided thresholds.

system being considered, a number of comparisons can be made. First, by comparing the aided and unaided results within each frequency region, we can assess the provision of the frequency/gain characteristics in terms of functional gain. At 1000 Hz, for example, the comparison of the aided (25-dB SPL) and unaided (75-dB SPL) threshold values reveals that a functional gain of 50 dB has been provided by this amplification system. These functional gain values are determined for each frequency region in which the comparative data are available. It can be observed that substantial functional gain has been obtained within all frequency regions assessed.

A second and necessary comparison is made between the target aided thresholds and the measured aided thresholds. It can be recalled that the target aided thresholds are generated during the selection stage and represent what we expect aided performance to be if we have provided the child with the desired frequency/

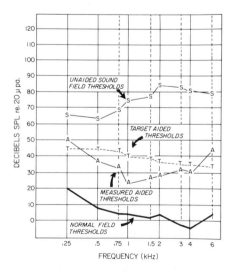

Fig. 6-13. Illustration of the actual aided and unaided soundfield thresholds, in decibels SPL, for the case example shown in relation to the target aided thresholds.

gain characteristics. As can be observed, some mismatch exists between these target aided threshold values and the aided thresholds that were obtained. When the target–measured aided threshold differences are of the magnitude of 10 dB or greater in either direction, they are interpreted to reflect the extent to which the amplification system's frequency/gain real-ear characteristics deviate from the desired performance.

As can be seen in Figures 6-12 and 6-13, the measured and target aided threshold values at 1000 Hz differ by approximately 10 dB. For this example, then, the measured–target threshold comparison suggests that a greater amount of real-ear gain has been provided than what has been projected as appropriate by the selection model. By making the same comparison at 6000 Hz, it can be observed that the reverse situation has occurred. Specifically, the 10-dB target–measured aided threshold in this case suggests that the amplification system under evaluation has provided insufficient real-ear data given within this frequency region. The target aided thresholds, in decibels HTL, as a function of unaided soundfield thresholds can be found in Appendix D.

One variation of our evaluation approach is to compare the relative aided soundfield performance of a variety of instruments. Generally, the instrument that provides the greatest improvement in threshold with the least degree of irregularity as a function of frequency is the one chosen for the child (Schwartz and Larson 1977b). Although this approach may provide adequate results for some children, it fails to account for the possibility of providing too much gain in terms of the important interaction among gain, speech acoustics, and the output limiting dimensions. It is for this reason that we feel that the selection of frequency/gain characteristics for young children must be speech-spectrum-based and focus on the suprathreshold dimensions of speech perception.

We have attempted to illustrate this point in Figure 6-14 by plotting the ampli-

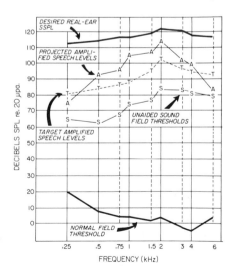

Fig. 6-14. Illustration of the mismatch between the desired levels of amplified speech and the projected levels of amplified speech that could be expected with the frequency/gain characteristics provided at the time of the evaluation.

fied speech output on an SPL scale with the hearing aid adjusted as it was during the evaluation. Although this amplification system certainly provides sufficient audibility of the speech signal within most frequency regions, it can be seen that the projected levels of amplified speech exceed our target levels by more than 10 dB within some frequency regions. This might be a desirable situation, in terms of speech perception, if we did not have to limit the hearing aid $SSPL_{90}$ output to reasonable levels. In considering the information presented in this figure, we must remind ourselves that the long-term speech spectrum has an intensity range within all frequency regions. With the frequency/gain characteristics provided by this system, we can expect some degree of saturation to occur with normal speech input levels. The unfortunate consequence will be the generation of a variety of distortion products. Thus the provision of appropriate frequency/gain characteristics must account for these important interactions at suprathreshold levels where speech perception occurs.

In view of the observed discrepancies between the target threshold values and the measured aided thresholds (Fig. 6-12 and 6-13), the evaluation has indicated the need for some reshaping of the frequency/gain characteristics. To bring the frequency/gain characteristics more in line with those we have selected for the child, a direct comparison is made between the obtained functional gain within each frequency region and the desired real-ear functional gain values generated during the selection process. These functional gain to desired gain differences, in decibels, are applied to the previously recorded coupler defined frequency/gain function; in this way we can observe how the system's coupler defined response needs to be modified to better achieve the child's functional gain requirements. This process is illustrated in Table 6-3. As shown here, the actual functional gain to desired functional gain differences, as determined for our case example, are subtracted from the previously recorded coupler gain values. This results in the desired frequency/gain function we wish to observe in the coupler. With this information, the frequency/ gain characteristics can be modified, using the electroacoustic analyzer, to achieve a more appropriate frequency response.

A sample of the computer generated output from the evaluation stage is presented in Figure 6-15. With the computer-assisted application of our approach, the clinician makes two separate data entries. First, the aided hearing thresholds are

Table 6-3

How Measured Functional Gain–Desired Real-Ear Gain Differences are Applied to the Original 2-cc Frequency/Gain Function in Determining Corrected Coupler Gain Values

	Frequency (kHz)								
	0.25	*0.5*	*0.75*	*1*	*1.5*	*2*	*3*	*4*	*6*
Measured coupler gain	16	20	25	41	37	46	42	41	34
Measured functional gain– desired gain difference	6	−6	−9	−16	−11	−9	−3	−5	10
Desired coupler gain	22	14	16	25	26	37	39	36	44

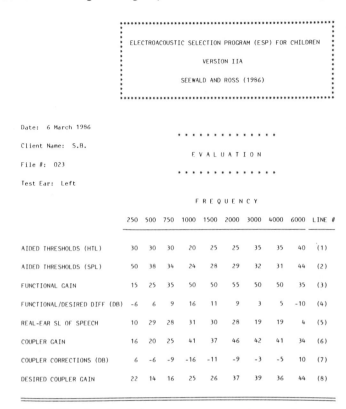

Fig. 6-15. Sample of the computer-generated output from the evaluation stage.

entered in dB HTL (line 1). Having entered these threshold values, the computer program generates the following information as a function of frequency:

- *Aided Thresholds (SPL)* (line 2): The values presented in this line are the aided thresholds converted from dB HTL to dB SPL.
- *Functional gain (decibels)* (line 3): The functional gain values presented in line 3 are computed by subtracting the aided soundfield threshold values (line 2) from the previously stored unaided soundfield thresholds. The result provides an estimate of the actual real-ear gain as a function of frequency.
- *Functional–desired gain difference (decibels)* (line 4): The values printed in this line are determined by calculating the difference between the functional gain values (line 3) and the desired gain values as determined during the selection stage. These values reflect the extent and direction to which the actual frequency/gain characteristics provided by the instrument deviate from those determined as appropriate during the selection stage. Positive values indicate the extent to which functional gain exceeds the desired gain values. In contrast, all negative values indicate the degree to which functional gain is less than the desired amount.

• *Real-ear SL of speech* (line 5): This line presents the sensation levels of the long-term average speech spectrum with the real-ear frequency/gain characteristics provided by the hearing aid under evaluation. These values are determined for each frequency region as follows: real-ear SL of speech = (desired SL of speech) + (functional − desired desired gain difference).

After this information has been printed, the clinician makes one final data entry. The *coupler gain* values (line 6) entered at this point are those that were obtained during the earlier electroacoustic analysis. Line 6 presents the frequency/gain characteristics as entered by the clinician. With these values entered, the computer program generates three additional lines of information, as follows:

• *Coupler corrections (decibels)* (line 7): The program couputes the difference between the desired gain values and the functional gain values (line 3) to provide an indication of the direction and extent to which the HA-2 coupler-defined response requires modification to produce a more appropriate real-ear frequency/gain response for the child. All positive values indicate the need to increase the coupler-defined response with all negative values indicating the need to reduce the coupler defined gain within that frequency region.

• *Desired coupler gain* (line 8): At this final step, the desired coupler frequency/gain function is developed by applying the coupler corrections (line 7) to the previously measured HA-2 coupler response (line 6). The result is the desired frequency/gain function as measured in the coupler, which should adequately place the average speech spectrum at the desired sensation levels within each frequency region.

With this computer-generated output, the program has produced a permanent record of all relevant information considered within the evaluation stage of the process.

What we have focused on within this section is the *initial* amplification selection and evaluation process. Certainly, as the child develops and becomes generally accustomed to amplification, we will be able to more precisely define the child's unique electroacoustic requirements and incorporate appropriate modifications into our initial recommendation. Nonetheless, what we have developed is a starting place that has been achieved systematically and can be replicated at appropriate intervals throughout the long-term amplification management program.

USE OF AMPLIFICATION

Establishing Full-Time Use and Consistency of Performance

At this point, the clinician has some workable estimate of the child's residual hearing status, active otologic pathology has been ruled out or treated, the output and gain characteristics have been selected appropriately, the clinician is convinced of the benefits and appropriateness of amplification for the child, the earmolds fit comfortably in the child's ears, and the parents have been enrolled in a systematic hearing aid orientation program, as will be described below. Given these assumptions, and the acceptance of the parents that has been developed through information, guidance, and support, the child is likely to make a good initial adjustment to amplification.

In our experience, the initial adjustment to amplification is more difficult for the parents than for the child. An insecure and fearful adult, who approaches the child with hearing aids in a tentative and uncertain manner, can easily convey such trepidations to the child. Approached authoritatively and positively, most children will accept amplification in much the same way they accept being changed, feel dressed, and so on. Involved recipes are not followed in preparing the young child to utilize amplification. The goal is to place the hearing aids on the child and keep them on all day everyday. Formulas that require 5 or 10 minutes of use daily, which is then increased over time, bring too much attention to bear on the hearing aids themselves. The hearing aids, at least for some children, can then too easily become a point of dispute with parents. We prefer to view the hearing aids as an accepted and integral part of the child and communicate this attitude to the child and the parents. We do not put ourselves in the position where the child is given an option to wear or not wear the hearing aids; what if that child says no?

None of our efforts to provide an appropriate electroacoustic system to hearing-impaired children will do any good, however, if the hearing aids do not work or, when working, do not work properly. The record, insofar as children are concerned, is simply deplorable. Beginning with Gaeth and Lounsbury's article in 1966, in which they report that at the most only 50 percent of the hearing aids of 134 children could be considered adequate (Gaeth and Lounsbury 1966), the same dismal picture has been repeated in study after study (Ross 1977b). It seems, if you will excuse this polemic cliché, easier to walk on the moon than to design "child-proof" hearing aids. Actually, the 50 percent estimate of operational hearing aids quoted above is somewhat optimistic when one considers that some portion of hearing-impaired children who should have hearing aids do not (Shepard et al. 1981); that many of those who do, do not use them (Karchmer and Kirwin 1977); that the acoustic situation in which they are worn precludes reception of an intelligible signal; and that the electroacoustic adjustments of hearing aids frequently leave much to be desired. The inescapable conclusion of this sad litany is that *for most hearing-impaired children, the effective use of residual hearing is a myth shrouded with good intentions.*

In our view, the situation described above has resulted largely from the limited role audiologists have often played in the long-term auditory management of hearing-impaired children. We are aware of many clinical settings in which significant interaction between the family and audiologist is reduced to annual or semiannual "recheck" encounters after the initial amplification recommendation has been made. Such a "service" model fails to recognize the ongoing audiologic needs of hearing-impaired children and their families and reflects an extremely limited self-perception of the professional role of the audiologist.

During the period following the initial amplification selection and evaluation process, a major role of the audiologist is to initiate a comprehensive hearing aid orientation and amplification monitoring program. There is much that the parents and other managing adults will need to know regarding the management and application of amplification if we are to expect consistent and optimal use of the child's residual hearing. We suspect that some of the "nuts and bolts" aspects of hearing aid orientation are often perceived as being unworthy of the attention of a true "professional." In our judgment, however, more of our good intentions and theoretically sound advice have foundered on apparent trivia than perhaps any other factor.

The hearing aid orientation program is not a single event in time, but a process during which information is systematically introduced over time. It has as its goal the consistent and optimal use of amplification. It is no less important than the audiologic assessment or the selection and evaluation of amplification and can be viewed as a basic and essential requirement for all other aspects of the child's habilitation program.

Although the topics of hearing aid orientation and postfitting counseling are presented in detail in Chapter 10, the following paragraphs provide a brief overview of the primary components of our hearing aid orientation and amplification monitoring program for young hearing-impaired children.

Demonstration and practice in fitting the hearing aids. The parents will need to be shown and have guided practice in placing the instruments on the child. For example, the clinician should demonstrate how to position the earmold in the child's ear and, with the audiologist present, the parents should, in turn, be provided with the time to develop their skills and confidence in performing this maneuver. Throughout the hearing aid orientation process, we take the point of view that no detail should be assumed too trivial for explanation and demonstration.

Information and demonstration regarding the operation and proper care of the hearing aids. The parents should develop an understanding of the major component parts, controls, and operation of the hearing aid. For example, the switch positions and controls on the instrument should be fully explained with the specific ones used by the child noted. Volume controls should be marked for easy replication of gain settings. The battery compartment should be identified and the parents shown how to replace a battery, and so on. As with the fitting of the instrument, it is important to observe the parent working with the hearing aid. It is not sufficient to provide parents with a 5-minute demonstration, which might include an overwhelming number of new concepts and terms, and to assume that all has been understood. We must provide the sufficient time and conditions such that the parent feels comfortable in asking for clarification and additional information.

Information regarding the choice of a specific system for the child. Although we developed this point within an earlier section, we want to reemphasize the importance of having the parent understand the rationale for why a specific system has been recommended for their child. Parents often wonder why, for example, a postauricular and not an in-the-ear instrument has been recommended or why a binaural fitting has been applied. These are often most important concerns of parents and deserve adequate consideration within the hearing aid orientation process.

Demonstration and practice in monitoring performance and troubleshooting problems. The rationale for this component of the program is clear from the consistent findings of studies regarding the performance characteristics of children's hearing aids. The routine monitoring of hearing aid performance by parents and other managing adults is essential if we are to make any reasonable assumptions regarding the young child's use of amplification in daily auditory-linguistic activity. Likewise, the parent will need to be able to troubleshoot the various, and unfortunately frequent, problems associated with hearing aid function. Monitoring and troubleshooting procedures have been described in detail by Ross et al. (1982) and Boothroyd (1982).

The nature of the amplification monitoring program will depend on the individual child's habilitation program and the availability of professional support. For example, once the child has been enrolled in a formal educational program, it is expected that, at a minimum, the teacher-clinician will perform daily visual and listening examinations of the child's personal and educational amplification systems (Ross et al. 1982). Additionally, for young hearing-impaired children, a complete electroacoustic analysis, performed monthly by the audiologist, or more frequently when performance difficulties are suspected, is strongly advised (Bess and McConnell 1981). Ultimately, we want to see audiologists more actively involved in the design and on-site performance monitoring aspects of this critical dimension of the child's auditory management program. Unfortunately, it remains more the exception than the rule that the audiologist is directly involved in the child's habilitation program beyond routine audiologic reevaluations within the clinical setting. Regardless of the nature of the audiologist's "homebase," it is, in our perception, well within every audiologist's scope of practice and responsibility to participate actively in the child's habilitation program within the child's environment if there is to be a well-coordinated effort. Until audiologists consider activities such as on-going consulting, monitoring of home and classroom environmental conditions, and monitoring of performance of the child's amplification to be within their scope of practice, the concept of auditory management will continue to be little more than illusion.

Information regarding the benefits and limitations of amplification. The goal of this aspect of the hearing aid orientation process is for parents to develop *realistic* expectations of what amplification will and will likely not do for their child. We have encountered parents whose expectations of amplification have ranged anywhere along the continuum from viewing the hearing aid as a complete solution to the child's problems to questioning the usefulness of a hearing aid at all since their child is "deaf." Understanding of the relative benefits and limitations of amplification often develops slowly over time but can be facilitated by ongoing discussion with the audiologist during the early stages.

Despite our own enthusiasm for and commitment to the amplification program, it is important, as Boothroyd (1982) points out, that parents not be misled into believing that the hearing aids will completely eliminate the problem. The advantages and limitations of amplification for the young child with sensorineural hearing impairment must be considered realistically and objectively. Boothroyd (1982) has provided examples of some clearly illustrated handout materials that are helpful to parents in understanding the general benefits and limitations of amplification.

Information regarding the effects of environmental factors in using amplification. In addition to helping parents to understand the interaction between their child and the hearing amplification, the parents also will need to understand and become sensitive to the effects of environmental factors, such as noise, distance, and reverberation, on the child's ability to use amplification. For example, it is important for parents to understand that hearing aids do not, in their current form, selectively amplify the speech signal and somehow eliminate unwanted environmental sound from reaching the child's ear. We have found it to be particularly useful to employ recorded simulations that have been developed to illustrate the individual and combined effects of environmental factors on speech intelligibility. This point will be developed more fully below.

Environmental Considerations

The primary purpose of amplification is to bring the desired acoustic signal within the child's residual hearing capacity. The entire rationale of an auditory approach to speech and language development rests on this factor. As a prerequisite, the speech signal must be perceived in order for it to be used in the course and sequence of auditory-linguistic development. This cannot occur when the speech signal is constantly being buried in a noisy background.

It is an unfortunate fact that the hearing-impaired listener, particularly one with a sensorineural hearing loss, is more susceptible to the effects of noise and reverberation on speech perception than is the normal hearing individual (Finitzo-Hieber and Tillman 1978, Hawkins and Yacullo 1984). As Tillman et al. (1970) state:

It is virtually impossible for a person with normal hearing to appreciate the handicaps to everyday listening that are experienced by the sensorineural patient because of such overmasking. . . . There are undoubtedly many times when hearing aid users cannot understand their companions even though all signals are sufficiently amplified and the background competition is so slight that a person with normal hearing would disregard it easily.*

*Reproduced from Tillman TW, Carhart R, Olsen WO: Hearing aid efficiency in a competing speech situation. J Speech Hearing Res 13:809, 1970. With permission.

These authors provide evidence to demonstrate that there is about a 30-dB spread between comparable conditions where listeners with normal hearing and those with sensorineural hearing loss could achieve a 40 percent intelligibility score. The listeners with normal hearing obtained this score at a signal-to-noise (S/N) ratio of − 12 dB, whereas the hearing-impaired subjects required a + 18-dB S/N ratio before they could achieve this same 40 percent correct score. Related findings were reported by Gengel (1971), who showed that S/N ratios of +15 to +20 dB were necessary in order for a hearing-impaired subject to achieve a maximum intelligibility score for aided listening under noise conditions. At + 10 dB and less, his subjects reported that listening required so much effort they would rather not use their hearing aids at all.

If hearing-impaired adults with existing language competencies are unable to recognize speech signals under only moderately adverse conditions, how can children be expected to exploit these amplified speech signals for their language and speech development? The answer is, unfortunately, that they cannot. Rarely does it appear that there has been sufficient awareness where it counts, in our homes, clinics, and schools, of the deleterious effects of noise and reverberation on speech perception. One of us (M. Ross), who wears a hearing aid, has often visited schools and clinics and had difficulty understanding the teacher's speech at the same time that the children were supposed to be listening and learning by means of this same speech signal!!

Although we live in an increasingly noisy world, it does not have to be noisy all of the time in the child's environment. It is possible to reduce noise levels at homes and schools, keeping in mind the admonition of Tillman et al. (1970) that acceptable noise levels for listeners with normal hearing may not be acceptable for hearing-impaired persons. One simple remedial measure to improve the S/N ratio is almost always possible, and that is to reduce the distance between the talker and the microphone of the hearing aid. Research on this effect, under various conditions, has been summarized elsewhere (Borrild 1978, Ross 1978). By providing the child with the best possible S/N ratio and clearly distinguishing foreground speech from background sounds, we can ensure, at the least, that the raw material of an auditory approach to speech and language development is available to the child. Without this provision, the child is supplied with the visible indication of the handicap, the hearing aid, but with no assurance that it can do the job for which it was designed.

The quality of the amplified sound reaching a child's ear is not only a product of the electroacoustic characteristics and the background sounds but also is reflected by the content of the speech signal arriving at the hearing aid microphone. The concept of optimal amplification must, of necessity, encompass optimal input. The quality and quantity of spoken language directed to a hearing-impaired child differs from that directed to the child's peers with normal hearing (Arnold and Tremblay 1979, Seewald and Brackett 1984). This is not a volitional or conscious policy, but, rather, seems to be a reaction to the child's inability to reinforce verbal communication with an appropriate response. As a consequence, the hearing-impaired child, while requiring enriched language experiences, actually receives a less satisfactory input than do that child's hearing peers (Goss 1970, Mogford et al. 1979). Only brief mention is made here of the vital area of the quality and quantity of language directed to the hearing-impaired child. This brief treatment reflects the nature of this volume rather than the significance of the area. Van Uden (1970) forcefully expressed the need of hearing-impaired children for intensive and increased language exposure, which is related to their maturation level and current experiences. Relevant conversation is the key. As Brown and his colleagues (1969) point out:

> It seems likely that the many kinds of grammatical exchange occurring in discourse will prove to be the richest data available to the child in his search for a grammar. We suspect that the changes sentences undergo as they shuttle between persons in conversation are . . . the data that most clearly expose the underlying structure of language. †

In other words, we must talk to children about what we and they are doing, always keeping in mind their interest and age level, and then listen for their responses and either expand or expatiate accordingly.

ADDITIONAL CONSIDERATIONS

Binaural Hearing Aids for Children

Binaural hearing aids per se are discussed in Chapter 7. In this section, we will briefly discuss some unique aspects of this approach as it pertains to young hearing-impaired children. In our judgment, supported by our interpretation of the evidence and our accumulated clinical experience, there is little doubt that *most hearing-impaired children can be helped more with binaural than with monaural hearing aids*. It has taken years of research to clarify the relative advantages of binaural hearing aids for adults (Ross 1980). As related to children, it has been more difficult to objectively and unambiguously demonstrate binaural advantages. In an attempt to circumvent the measurement problem, a number of investigators have interviewed parents and teachers, or employed rating scales to distinguish between binaural and monaural hearing aid functioning (Bender and Wiig 1960, Lewis and Green 1962, Luterman 1969, Ross et al. 1974). In all of these reports, it was noted that *superior receptive and expressive behavior was associated with binaural amplification*.

In our opinion, a key consideration in early binaural fitting for hearing-impaired children relates as much to preventive as to performance considerations. One reason why early amplification in general is stressed is the attempt to preclude auditory sensory deprivation effects from occurring. It is reasonable to believe that the same logic holds regarding binaural amplification: the longer the central audi-

---

†Reproduced from Brown R, Cazden CB, Bellugi U: The child's grammar from I to III, in Hill JP (ed): 1967 Minnesota Symposia on Child Psychology. Minneapolis, University of Minnesota Press, 1969, p 72. With permission.

tory system is deprived of patterned, binaural auditory input, the less likely it is that the full potential of the binaural system will be realized. A recurring clinical observation is that of clients with bilaterally symmetrical hearing losses who present superior speech discrimination scores in the monaurally aided ear. This clinical observation has been recently corroborated experimentally by Silman et al. (1984). This not only serves to illustrate the observations of Patchett (1977), Clopton and Winfield (1976), and Webster and Webster (1977) regarding the behavioral, physiological, and morphological consequences of auditory sensory deprivation in general, but it also has special implications for binaural functioning. Silverman and Clopton (1977) and Clopton and Silverman (1977) observed that units in the inferior colliculus are activated by clicks delivered to the contralateral ear and suppressed by ipsilateral clicks. When the rats used in their study were deprived of sound monaurally shortly after birth for a period of 3–5 months, the ipsilateral clicks could no longer suppress contralateral activity and thus abolished this evidence of binaural interactions. This may be the underlying reason why, with human subjects, Beggs and Foreman (1981) found that *a prolonged delay in providing binaural amplification could result in an inability to localize the source of sounds.*

It seems to us that as it relates to children, the presumption should be in their favor. That is, there is a greater likelihood that a delay in binaural amplification (as well as sound amplification generally) would limit their ultimate binaural auditory behavior than that it would have no effect. We simply cannot wait until all the evidence comes in before we make a clinical decision.

We would suggest binaural amplification even if a child displayed divergent threshold configurations in both ears (Franklin 1981, Rand 1974). We would ascribe many of the failures we have had with such children to the lengthy delay before binaural fittings were tried, that is, to the possibly irreversible sensory deprivation effects that may have ensued. This is not to say that binaural amplification should not be attempted on an older child. First, the advantages may not be apparent until after a fairly lengthy trial (Fisher 1964). Second, there are binaural advantages that do not depend on binaural interactions as such, but simply relate to the location of a hearing aid on either side of the head. Third, we may not be dealing with an all-or-nothing situation; some gains are better than none, and some interactive dimensions, such as loudness summation, may be possible whereas others, such as localization, may be absent. Finally, a clinician should always test recommendations against results. Beginning with the presumption that the normal situation is binaural, the clinician should continually observe the child to validate and, if necessary, modify the recommendations.

One final point about binaural amplification for children. In or out of school, they are going to be exposed to potentially disturbing noise and reverberant conditions as they attempt to learn speech and language skills. In schools, FM auditory training systems will enhance the speech to noise ratio. But whether they employ FM systems or not, the provision of directional microphones on the hearing aids, with or without the FM system, can serve to further enhance the speech-to-noise ratio (Hawkins 1984, Hawkins and Yacullo 1984). The research results in this regard are fairly unambiguous; except in perhaps the most reverberant situations, binaural hearing aids with directional microphones will improve speech recognition ability.

Cochlear Implants and Vibrotactile Systems

At the time when the second edition of this chapter was prepared, no child had been implanted with a cochlear prosthesis, and vibrotactile systems were limited to the waveform information provided by a simple bone vibrator. As of May 1986, 220 children had been implanted with a single-channel device. By the time this chapter is printed, this figure will undoubtedly be much greater. Vibrotactile systems also, possibly in an effort to discover a noninvasive alternative to implants, are experiencing a resurgence of interest. Both of these systems are considered as alternatives to traditional hearing aid amplification. Because one selection criterion of both requires poorer performance with a hearing aid than is possible with either system, some comments are appropriate in a chapter dealing with amplification for young children.

At the outset, we should point out that we are encouraged by the results obtained with either single- or multichannel implants for adventitiously deaf adults (Millar et al 1984, Parkins and Anderson 1983). One of us (M. Ross) personally witnessed open set recognition of spondee words and sentences by a multichannel recipient who, prior to the implant, could be communicated with through only a sign-language interpreter. The literature describes other such "stars" as well as those receiving less, but still extremely valuable auditory assistance through a cochlear implant. These individuals all had long histories of normal auditory development in common prior to the onset of the hearing loss. The situation is different for children, even for those with adventitious losses dating from an early age.

The rationale for implanting children is straightforward: it is an attempt to preclude auditory sensory deprivation from occurring, to provide auditory-linguistic information during the early years of speech and language development, and to reduce the psychological effect of the deafness upon the child (Berliner and Eisenberg 1985). It is still too early in the history of cochlear implants with children to judge whether these purposes have been achieved. The doubts that have been expressed, sometimes forcibly, (Pickett and McFarland 1985, Simmons 1985) are countered by the careful research of the proponents, which show definite improvement in auditory responses, although usually minimal, and some increase in speech and language development (Kirk and Hill-Brown 1985, Thielemeir et al. 1985).

No one recommending such a procedure does so without the most careful evaluation and preparation of the children and their parents. Nevertheless, specifically from an audiologic perspective, a number of issues and questions have been raised. The first deals with the relative merits of a single- versus a multichannel electrode. To our knowledge, no child has received a multichannel electrode, so it is necessary to consider the comparisons made with adults as the best information we have. According to Pickett and McFarland (1985), who extensively reviewed and analyzed the relevant literature, single word recognition is on average better with a multichannel electrode while the results with sentence material show similar results for the best subjects using both types of systems. The results with sentences, however, are much more heavily dependent on stored linguistic knowledge than would be true for monosyllabic words; thus the superiority of the multichannel system for word recognition suggests possible advantages in the linguistic development of children compared to the single-channel system. The point has been made, however, that multichannel systems are in a state of rapid changes and that the time-limited auditory and linguistic stages of a child cannot be delayed too long without permanent deleterious effects. Perhaps by the time this chapter is published, multichannel cochlear implants will have been applied with children, with direct comparisons then possible.

The alternative to a cochlear implant of a vibrotactile system has not been sufficiently explored. Pickett and McFarland (1985) also compare performance with implants to that of well-practiced normal hearing subjects and conclude that they are not exceedingly different. The studies accomplished with deaf children (Friel-Patti and Roeser 1983; Goldstein et al. 1983; Goldstein and Proctor 1985) demonstrate increased vocalizations, vocabulary enhancement, and improved speech recognition compared to their performance without the vibrotactile system. It is not possible to directly compare the results of these studies to those obtained with implanted children (Kirk and Hill-Brown 1985, Thielemeir et al. 1985). Improvement was noted with the consistent use of both systems, particularly as an aid to speech reading. Given the rapid technological improvements in vibrotactile systems (Goldstein and Proctor 1985), one can assert that this topic is a vital area for future research.

The issue that will engage audiologists most directly is that of subject selection. Recall that only children considered basically nonaidable are candidates for either device. It must be shown that aided performance is poorer than what would be expected with an implant before surgery can be recommended. It is, therefore, imperative that the amplification provided a child be optimally adjusted for the hearing loss, and furthermore that the child be given the same intensive auditory training program ordinarily scheduled as a postimplant procedure, before the child is implanted. We do not believe that this has been given sufficient informed attention.

For example, in the selection criteria given in Thielemeir et al. (1985), the children are evaluated with hearing aids with an $SSPL_{90}$ no greater than 132-dB SPL. The children's mean hearing losses, in SPL, were 123, 126, 129.6, 129.7, and 129.8 dB at 250, 500, 1000, 2000, and 4000 Hz, respectively. As is obvious, at the maximum output, with the aid in saturation, the possible degree of aided sensation level is extremely limited. It really is rather odd. These children had been considered potential candidates for cochlear implants precisely because their residual hearing was thought to be nonfunctional. They were then fitted with hearing aids whose output limitations reflect our concern about producing threshold shifts in children *with moderate and severe hearing losses*. Children who are potential implant candidates have nothing to lose and possibly a lot to gain by increasing the hearing aid output and then working systematically on increasing this level, as is now done with the implant in an attempt to increase the dynamic range. By maximizing speech audibility in this fashion, we would predict that more hearing-impaired children who are considered potential implant candidates would demonstrate better performance with a hearing aid than they could achieve with the current generation of cochlear implants.

Finally, children who are receiving, or who have received implants, undergo a carefully sequenced pre- and postauditory performance evaluation and extensive auditory training experiences. This is admirable and we have no reservations about these activities. We do find it rather unfortunate, however, that as a profession, we have not applied these same careful procedures to children who are being fitted with conventional hearing aids. It does seem to belie our often indignant and emotional claims for professional autonomy when it appears that we can only make our full nonmedical contribution to a child in a medical setting.

CONCLUSION

In our judgment, the proper selection and use of amplification is the single most effective tool available to us in our habilitative efforts with young hearing-impaired children. We would not minimize the importance of parent counseling or any type of therapeutic endeavor. These will often set limits to the success of our efforts. Amplification, however, is the only therapeutic tool specifically focused on the problem—the hearing loss itself. It is, after all, the hearing loss that is the responsible agent for observed speech, language, and educational deviances. The effective exploitation of residual hearing will minimize these developmental deviances and ensure the maximum effectiveness of other therapeutic endeavors.

We have presented the view that fitting amplification to a young child requires the systematic application of time, information, sensitivity, and experience. To be most effective, the parents and the child should be enrolled in an educational program directly associated with the audiology clinic. This association would facilitate the process of systematic, ongoing evaluation and modification that is generally required in the management of young children. Our primary goal with amplification is to provide the child with the maximum auditory information in a manner that is consistent with that child's residual hearing. We can expect, once this is accomplished, that that child will prove to be a much superior "learner" of speech and language than we could ever possibly be as "teachers." Clinicians will rarely make better use of their time or accomplish a more worthwhile objective than by making this possibility a reality.

ACKNOWLEDGMENT

We express our appreciation to Carole Tomassetti, Mark K. Spiro, and Patricia Stelmachowicz for their contributions to this work.

REFERENCES

Arnold D, Tremblay A: Interaction of deaf and hearing preschool children. J Communication Disorders 12:245–251, 1979

Beggs WD, Foreman DL: Sound localization and early auditory experience in the deaf. Br J Audiol 14:41–48, 1981

Bender R, Wiig E: Binaural hearing aids in young children. Volta Rev 62:113–115, 1960

Benson RW, Hirsh IJ: Some variables in audio spectrometry. J Acoust Soc Am 25:449–505, 1953

Berger, KW: Prescription of hearing aids: A rationale. J Am Audiol Soc 2:71–78, 1976

Berlin CI: I.D. and management of hearing-impaired infants and neonates. Hearing Instruments 36:43–45, 1985

Berliner KI, Eisenberg LS: Methods and issues in the cochlear implantation of children: An overview. Ear Hearing 6:6S–13S, 1985

Bess FH, McConnell FE: Audiology, Education and the Hearing-Impaired Child. St. Louis, CV Mosby, 1981

Boothroyd A: Distribution of hearing levels in Clarke School for the Deaf students. SARP #3 Clarke School for the Deaf, Northampton, MA, 1972

Boothroyd A: Speech perception and sensorineural hearing loss, in Ross M, Giolas TG (eds): Auditory Management of Hearing-Impaired Children. Baltimore, University Park Press, 1978, pp 117–144

Boothroyd A: Hearing Impairments in Young Children. Englewood Cliffs, NJ, Prentice-Hall, 1982, pp 96–114

Borrild K: Classroom acoustics, in Ross M, Giolas TG (eds): Auditory Management of Hearing-Impaired Children. Baltimore, University Park Press, 1978, pp 145–180

Braida LD, Durlach NI, Lippmann RP, et al: Hearing Aids—Review of Past Research on Linear Amplification, Compression Amplification and Frequency Lowering. Washington, DC, ASHA Publications, 1979

Brown R, Cazden CB, Bellugi U: The child's grammar from I to III, in Hill JP (ed): 1967 Minnesota Symposia on Child Psychology. Minneapolis, University of Minnesota Press, 1969

Byrne D: The speech spectrum—some aspects of its significance for hearing aid selection and evaluation. Br J Audiol 11:40–46, 1977

Byrne D: Selection of hearing aids for severely deaf children. Br J Audiol 12:9–22, 1978

Byrne D: Selective amplification: Some psychoacoustic considerations, in Bess FH, Freeman BA, Sinclair JS (eds): Amplification in Education. Washington, DC, AG Bell, 1981, pp 260–285

Byrne D: Theoretical approaches for hearing aid selection, in Studebaker GA, Bess FH (eds): The Vanderbilt Hearing Aid Report. Upper Darby, PA, Monographs in Contemporary Audiology, 1982, pp 175–179

Byrne D, Dillion H: The National Acoustic Laboratories' (NAL) new procedure for selecting the gain and frequency response of a hearing aid. Ear Hearing 7:257–265, 1986

Byrne D, Fifield D: Evaluation of hearing aid fittings for infants. Br J Audiol 8:47–54, 1974

Byrne D, Tonisson W: Selecting the gain of hearing aids for persons with sensorineural hearing impairments. Scand Audiol 5:51–62, 1976

Castleton LV: Children's fittings: Part II: Acoustic modifications. Hearing Instruments 36:33, 44, 1985

Clopton BM, Winfield JA: Effect of early exposure to patterned sound on unit activity in rat inferior colliculus. J Neurophysiol 39:1081–1089, 1976

Clopton BM, Silverman MS: Plasticity of binaural interaction: II. Critical period and changes in midline response. J Neurophysiol 40:1275–1280, 1977

Cox RM: Using ULCL measures to find frequency/gain and SSPL90. Hearing Instrumentats 34:17–21, 39, 1983

Cox RM: A structured approach to hearing aid selection. Ear Hearing 6:226–239, 1985

Cox RM, Bisset JD: Prediction of aided preferred listening levels for hearing aid gain prescription. Ear Hearing 3:66–71, 1982

Danaher EM, Wilson MP, Pickett JM: Backward and forward masking in listeners with severe sensorineural hearing loss. Audiology 17:324–338, 1978

Dunn HK, White SD: Statistical measurements on conversational speech. J Acoust Soc Am 11:278–288, 1940

Elliot LL: Descriptive analysis of audiometric and psychometric scores of students at a school for the deaf. J Speech Hearing Res 10:21–40, 1967

Erber NP: Speech-envelope cues as an acoustic aid to lipreading for profoundly deaf children. J Acoust Soc Am 51:1224–1227, 1972

Erber NP: Body-baffle and real-ear effects in the selection of hearing aids for deaf children. J Speech Hearing Disorders 38:224–231, 1973

Erber NP, Witt LH: Effects of stimulus intensity on speech perception by deaf children. J Speech Hearing Disorders 42:271–278, 1977

Finitzo-Hieber T, Tillman TW: Room acoustics effect on monosyllabic word discrimination ability for normal and hearing-impaired children. J Speech Hearing Res 21:440–458, 1978

Fisher B: An investigation of binaural hearing aids. J Laryngol Otol 78:658–668, 1964

Franklin B: Split-band amplification: A HI/LO hearing aid fitting. Ear Hearing 2:230–233, 1981

Friel-Patti S, Roeser R: Evaluating changes in the communication skills of deaf children using vibrotactile stimulation. Ear Hearing 4:31–40, 1983

Fry DB: The role and primacy of the auditory channel in speech and language devlopment, in Ross M, Giolas TG (eds): Auditory Management of Hearing-Impaired Children. Baltimore, University Park Press, 1978, pp 15–43

Gaeth JH, Lounsbury E: Hearing aids and children in elementary schools. J Speech Hearing Disorders 31:282–289, 1966

Gengel RW: Acceptable speech-to-noise ratios for aided speech discrimination by the hearing impaired. J Audiol Res 11:219–222, 1971

Gengel RW, Pascoe D, Shore I: A frequency-response procedure for evaluating and selecting hearing aids for severely hearing impaired children. J Speech Hearing Disorders 36:341–353, 1971

Goldstein M, Proctor A, Bulli L, et al: Tactile stimulation in speech reception: Experience with a non-auditory child, in Hochberg I, Levitt H, Osberger MJ (eds): Speech of the Hearing Impaired. Baltimore, University Park Press, 1983, pp 147–166

Goldstein MH, Proctor A: Tactile aids for profoundly deaf children. J Acoust Soc Am 77:258–265, 1985

Goodman AI: Residual capacity to hear of pupils in schools for the deaf. J Laryngo Otol 63:551–662, 1949

Goss, RN: Language used by mothers of deaf children and mothers of hearing children. Am Ann Deaf 115:93–96, 1970

Green KW, Margolis RH: Detection of hearing loss with ipsilateral acoustic reflex thresholds. Audiology 22:471–479, 1983

Hall JW: Acoustic reflexes and auditory evoked responses in hearing aid evaluation. Semin Hearing 6:251–277, 1985

Harford ER: The use of a miniature microphone in the ear canal for the verification of hearing aid performance. Ear Hearing 1:329–337, 1980

Harford ER, Leijon A, Liden G, et al: A simplified real ear technique for verifying the maximum output of a hearing aid. Ear Hearing 4: 130–136, 1983

Hawkins DB: Overamplification: A well documented case report. J Speech Hearing Disorders 47:382–384, 1982

Hawkins DB: Comparisons of speech recognition in noise by mildly-to-moderately hearing-impaired children using hearing aids and FM systems. J Speech Hearing Disorders 49:409–418, 1984

Hawkins DB, Haskell GB: A comparison of functional gain and 2 cm^3 coupler gain. J Speech Hearing Disorders 47:71–76, 1982

Hawkins DB, Schum DJ: Relationships among various measures of hearing aid gain. J Speech Hearing Disorders 49:94–97, 1984

Hawkins DB, Yacullo WS: Signal-to-noise advantage of binaural hearing aids and directional microphones under different levels of reverberation. J Speech Hearing Disorders 49:278–286, 1984

Hawkins DB, Montgomery AA, Prosek RA, et al: Examination of two issues concerning functional gain measurements. Convention of the American Speech-Language-Hearing Association, Washington, DC, 1985

Hawkins DB, Mueller HG: Some variables affecting the accuracy of probe tube microphone measurements. Hearing Instruments 37:8–12, 1986

Hecox KE: Role of auditory brain stem response in the selection of hearing aids. Ear Hearing 4:51–55, 1983

Hine WD: How deaf are deaf children? Br J Audiol 7:41–44, 1973

Huizing HC: Deaf mutism: Modern trends in treatment and prevention. Ann Otol Rhinol Laryngol 5:74–106, 1959

Humes LE, Bess FH: On the potential deterioration in hearing due to hearing aid usage. J Speech Hearing Res 46:3–15, 1981

Jablin MA: Computer-based insertion-gain measurements: A reality. Hearing J 37:13–16, 1984

Jacobson JT (ed): The Auditory Brainstem Response. San Diego, College-Hill Press, 1985

Jirsa R, Norris WT: Relationship of acoustic gain to aided threshold improvement in children. J Speech Hearing Disorders 43:348–352, 1978

Kamm C, Dirks DD, Mickey MR: Effect of sensorineural hearing loss on loudness discomfort level and most comfortable loudness judgements. J Speech Hearing Res 21:668–681, 1978

Karchmer MA, Kirwin L: The use of hearing aids by hearing impaired students in the United States. Series S, No. 2, Washington, DC. Gallaudet College, Office of Demographic Studies, 1977

Kileny P: Auditory brainstem responses as indicators of hearing aid performance. Ann Otol Rhinol Laryngol 91:61–64, 1982

Killion MC, Monser EL: CORFIG; coupler response for flat insertion gain, in Studebaker GA, Hochberg I (eds): Acoustical Factors Affecting Hearing Aid Performance. Baltimore, University Park Press, 1980, pp 149–168

Kirk KI, Hill-Brown C: Speech and language results in children with a cochlear implant. Ear Hearing 6:36S–47S, 1985

Kuhn GF: Some effects of microphone location, signal bandwidth, and incident wave field in the hearing-aid input signal, in Studebaker GA, Hochberg I (eds): Acoustical Factors Affecting Hearing Aid Performance. Baltimore, University Park Press, 1980, pp 55–80

Leijon A, Eriksson-Mangold M, Bech-Karlsen A: Preferred hearing aid gain and bass-cut in relation to prescriptive fitting. Scand Audiol 13:157–161, 1984

Leister CM, Claus-Parodi ST: Real ear measurement: The time has come. Hearing Instruments 37:23–27, 1986

Levitt H: The acoustics of speech production, in Ross M, Giolas TG (eds): Auditory Management of Hearing-Impaired Children. Baltimore, University Park Press, 1978, pp 45–115

Levitt H: Speech discrimination ability in the hearing impaired: Spectrum considerations, in Studebaker GA, Bess FH (eds): The Vanderbilt Hearing Aid Report. Upper Darby, PA, 1982 pp 32–43

Lewis D, Green R: Value of binaural hearing aids for hearing impaired children in elementary schools. Volta Rev 64:537–542, 1962

Libby ER: State-of-the-art of hearing aid selection procedures. Hearing Instruments 36:30–38, 62, 1985

Ling D: Auditory coding and recoding: An analysis of auditory training procedures for hearing-impaired children, in Ross M, Giolas TG (eds): Auditory Management of Hearing-Impaired Children. Baltimore, University Park Press, 1978, pp 181–218

Lippmann RP, Briada LD, Durlach NI: Study of multichannel amplitude compression and linear amplification for persons with sensorineural hearing loss. J Acoust Soc Am 69:524–534, 1981

Luterman D: Binaural hearing aids for preschool deaf children. Maico Audiological Series 8(3), 1969

Luterman D: Counselling Parents of Hearing-Impaired Children. Boston, Little Brown, 1979

Luterman D: Counselling the Communicatively Disordered and Their Families. Boston, Little Brown, 1984

Macrae JH: Personal communication, 1985

Madell JR, Gendel JM: Earmolds for patients with severe and profound hearing loss. Ear Hearing 5:349–351, 1984

Mahoney TM: Auditory brainstem response hearing aid applications, in Jacobson JT (ed): The Auditory Brainstem Response. San Diego, College-Hill Press, 1985, pp 349–370

Matkin ND: Wearable amplification: A litany of persisting problems, in Jerger J (ed): Pediatric Audiology. San Diego, College-Hill Press, 1984, pp 125–145

McCandless GA: Special considerations in evaluating children and the aging for hearing aids, in Rubin M (ed): Hearing Aids. Baltimore, University Park Press, 1976, pp 171–182

McCandless GA, Lyregaard P: Prescription of gain/output (POGO) for hearing aids. Hearing Instruments 34:16–21, 1983

Millar JB, Tong YC, Clark GM: Speech processing for cochlear implant prostheses. J Speech Hearing Res 27:280–296, 1984

Mogford K, Gregory S, Keay S: Picture book reading with mother: A comparison between hearing-impaired and hearing children at 18 and 20 months. J Br Assoc Teach Deaf 3:43–45, 1979

Montgomery GW: Analysis of pure-tone audiometric responses in relation to speech development in the profoundly deaf. J Acoust Soc Am 41:53–59, 1967

Morgan DE, Dirks DD, Bower DR: Suggested threshold sound pressure levels for frequency modulated (warble) tones in the sound field. J Speech Hearing Disorders 44:37–54, 1979

Moses KL, Van Hecke-Wulatin M: The socio-emotional impact of infant deafness: A counselling model, in Mencher GT, Gerber SE (eds): Early Management of Hearing Loss. Orlando, FL, Grune & Stratton, 1981, pp 243–278

Murry N, Byrne D: Predicting optimal frequency response characteristics of hearing aids from hearing thresholds. Coolangatta, Queensland: Paper presented at Conference of the Audiological Society of Australia, 1984

Nelson-Barlow NL, Auslander MC, Rines D, et al: Probe-microphone measures in hearing-impaired children and adults. Paper presented at Convention of the American Speech-Language-Hearing Association, Washington, DC, 1985

Nielsen HB, Rasmussen SB: New aspects in hearing aid fittings. Hearing Instruments 35:18–20, 1984

Northern JL, Downs MP: Hearing in Children (ed 3). Baltimore, Williams & Wilkins, 1984, pp 93–177

Olsen WO: The influence of harmonic and intermodulation distortion on speech intelligibility. Scand Audiol Suppl 1:109–125, 1971

Orchik DJ, Mackimmie KS: Immittance audiometry, in Jerger J (ed): Pediatric Audiology. San Diego, College-Hill Press, 1984, pp 45–70

Parkins CW, Anderson SW: Cochlear prostheses: An international symposium. Ann NY Acad Sci 405, 1983

Pascoe DP: Frequency responses of hearing aids and their effects on the speech perception of hearing-impaired subjects. Ann Otol Rhinol Laryngol 84(suppl 23):xi–40, 1975

Pascoe DP: An approach to hearing aid selection. Hearing Instruments 29:12–16, 36, 1978

Pascoe DP, Niemoeller AF, Miller JD: Hearing aid design and evaluation for a presbycusic patient. Los Angeles: Paper presented at Eighty-sixth Meeting of the Acoustical Society of America, 1973

Patchett TA: Auditory pattern discrimination in albino rats as a function of auditory restriction at different ages. Devel Psychol 13:168–169, 1977

Pearsons KS, Bennett RL, Fidell S: Speech Levels in Various Environments. Report No. 3281. Cambridge, MA, Bolt Beranek and Newman, 1976

Pickett JM, McFarland W: Auditory implants and tactile aids for the profoundly deaf. J Speech Hearing Res 28:134–150, 1985

Popelka GR: Hearing Assessment with Acoustic Reflex. Orlando, Fl, Grune & Stratton, 1981

Preves DA: Levels of realism in hearing aid measurement techniques. Hearing J 7:13–15, 1984

Punch JL, Montgomery AA, Schwartz DM, et al: Multidimensional scaling of quality judgements of speech signals processed by hearing aids. J Acoust Soc Am 68:458–466, 1980

Punch JL, Beck LB: Relative effects of low-frequency amplification on syllable recognition and speech quality. Ear Hearing 7:57–62, 1986

Rand TC: Dichotic release from masking for speech. J Acoust Soc Am 55:678–680, 1974

Rines D, Stelmachowicz PG, Gorga MP: An alternate method for determining functional gain of hearing aids. J Speech Hearing Res 27:627–633, 1984

Rintleman WF, Bess FH: High-level amplification and potential hearing loss in children, in Bess FH (ed): Childhood Deafness: Causation, Assessment and Management. Orlando, FL, Grune & Stratton, 1977, pp 267–293

Ross M: Hearing aid selection for preverbal hearing-impaired children, in Pollack M (ed): Amplification for the Hearing-Impaired (ed I). Orlando, FL, Grune & Stratton, 1975, pp 207–242

Ross M: Binaural versus monaural hearing aid amplification for hearing-impaired individuals, in Bess FH (ed): Childhood Deafness: Causation, Assessment and Management, Orlando, FL, Grune & Stratton, 1977a

Ross M: A review of studies on the incidence of hearing aid malfunctions. In the condition of hearing aids worn by children in a public school program. HEW Publication No. (OE)77-05002. Washington DC, US Govt Printing Office, 1977b, pp 1–9

Ross M: Classroom acoustics and speech intelligibility, in Katz J (ed): Handbook of Clinical Audiology (ed 2). Baltimore, Williams & Wilkins, 1978, pp 469–478

Ross M: Binaural versus monaural hearing aid amplification for hearing-impaired individuals, in Libby ER (ed): Binaural Hearing and Amplification. Chicago, Zenetron, 1980, pp 1–23

Ross M: Amplification: Tool for language skills. Topics Lang Disorders 2:29–45, 1982

Ross M, Brackett D, Maxon AB: Hard of Hearing Children in Regular Schools. Englewood Cliffs, NJ, Prentice-Hall, 1982

Ross M, Duffy RJ, Cooker HS, et al: Contribution of the lower audible frequencies to the recognition of emotions. Am Ann Deaf 118:37–42, 1973

Ross M, Giolas TG: Management of Hearing-Impaired Children: Principles and Prerequisites for Intervention. Baltimore, University Park Press, 1978

Ross M, Hunt MF, Kessler M, et al: The use of a rating scale to compare binaural and monaural amplification with hearing-impaired children. Volta Rev 76:93–99, 1974

Schwartz DM, Larson VD: Hearing aid selection and evaluation procedures in children, in Bess FH (ed): Childhood Deafness: Causation, Assessment and Management. Orlando, FL, Grune & Stratton, 1977b, pp 217–233

Schwartz DM, Surr RK, Montgomery AA, et al: Performance of high-frequency-impaired listeners with conventional and extended high frequency amplification. Audiology 18:157–174, 1979

Seewald RC, Brackett D: Spoken language modifications as a function of the age and hearing ability of the listener. Volta Rev 86:20–35, 1984

Seewald RC, Ross M, Spiro MK: Selecting amplification characteristics for young hearing-impaired children. Ear Hearing 6:48–53, 1985

Shapiro I: Hearing aid fitting by prescription. Audiology 15:163–173, 1976

Shaw EA: The acoustics of the external ear, in Studebaker GA, Hochberg I (eds): Acoustical Factors Affecting Hearing Aid Performance. Baltimore, University Park Press, 1980, pp 109–125

Shepard NT, Gorga MP, Davis JM, et al: Characteristics of hearing-impaired children in the public schools: Part I—Demographic data. J Speech Hear Disorders 46:123–129, 1981

Silman S, Gelfand SA, Silverman CA: Late-onset auditory deprivation: Effects of monaural versus binaural hearing aids. J Acoust Soc Am 76:1357–1362, 1984

Silverman MS, Clopton BM: Plasticity of binaural interaction: I. Effect of early auditory deprivation. J Neurophysiol 40:1266–1274, 1977

Simmons FB: Cochlear implants in young children: Some dilemmas. Ear Hearing 6:61–63, 1985

Skinner MW: Audibility and intelligibility of speech for listeners with sensorineural hearing loss, in Yanick P (ed): Rehabilitation Strategies for Sensorineural Hearing Loss. Orlando, FL, Grune & Stratton, 1979, pp 159–184

Skinner MW: Speech intelligibility in noise-induced hearing loss: Effects of high-frequency compensation. J Acoust Soc Am 67:306–317, 1980

Skinner MW, Karstaedt MM, Miller JD: Amplification bandwidth and speech intelligibility for two listeners with sensorineural hearing loss. Audiology 21:251–268, 1982a

Skinner MW, Pascoe DP, Miller JD, et al: Measurements to determine the optimal placement of speech energy within the listener's auditory area: A basis for selecting amplification characteristics, in Studebaker GA, Bess FH (eds): The Vanderbilt Hearing Aid Report. Upper Darby, PA, Monographs in Contemporary Audiology, 1982b, pp 161–196

Stelmachowicz PG, Larson LL, Johnson DE, et al: Clinical model for the audiological management of hearing-impaired children. Semin Hearing 6:223–237, 1985

Sweetow RW: Temporal and spread of masking effects from extended low frequency amplification. J Audiol Res 17:161–170, 1977

Thielemeir MA, Tonokawa LL, Peterson B, et al: Audiological results in children with a cochlear implant. Ear Hearing 6:27S–35S, 1985

Tillman TW, Carhart R, Olsen WO: Hearing aid efficiency in a competing speech situation. J Speech Hearing Res 13:789–811, 1970

Tonisson W: Measuring in-the-ear gain of hearing aids by the acoustic-reflex method. J Speech Hearing Res 18:17–30, 1975

Triantos TJ, McCandless GA: High frequency distortion. Hearing Aid J 27:9, 38, 1974

Turner CW, Holte LA: Evaluation of FM amplification systems. Hearing Instruments 36:7–12, 56, 1985

van Uden A: A World of language for deaf children, Part I (ed 2). Rotterdam, The Netherlands, Rotterdam University Press, 1970

Walker G, Dillon H, Byrne D: Soundfield audiometry: Recommended stimuli and procedures. Ear Hearing 5:13–21, 1984

Webster DB, Webster M: Neonatal sound deprivation affects brain stem auditory nuclei. Arch Otolaryngol 103: 392–396, 1977

Wetzell C, Harford ER: Predictability of real ear hearing aid performance from coupler measurements. Ear Hearing 4:237–242, 1983

Wilson WR, Thompson G: Behavioural audiometry, in Jerger J (ed): Pediatric Audiology. San Diego, College-Hill Press, 1984, pp 1–44

Worthington DW, Peters JF: Electrophysiologic audiometry, in Jerger J (ed): Pediatric Audiology. San Diego, College-Hill Press, 1984, pp 95–124

Worthington DW, Stelmachowicz PG, Larson LL: Audiologic evaluation, in Osberger MJ (ed): Language and Learning Skills of Hearing Impaired Students. Washington DC, ASHA Publications, 1985

Appendix A

Desired Real-Ear Gain Values (in dB) for Nine Frequency Regions as a Function of
Soundfield Threshold (dB HTL) for FM Tones

Soundfield*	Frequency (Hz)								
Threshold (dB HTL)	250	500	750	1000	1500	2000	3000	4000	6000
20	0	−9	−9	−6	−3	4	3	−2	1
25	4	−5	−4	−2	2	8	7	3	6
30	8	−1	0	3	6	12	11	7	10
35	13	4	4	7	10	16	15	11	15
40	17	8	8	11	15	20	19	16	19
45	21	11	12	15	19	24	23	20	23
50	25	15	16	19	22	27	26	23	27
55	28	19	19	23	26	31	30	27	31
60	32	22	23	27	29	34	33	30	35
65	35	25	26	31	33	37	36	34	38
70	39	29	29	34	36	40	39	37	42
75	42	32	32	37	39	43	42	40	45
80	45	35	35	41	42	46	45	43	48
85	50	37	38	44	44	48	47	45	51
90	55	40	41	47	47	51	50	48	54
95	60	42	42	49	48	52	51	49	57
100	65	47	47	54	53	57	56	54	62
105	—	52	52	59	58	62	61	59	—
110	—	57	57	64	63	67	66	64	—

*Soundfield SPL reference values according to Morgan et al. (1979).

Appendix B

Desired Real-Ear Maximum SPL (in dB) for Nine Frequency Regions as a Function of
Soundfield Threshold (dB HTL) for FM Tones

Soundfield*	Frequency (Hz)								
Threshold (dB HTL)	250	500	750	1000	1500	2000	3000	4000	6000
20	102	101	99	97	100	103	99	96	97
25	104	103	101	99	102	105	102	99	99
30	106	105	103	101	104	107	103	101	101
35	108	107	105	103	106	109	105	103	103
40	110	109	107	105	108	110	107	105	105
45	112	111	109	107	110	112	109	106	107
50	114	113	111	109	112	114	111	108	109
55	116	114	112	111	113	115	112	110	111
60	117	116	114	113	115	117	114	112	113
65	119	117	116	115	116	119	115	113	114
70	121	119	117	116	118	120	117	115	116
75	122	120	119	118	119	121	118	116	118
80	124	122	120	119	121	123	119	117	119
85	126	123	121	121	122	124	121	119	121
90	128	124	122	122	123	125	122	120	122
95	131	125	123	123	124	126	122	120	123
100	133	127	126	126	126	128	125	123	125
105	—	130	128	128	128	130	127	125	—
110	—	132	130	130	131	133	129	127	—

*Soundfield SPL reference values according to Morgan et al. (1979).

Appendix C

Desired HA-2 Coupler SSPL$_{90}$ for Nine Frequency Regions as a Function of Soundfield Threshold (dB HTL) for FM Tones

Soundfield* Threshold (dB HTL)	Frequency (Hz)								
	250	500	750	1000	1500	2000	3000	4000	6000
20	102	99	97	95	92	92	94	90	97
25	104	101	99	97	94	94	96	92	99
30	106	103	101	100	97	96	98	94	101
35	108	105	103	102	99	98	100	96	103
40	110	107	105	104	101	100	101	98	105
45	112	108	107	106	102	102	103	100	107
50	114	110	109	107	104	103	105	102	109
55	116	112	110	109	106	105	106	104	111
60	117	113	111	111	108	107	108	105	113
65	119	115	114	113	109	108	109	107	114
70	121	116	115	114	111	110	111	108	116
75	122	118	117	116	112	111	112	110	118
80	124	119	118	117	113	112	113	111	119
85	126	121	119	119	115	113	115	112	121
90	128	122	120	120	116	115	116	113	122
95	131	123	121	121	116	115	116	114	123
100	133	125	124	124	119	117	119	116	125
105	—	127	126	126	121	120	121	119	—
110	—	130	128	128	123	122	123	121	—

*Soundfield SPL reference values according to Morgan et al. (1979).

Appendix D

Aided Soundfield Threshold Target Values (in dB HTL) for Nine Frequency Regions as a Function of Soundfield Unaided Threshold Values

Soundfield*	Frequency (Hz)								
Threshold (dB HTL)	250	500	750	1000	1500	2000	3000	4000	6000
20	20	29	29	26	23	16	17	22	19
25	21	30	29	27	23	17	18	22	19
30	22	31	30	27	24	18	19	23	20
35	22	31	31	28	25	19	20	24	20
40	23	32	32	29	25	20	21	24	21
45	24	34	33	30	26	21	22	25	22
50	25	35	34	31	28	23	24	27	23
55	27	36	36	32	29	24	25	28	24
60	28	38	37	33	31	26	27	30	25
65	30	40	39	34	32	28	29	31	27
70	31	41	41	36	34	30	31	33	28
75	33	43	43	38	36	32	33	35	30
80	35	45	45	39	38	34	35	37	32
85	35	48	47	41	41	37	38	40	34
90	35	50	49	43	43	39	40	42	36
95	35	54	53	46	47	43	44	46	39
100	35	54	53	46	47	43	44	46	39
105	—	54	53	46	47	43	44	46	—
110	—	54	53	46	47	43	44	46	—

*Soundfield SPL reference values according to Morgan et al. (1979).

Kenneth W. Berger

7

Prescriptive Hearing Aid Selection Strategies

In recent years a number of approaches to hearing aid selection have been proposed that utilize formulas to determine desired gain and output. Their use has generated controversy and misunderstanding. In this chapter, Ken Berger presents a comprehensive overview of this subject, describing the prominent prescriptive approaches and how they are utilized. Ken also discusses the use of computers to assist in the selection process. Regardless of whether you are a proponent of selection by formula, this chapter will clarify many misconceptions and objectively present the issues involved.

MCP

Hearing aid prescriptive—or descriptive—methods employ some a priori determination of the gain and frequency response presumed to be appropriate for a given hearing loss pattern. They also involve a method of determining whether the predicted aided response was actually obtained. Thus, unlike other hearing aid fitting methods, the prescriptive ones make a prediction of a specific desired aided response, and, after the fitting is completed, provide for an aided check to determine whether this response was obtained. The aided check may consist of aided determination of thresholds or most comfortable loudness level (MCL) (both of which are referred to as *functional gain* when compared with unaided test results) or, more recently, functional gain can be determined by differences between unaided and aided measures by using a probe tube technique (Nielsen 1984).

Most of the prescriptive methods involve formulas in their gain-frequency response determination, and, fortunately, formula-based prescriptions are readily

AMPLIFICATION FOR THE HEARING-IMPAIRED, THIRD EDITION   ISBN 0-8089-1886-9
Copyright © 1988 by Grune & Stratton, Inc.

computerized. Some prescriptive methods involve the hearing threshold level (HTL), others the MCL. Either may or may not also include uncomfortable loudness level (UCL) data to prescribe the saturation sound pressure level (SSPL). Virtually all contemporary prescriptive methods shape the frequency response in some way, usually in reference to the speech spectrum as overlaid on either the threshold of sensitivity or the MCL. Therefore, the gain portion of the prescription is for gain-by-frequency, or in other words, a gain-frequency response.

Prescriptive methods received considerable professional attention and debate in the 1940s, but the popularity of the few available methods then waned. Beginning in the 1970s there has been a renewed interest in prescriptive methods, specifically in the formula-based ones. These cannot only be computerized, but also hearing aid makes and models that approximate the prescription can be located from a data bank of instruments listed in the computer program.

EARLY FITTING METHODS

From the few pre-1940 published reports that are available on the subject of hearing aid selection and fitting, it can be concluded that most "fitting" was on a trial-and-error basis. Persons purchasing a preelectric device tried several of them at the office selling them, choosing the one that either provided the best sound or the one that was most cosmetically acceptable. With the introduction of the electric (i.e., carbon) hearing aid in the first decade of this century, one sees a few efforts to more precisely relate the amplifier to the hearing loss. In 1905, Miller Reese Hutchison patented a master hearing aid device. He also is credited with developing the first electric hearing aid.

The Hutchison master hearing aid unit consisted of a number of transmitters (i.e., carbon microphones) and magnetic earphones. Each of the transmitters and earphones had different electroacoustic characteristics, and therefore the sound of various combinations could be evaluated informally. There is no record that the Hutchison device was actually marketed, perhaps because the idea, while good, was premature. In 1913 Eric T. Hincks of England patented a similar device, which permitted adjusting battery voltage as well as gain. In 1923 Edgar D. Tillyer of Southbridge, Massachusetts filed a patent for what today is considered selective amplification. Tillyer's idea was to employ various filter networks with vacuum tube hearing aids. Vacuum tubes had just appeared on the market in table model instruments but would not replace carbon hearing aids for another twenty years (Berger 1984, Lybarger 1978).

A 1938 patent application by Samuel Lybarger was for a master hearing aid in which carbon boosters (i.e., amplifiers) were included so as to increase gain as well as alter frequency response. Low-frequency response characteristics were controlled by the choice of microphone, middle-frequency response by earphone choice, and high-frequency response by carbon amplifier choice. The Lybarger patent resulted in a device called the *Selex-A-Phone*, which was used as a fitting tool by many Radioear dealers for almost a decade.

For the 1930s and into the 1940s there is no known published record of detailed descriptions, or of any experimental data, regarding hearing aids chosen or fitted by any method. Presumably persons fitting hearing aids employed one of the early master hearing aids for this purpose, or merely based their choice on some rather general observation of the person's threshold pattern.

COMPARISON PROCEDURES

The first major change in selecting hearing aids came in the 1940s. In a series of articles Carhart described a hearing aid elevation procedure which is now referred to as the comparison method (Carhart 1946a; Carhart and Thompson 1947). This procedure was used with hearing impaired military personnel at the close of World War II.

The comparison procedure primarily involved obtaining certain speech audiometric test results while the person was wearing one of a series of hearing aids. The instrument that produced the best scores was issued to the serviceman. In the military program, speech and hearing therapy as well as extended counseling was an inherent part of the procedure, as was the person wearing some of the hearing aids in assorted environments. It may be recalled that at that time there were fewer hearing aid manufacturers than today, and only one hearing aid type—the body aid.

Soon, the comparison procedures were incorporated into the rapidly growing number of university programs in a new academic field called *audiology*. Although a few community agencies scattered around the United States and England employed what would later be called *audiologists,* the impetus came in the mid-1940s as a result of the work in the military hospitals. As might be expected, the time involved in the comparison procedure was drastically reduced in its civilian version.

The comparison procedure in its modified form seems to have been the most popular hearing aid selection method among audiologists until the 1980s. In spite of its popularity over a span of 35 years, the comparison method produced little published research pertaining to either its reliability or its validity.

A number of factors involved with aided hearing can be measured, such as (1) change from unaided threshold or MCL, (2) an SSPL as related to the individual's UCL, and (3) word discrimination scores obtained in quiet or in noise. The comparison procedure considered all three factors, but there was a decided emphasis on word discrimination scores.

In addition to the foregoing, there are other and more subjective factors that are more difficult to determine. These include (1) success or failure with amplification, (2) client acceptance of the hearing aid, and (3) satisfaction or happiness with the hearing aid. The latter probably encompasses the first two factors. These subjective factors can be documented to some extent by anecdotal information, but, as might be expected, there have been many more published reports on the aided (or aided vs unaided) audiometric test results than on the more subjective factors.

THE FIRST PRESCRIPTIVE APPROACHES

The Tillyer patent mentioned above, and a few other similar ones, ushered in the concept of selective amplification. Soon a number of selective amplification ideas appeared, although none had wide appeal or usage. Watson and Knudsen (1940) were critical of the fitting procedures employed before 1940. They were especially critical of what today is often referred to as "pure" selective amplification (they called it "uncontrolled" selective amplification); i.e., an amount of gain at each measured frequency equal to the amount of hearing loss. According to that method, if a person had a threshold of 50 dB at 500 Hz and 60 dB at 1000 Hz, for example, the goal was 50 dB of gain at 500 Hz and 60 dB gain at 1000 Hz. This, of course, overpowered the listener. One variation was to employ gain at each frequency equal to the hearing loss minus a constant, while another variation bisected the threshold of sensitivity and the threshold of discomfort to determine the required gain.

Selective amplification was criticized by Watson and Knudsen (1940) as ignoring the levels needed to make the various speech sounds audible, as well as ignoring the loudness function of sensory losses. Nor did they consider uniform amplification to be appropriate, that is, equal amplification at all frequencies (Watson 1939). Rather, their goal was "true selective amplification," which was "a controlled variation from uniform amplification over the entire speech range."

Watson-Knudsen Method

In place of "pure" selective amplification, Watson and Knudsen suggested a method based on a "most comfortable equal loudness curve." To accomplish this they recommended determining air and bone conduction thresholds, then a most comfortable equal loudness curve. The latter was obtained by determining the most comfortable listening level for a 1000-Hz puretone, and then obtaining an equal loudness contour for other prescribed frequencies by using the 1000-Hz MCL as a reference for loudness balancing.

From this information a formula was employed to determine the required amplification at the prescribed frequencies:

$$Gf = HLf - (Drf - Df) + K$$

where Gf is the desired (required) gain at a frequency, HLf is the hearing level at that frequency, Drf is the difference between MCL in decibels HL and the hearing threshold level for a pure-tone at a reference frequency, Df is the difference between

MCL in decibels HL and the hearing threshold level at the test frequency, and K is a constant.

The published description of their method by Watson and Knudsen is such that the basis for the constant employed in their formula cannot be determined at this time. Other weaknesses of their method were that it was time-consuming and difficult for many listeners to make accurate loudness judgments from 1000 Hz to the other frequencies.

Fletcher Formula

A formula for hearing aid fitting was published in 1954 by Harvey Fletcher. This was based on the Articulation Index and the threshold pattern, including air–bone gap. His formula was as follows:

$$R \text{ (Response)} = Bc + rBn$$

where Bc was the conductive component in decibels, Bn is the sensorineural component, and r is a correction factor. The Fletcher prescription method seems to have attracted few adherents and is not used today, to my knowledge.

Half-Gain Rule

In 1953 Samuel F. Lybarger published his fitting procedure. This has come to be known as the *one-half gain rule;* however, in his procedure he also accounted for output and frequency response. Considerable experimental evidence has subsequently accumulated to confirm the validity of the one-half gain rule (Berger et al. 1980, Brooks 1973, Byrne and Fifield 1974, Martin 1973). That is, a person with a 70-dB average hearing threshold level will usually choose to set the volume control to provide about 35 dB of gain, and the person with a 50-dB HTL will choose approximately 25 dB of gain.

Lybarger's publication was little known outside the Radioear dealership organization, of which he was a part. Nor did the 1963 revision obtain general acceptance. Lybarger presented the procedure at the ASHA convention in 1957, but again, there was little acceptance from audiologists. As may be seen, until it was "rediscovered" in England, Australia, and the United States in the 1970s by a number of clinicians, the one-half gain rule had few adherents. Now, almost two decades later, however, several clones, modifications, and refinements have appeared, sometimes without acknowledgment of their predecessor.

The Lybarger prescription, as noted, employs a one-half gain rule based on threshold data. His method also included a one-fourth rule for the SSPL (then called *output*) portion of the prescription. Maximum gain was comprised of *operating gain* (which is referred to by others as *use gain,* or *preferred gain,* or *effective gain*) plus *reserve gain.* Operating gain was based on the assumption that typical speech from a speaker 1 m in front of the listener averages 65-dB SPL, and if at all practical, this speech should be amplified into the hearing impaired individual's comfortable range. His formula for operating gain, using air conduction and bone conduction threshold data, was as follows:

$$\frac{A\,C\,loss}{2} + \frac{A\,C - B\,C\,loss}{4} + 5\,dB$$

The air and bone conduction loss data, in decibels, were for the average of 500, 1000, and 2000 Hz. It may be seen that the formula increased the gain in cases of conductive losses by one-fourth of the air-bone gap. When binaural amplification was to be employed the constant $+5$ was changed to -10. To the operating gain was added an arbitrary 15 dB for reserve gain. This amount of reserve gain was probably appropriate for the body-type hearing aids used when the procedure was published, but less reserve gain is needed for the more recent ear-level models. In Lybarger's 1963 revision the frequency response was plotted according to whether the threshold was rising, falling, flat, and so on.

Wallenfels Approach

A selective amplification procedure recommended by Wallenfels (1967) borrowed partially from Victoreen (see below) and involved four steps. Step 1 was to obtain a pure-tone audiogram and convert threshold data to SPL. Step 2 was to make a "recruitment calculation" by determining the client's UCL at various frequencies and converting these values to SPL. He recommended against using pure tones for the UCL determination, preferring narrowband noise.

Step 3 was accomplished by the clinician bisecting the threshold of sensitivity and UCL at 1000 Hz and drawing a line between 1000 and 4000 Hz. An approximate formula would be:

$$G = \frac{NBNT + UCL}{2}$$

where the desired gain (G) equals the narrowband noise threshold at either 1000 or 4000 Hz and UCL represents the uncomfortable loudness level at that frequency. Below 1000 Hz a cut "of various proportions" was made, depending "to a large degree [on] how much trouble our new user will have in getting used to" the hearing aid. In step 4, Wallenfels subtracted 65 dB from the client's MCL to determine the amount of amplification needed. The Wallenfels procedure is discussed in some textbooks but seems to have had little clinical acceptance.

Kee Method

A modification of the Wallenfels method was made by Kee (1972), who employed the pure-tone threshold as plotted in SPL and then obtained three comfort judgments: too loud to be comfortable, comfortable, and too soft to be comfortable.

Kee's third step was to prescribe hearing aid gain by the difference between the MCL and 65 dB at each test frequency. It may be noted that Kee avoided the mistake of assuming the bisection of threshold of sensitivity and UCL represented the MCL. Kee did not involve the UCL for SSPL prescription, however, and did not report whether he included reserve gain in his suggested procedures.

Victoreen Method

In 1960, John A. Victoreen published his book *Hearing Enhancement* (Victoreen 1960) which was an expansion of some of his earlier writings published by Vicon Instrument Corporation. The book was completely revised in 1973 as *Basic Principles of Otometry* (Victoreen 1973). In the latter book Victoreen described a fitting method employing comfortable judgments made by the client while listening to damped wave train (DWT) signals. The DWT is a sound that decreases in amplitude (e.g., 0.90) with each succeeding cycle. The damped sinusoid wave train was stated to have advantages over pure tones; for example, it more nearly representing the duration of a consonant sound, and not being susceptible to standing waves in the soundfield.

In using the damped wave train the client is to respond only "soft" or "loud" to each presentation of trains. The midpoint between the responses to "soft" and "loud" is, then, the MCL, or as Victoreen termed it, "Most Comfortable Loudness Pressure" for that frequency. The MCL is plotted at 10 frequencies. The client's MCL is then compared with the "normal" or "standard" MCL of 72-dB SPL for a DWT, which was determined by Victoreen with six young men for damped wave trains. If the client's MCL is below that norm, a hearing aid is indicated. At that point an actual hearing aid of the make and model to be prescribed is placed on the client and the MCLs are again determined. Differences between the measured aided MCLs are then prescribed at each test frequency.

More recently, some of those using the Victoreen method decrease the gain at 500 Hz and below from the level that would be predicted from the measured MCL, so as to avoid the upward spread of masking. After the person's own hearing aid has been fitted, the aided MCLs are again determined. Variations no greater than 4 dB, and usually within 2 dB, from those prescribed have been reported (Melen 1977). Although UCLs with the DWT are obtained, an SSPL of 130 dB is considered appropriate for most clients. In his book, Victoreen is critical of hearing aids with automatic gain control and of earmolds other than the standard closed variety.

The Victoreen method has had some acceptance by clinicians in the United States and abroad. Disadvantages are that a DWT apparatus is needed, that the make and model of hearing aid to be purchased by the client needs to be on hand, and that the more recent custom in-the-ear (ITE) and canal type aids make the comparison tedious if not impossible.

Some clinicians have been critical of the Victoreen method, in particular his penchant for coining new terms to approximate those already standardized. However, Victoreen should be credited with giving renewed emphasis to psychoacoustic measurements for the purposes of hearing aid fitting as opposed to audiometric measurements for diagnostic-medical purposes. Thus he created a renewed climate for debate on the scientific fitting of hearing aids.

Summary

The various prescriptive methods mentioned above appeared primarily as written rationales plus procedures that were often far from complete. Other than an occasional description of an "interesting case study," the various methods did not include results or reliability studies of clients who were fitted with their particular method. Most of the current prescriptive methods, likewise, do not include much, if any, group data resulting from fittings. Thus the user of the methods must rely on the presumed logic of the methods or on the reputation of their developers. One other observation should be made. It will be noticed that the current prescriptive methods, like the earlier ones briefly described above, do not directly involve word discrimination scores as part of the prescriptive criteria. The reason for this, presumably, is the poor test-retest reliability of word discrimination scores for prescriptive purposes.

CURRENT PRESCRIPTIVE METHODS

In addition to the Lybarger and Victoreen methods, a number of other prescriptive procedures have attained some degree of acceptance with clinicians. Some of these methods have been published in detail, while others have appeared only in general outline form. Some have now built up considerable case history data, while others have not. A brief description of these methods follows.

As noted earlier, prescriptive methods in use today are, for the most part, concerned primarily with gain by frequency. The two common variations of current methods are those that employ threshold data and those that employ MCL data. Each may be stated in a generalized formula. The formulas for gain-frequency response based on hearing threshold level are almost always a variation of (Byrne 1982):

Gain needed for comfortable listening* = an arbitrary factor (commonly ~ 0.5) times HTL

The formulas for gain-frequency response based on unaided comfort level are most usually a variation of:

Gain = unaided MCL minus a constant†

---

*Determined by the client's volume control setting preference.
†Usually 60–70 dB, which represents the average intensity of speech in SPL.

Shapiro Method

The Shapiro method appears to be a merging of some of the Victoreen ideas with those of Kee (1972) and Shapiro (1976). In one of his studies, Shapiro found that by bisecting the threshold of sensitivity and the UCL, the MCL could be approximated for 3000 and 4000 Hz, but that the MCL was at a higher level for the lower frequencies. Shapiro then recommended a four-step procedure for selecting the amplifier characteristics.

The first two steps involved determining the MCL and UCL with pulsed narrowband noise for the octaves from 250 to 4000 Hz, plus 3000 Hz. From this information the ear with the largest dynamic range and the highest UCL could be determined and was the ear to be fitted. In the third step he subtracted 60 dB from the MCLs at 1000, 2000, 3000, and 4000 Hz to determine the operating gain. Gain at 500 Hz was to be that of 1000 Hz minus 10 dB. For reserve gain Shapiro added 10 dB at each frequency, and he determined the SSPL by averaging the UCLs at 500, 1000, and 2000 Hz.

Pascoe Method

Pascoe (1975) came to the conclusion, based on experimental evidence with six hearing-impaired subjects, that the best word discriminating scores were obtained with amplifiers that provided an aided uniform hearing level. This response appeared to be superior to that of a simulated commercially available hearing aid, the aid the subject was wearing, uniform functional gain, and gain that rose 6 dB per octave. The resulting recommendation by Pascoe was:

$$FG = NBT - NNBT$$

where FG is the desired functional gain at a given one-third octave band of noise, NBT is the client's threshold for that noise, and NNBT is the normal average threshold for that noise. Subsequently, Pascoe published a study showing that the gain-frequency response needed to have a two-humped shape for best fitting. One hump of added gain was below 1000 Hz and the other, above 1000 Hz. This two-humped shape was considered vital because experimentation with subjects in sound-field showed that as speech stimuli are made softer and softer, the last two frequency areas to become inaudible are those just mentioned (Pascoe 1978).

More recently Pascoe has modified his fitting procedure so that it contains some of the elements of the Victoreen method. That is, it includes a gain-frequency response that is determined by having the subject indicate varying degrees of loudness when presented with discrete frequency test stimuli (Pascoe 1980, Skinner et al. 1982).

Byrne Method

Byrne, along with his co-workers at the National Acoustics Laboratory in Australia, has been active in researching hearing aid needs and similar requirements. Through research they found that gain amounting to 4.6 dB for every 10-dB increase in hearing loss provided optimal amplification. It may be noted that this figure is only slightly different from the 5 dB for every 10-dB increase in hearing loss noted earlier in Lybarger's one-half gain rule.

Byrne then made a correction for equal loudness from a 60-phon contour, and applied these corrections to the required gain at frequencies from 250 to 4000 Hz. To simplify these determinations a table was published, making the clinician's job relatively easy in prescribing gain-frequency response. Built into the table was information from the frequency response of Australian speech, that is, the long-term speech spectrum, analyzed by third-octave bands. A major contribution of Byrne and his co-workers was to incorporate the speech spectrum in the gain-frequency response formula rather than using a constant correction of 60 or 65 dB as representative of speech (Byrne 1976, 1982; Byrne and Fifield 1974; Byrne and Tonisson 1976).

The speech spectrum shows a peak of energy at around 500 or 550 Hz, with a gradually decreasing amount of energy in speech up to about 10,000 Hz. In addition, Byrne's tabular data make the clinician's prescribing job easier than having to mathematically work out each portion of the gain formula by frequency. In their tables the Australian group included 15 dB of reserve gain. Byrne and his co-workers have been active in experimentally testing various prescriptive ideas and of refining their own method as well as testing fitting procedures in general.

Following several experimental studies, Byrne's formula was modified. The revised formula permits calculating real-ear gain (i.e., insertion gain or functional gain), with 15 dB of reserve gain (Byrne and Dillon, 1986). The revised formula is as follows:

$$G_{250} = X + 0.31\, H_{250} - 17$$
$$G_{500} = X + 0.31\, H_{500} - 8$$
$$G_{750} = X + 0.31\, H_{750} - 3$$
$$G_{1K} = X + 0.31\, H_{1K} - 1$$
$$G_{1.5K} = X + 0.31\, H_{1.5K} + 1$$
$$G_{2K} = X + 0.31\, H_{2K} - 1$$
$$G_{3K} = X + 0.31\, H_{3K} - 2$$
$$G_{4K} = X + 0.31\, H_{4K} - 2$$
$$G_{6K} = X + 0.31\, H_{6K} - 2$$

where G is the insertion gain in decibels at the indicated frequency, X is 0.05 times the sum of hearing thresholds for three frequencies (500, 1000, and 2000 Hz) under ISO (1964) audiometer calibration, and H is the hearing threshold level at the indicated frequency, in each case multiplied by 0.31. Byrne and Dillon also presented calculations for 2-cc coupler gain approximating the level that would be obtained under the real-ear gain formula.

The revised prescription formulas by Byrne and his coworkers are available in three slide charts: for ITE aids, for behind-the-ear (BTE) aids, and for body aids. One side of each slide chart pertains to the insertion gain required to reach the prescribed aided thresholds, and the other side of the slide chart is for the same purpose but the gain is that for a 2-cc coupler.

Berger Method

Berger (1976) presented a rationale for hearing aid prescription including steps from guidelines for choosing the hearing aid candidate, through the specific electro-acoustic characteristics presumed to provide optimum amplification for a given hearing loss. Included was provision for binaural fittings and for conductive hearing losses. The Berger method is a modification of the work of Lybarger, in that the basic one-half gain role is applied to specific frequencies rather than the average of the speech frequencies, and operating gain (OG) is slightly greater than one-half of the hearing loss. The basic operating gain-frequency response is as follows:

$$\frac{\text{HTL at 500 HZ}}{2}; \quad \frac{\text{HTL at 1000 Hz}}{1.6}; \quad \frac{\text{HTL at 2000 Hz}}{1.5};$$

$$\frac{\text{HTL at 3000 Hz}}{1.7}; \quad \frac{\text{HTL at 4000 Hz}}{2}$$

Later, the formula was expanded to include 6000 Hz for hearing losses that were mild or moderate, with a denominator of 2, and the denominator at 4000 Hz changed to 1.9. The various denominators in the formula were chosen to mirror the long-term speech spectrum as much as was considered practical. Another modification was to slightly reduce the gain at 500 Hz for mild hearing losses. Like the Byrne formula, this one was for closed earmolds. The OG formula is not the prescription but, rather, is used to predict the desired aided threshold. The maximum gain (MG) portion of the formula is:

$$MG = OG + 10\,dB \text{ reserve gain} + \text{correction factors}$$

(Berger et al. 1984). MG is presumed to approximate the coupler gain required to reach the predicted aided thresholds and retain reserve gain.

The correction factors to the formula are dependent on whether the microphone was located on the body (body aids), at ear level (BTE or eyeglass aids), or at the ear (ITE models). Correction factors for canal aids have not clearly emerged from published research. Perhaps canal aids can be prescribed by using ITE data (Hodgson and Wernick (1985) but require less reserve gain. Berger also gives correction factors to the gain-frequency response formula for binaural fittings, for conductive losses (adding 20 percent of the air–bone gap, as opposed to 25 percent in the Lybarger formula), and for open earmolds. An arbitrary 10 dB of reserve gain is recommended for all fittings.

In addition to gain-frequency response, the method necessitates the specification of SSPL. This is accomplished by determining the UCLs with pulsing discrete frequency stimuli, and then converting them to SPL to prescribe maximum permissible SSPL. In addition, from the operating gain and speech spectrum data a minimum desirable SSPL may be prescribed, allowing the clinician to find a hearing aid with SSPL anywhere between the two sets of data. Provision for automatic gain control (AGC) recommendation is included where the unaided dynamic range is smaller than considered appropriate for a conventional amplifier. Berger and his co-workers have published a number of reports on their successes and failures with the method, degree of accuracy expected, and other aspects of clinical experiences with the method (Berger and Hagberg 1982, Berger et al. 1982).

McCandless Method

McCandless (1976) was among the first to include a rationale for hearing aid need in his prescription. This was determined by administering a word discrimination test at 40-dB HL (considered the level of soft conversational speech), then "some form of discrimination test at 70–80 dB" (considered the level of loud conversational speech. If the discrimination score at 70 dB improved by at least 12 percent over that at 40 dB, it was assumed that the person could benefit from amplification.

By testing 200 hearing aid users it was found that no more than gain amounting to 50 percent of the hearing threshold level would be tolerated. The resulting prescription for adults with a sensory loss was *operating gain of one-half of the hearing threshold level and 10–15 dB of reserve gain.* Output depended on the hearing level; for 20-dB levels, output would be 95-dB SPL; for 40-dB levels, output would be 105-dB SPL; for 60-dB levels, output would be 115 dB; and so forth. For children the prescription was altered slightly for both gain and output.

Where UCLs could not be obtained the SSPL was determined by using "the beginning acoustic reflex" threshold (ART) data inasmuch as UCLs and ARTs were assumed to be nearly identical (McCandless 1976, McCandless and Miller 1972). It was reported that the use gain (i.e., operating gain) was found to be within 1 dB of what would be predicted from the acoustic reflex measures. For children the use gain was found to be less than 3 or 4 dB from that plotted by the prescription. McCandless cautioned that the preferred aided listening level is unlikely to change upward. In fact, he notes that in 98 percent of the subjects tested the preferred listening level was down, not up, after the first test.

Later, McCandless and Lyregaard (1983) published the rationale and procedures for a fitting method called *POGO (prescription of gain/output for hearing aids).* The method is for persons with sensorineural hearing losses. In the POGO method the required gain and SSPL are determined from thresholds and UCLs obtained at 500, 1000, and 2000 Hz. Once fitted with hearing aids, the clients are tested for functional gain by comparing aided and unaided warble tone or narrow-band noise thresholds.

After 5 months of trial in a clinical audiology setting, involving 48 hearing impaired adults, Smriga (1984) found this method to combine simplicity and practicality. In about 54 percent of the cases the obtained functional gain was within 5 dB of the prescribed gain at all test frequencies, 32 percent were within 10 dB, and for 14 percent the mismatch was greater than 10 dB. In another study, Lyregaard (1986) employed experienced hearing aid users, 39 of whom worn BTE hearing aids and 29 ITE aids. He found the predicted overall gain by the POGO method to be valid for the hearing aids in actual use, but, as expected, there were many individual differences.

A number of other hearing aid fitting methods, or discussions of specific fittings, have been described, such as those of Leijon et al. (1984), Ickes (1983), Cox (1981, 1983; Cox and Bisset 1982), Engebretson (Engebretson and Miller 1982, Engebretson et al. 1986), and Skinner (1976). Reviews of many current hearing aid fitting methods have been published (Humes 1986, Keith and Sininger 1972, Libby 1985, Williams and Webber 1985).

It would require a mammoth dedication of time, number of subjects, and a large assortment of hearing loss patterns to make a direct comparison of actual aided results between even a few of the prescriptive hearing aid methods. Not surprisingly, there has been no such study. Byrne (1987), however, employed six different methods by applying them to eight hearing loss patterns (low-frequency pattern, flat threshold, moderately sloping high-frequency loss, and steeply falling high-frequency loss, each of two magnitudes of overall loss). Byrne concluded that the various formulas do prescribe substantially different frequency response character-istics for some of the audiometric patterns. He also concludes that his comparisons of hearing loss pattern to prescriptive formulas did not settle the question of which formula was best. However, the reader can easily infer from Byrne's discussion that his bias is toward the formula developed at his own laboratory.

RELATIONSHIPS TO TEST EQUIPMENT

Prescriptive fitting methods entail relating the prescribed gain data (and often SSPL data) to electroacoustic measurements. Present published hearing aid stan-dards involve electroacoustic measurements made in the 2-cc coupler. It has long been known that the 2-cc coupler is an inexact representation of the ear canal when an earmold is in place. The so-called Harvard Report (Davis et al. 1947) noted this. On the other hand, a few overzealous writers have criticized the 2-cc coupler more than it deserves. The question should be whether measurements made in the 2-cc coupler can be related to an average real ear, and the jury is still out on that subject.

The Zwislocki coupler, developed in 1970, and the KEMAR manikin, devel-oped by Knowles Electronics in 1972, combined to provide a more meaningful measurement of hearing aid response than that from the 2-cc coupler. The Zwislocki coupler with KEMAR represents the median dimensions of an adult ear. Some technical data sheets published by hearing aid manufacturers include measurement data from KEMAR; however, as of this writing such is not part of a hearing aid standard. Refer to Chapter 2 for a discussion of measurements on KEMAR.

The latest development in test equipment for hearing aid fitting purposes is the probe tube assembly. The probe tube method permits rapid and accurate measurement, from the ear canal, of the frequency response of a hearing aid while being worn. This, compared with a measurement made without the hearing aid in place, permits specification of what is called *insertion gain*. Insertion gain equals overall gain (called *in situ gain*) minus external ear resonance. Test-retest reliability of probe tube measurements and possible problems with the probe tube in individual ears has received some, but as yet inadequate, examination by researchers. Further description of measurements by probe microphone may be found in Chapters 2 and 5.

None of the test apparatuses (2-cc coupler, Zwislocki coupler, or probe tube) replace fitting methods. Rather, the prescriptive methods employ one or more of these measurement techniques. Obviously the probe tube can be more accurate for this purpose since it involves a specific ear canal. Probe tube measures can also be used instead of functional gain measurements. Prescriptive formulas for operating gain based on threshold as measured in decibels HL may be converted to SPL and applied to probe tube measures; however, prescriptive formulas stated in terms of 2-cc coupler gain cannot be directly applied to probe tube measures. Aided–unaided comparisons of probe tube measures can, of course, be used to verify operating gain (also called *functional gain*). No known conversion factors have been published to relate MCL measures to probe tube measures.

Correction factors to change 2-cc coupler data to insertion gain data have been measured and also calculated (Lybarger and Teder 1986). Studies that have related functional gain to 2-cc coupler gain, and insertion gain to 2-cc coupler gain, have been summarized by Hawkins et al. (1987).

Gradually some research evidence on the subject of probe tube measures is appearing. For example, Hawkins (1987) found the mean insertion gain for ear probe measurements made by six experienced clinicians on the same subject to range from 2.2 dB at 1000 Hz to 7.0 dB at 6000 Hz. He concluded that probe microphone measurements have a number of advantages over functional gain measurements, as follows: (1) they are more time efficient, (2) speaker output limitations are not a problem even with severe hearing losses, (3) hearing aid circuit noise or ambient room noise does not affect the results even for subjects with normal or near-normal hearing, and (4) the measurement is less variable.

Libby (1987) points out some of the differences in hearing aid measurements by referring to three categories of gain-frequency response measurement. Class I is simulated gain, frequency response, and SSPL as measured per ANSI S3.22-1982. Class I measures are determined in a 2-cc coupler. Class II is a measurement of similar electroacoustic factors by determining them on KEMAR with its Zwislocki coupler. Class II is a simulation, closer to reality than class I, but still a median value of real ears. Class III is a real-ear measurement of the same electroacoustic factors on an actual person. Hearing aid specifications have been published under class I measurements, although some are now appearing under class II measurements. Class II measurements, to some extent, and class III measurements, completely, have the advantage of avoiding variations of the hearing aid wearer's head, pinna, and eardrum transfer effect.

COMPUTER PROGRAMS

Prescriptive hearing aid methods are comprised of formulas for gain-frequency response, and usually SSPL. Therefore, these are readily computerized. Sheeley (1984) lists an assortment of computer programs available for various hearing aid fitting methods. Smaldino (1985) made a detailed comparison of four computer-assisted hearing aid selection programs.

Some computerized programs not only result in a generic prescription but can also be used to search for entered data on specific hearing aid models. Thereby, the clinician can not only obtain the prescription proper, and print it out for record keeping, but also have the computer search for specific models approximating the prescription. The model data, of course, need to be entered into the computer program. An example of one computerized hearing aid prescriptive method is as follows (Berger et al. 1984, Gans et al. 1983). The capitalized messages are those asked by the computer, and examples of responses entered by the clinician are shown in parentheses:

WHAT IS THE NAME OF YOUR CLIENT?   (John Doe)

WHAT IS THE DATE OF THE FITTING?   (June 8, 1987)

ENTER TYPE OF AID DESIRED
1. BEHIND-THE-EAR
2. EYEGLASS
3. IN-THE-EAR
4. BODY   (1)

ENTER TYPE OF FITTING
1. MONAURAL
2. BINAURAL
3. CROS
4. BICROS   (1)

IS THIS AN OPEN EARMOLD FITTING? Y/N?   (N)

IS THIS FITTING FOR A YOUNG CHILD (OR A PERSON WITH A VERY SMALL EXTERNAL AUDITORY CANAL)? Y/N?   (N)

IS THERE MEASURABLE HEARING AT 1000 HZ? Y/N?   (Y)

IF ANY OF THE MEASUREMENTS WERE NOT OBTAINED, ENTER A '1'

ENTER HTL AT 500 HZ: ____ DB.   (30)
ENTER HTL AT 1000 HZ: ____ DB.   (40)

ENTER HTL AT 2000 HZ: ____ DB.	(45)
ENTER HTL AT 3000 HZ: ____ DB.	(55)
ENTER HTL AT 4000 HZ: ____ DB.	(60)
ENTER HTL AT 6000 HZ: ____ DB.	(65)
ENTER AIR-BONE GAP AT 500 HZ: ____ DB.	(0)
ENTER AIR-BONE GAP AT 1000 HZ: ____ DB.	(0)
ENTER AIR-BONE GAP AT 2000 HZ: ____ DB.	(0)
ENTER AIR-BONE GAP AT 4000 HZ: ____ DB.	(0)
ENTER UCL AT 500 HZ: ____ DB HL.	(100)
ENTER UCL AT 1000 HZ: ____ DB HL.	(105)
ENTER UCL AT 2000 HZ: ____ DB HL.	(110)
ENTER UCL AT 4000 HZ: ____ DB HL.	(100)

For most computers, as soon as the last bit of information just given is entered (in this example "100"), the computer immediately shows the generic prescription on the screen. The prescription of the example above would look like the following:

PRESCRIPTION FOR BEHIND-THE-EAR HEARING AID FOR JOHN DOE

MONAURAL FITTING 6-8-87

FREQUENCY	AIDED THRESHOLD	MAXIMUM GAIN	MINIMUM SSPL	MAXIMUM SSPL
500 HZ	21	19	84	111
1000 HZ	15	35	100	112
2000 HZ	15	42	104	119
3000 HZ	23	45		
4000 HZ	28	42	102	109
6000 HZ	33	43		

NOTE: MAXIMUM GAIN INCLUDES 10 DB OF RESERVE GAIN

As may be seen from this generic prescription, the predicted aided response is shown as "AIDED THRESHOLD". The 2-cc coupler gain presumed to approximate the aided threshold is shown as "MAXIMUM GAIN." As electroacoustic data obtained with KEMAR become available in hearing aid standards, the "MAXIMUM GAIN" portion of the prescription will be a little more accurate.

The third data column shows the minimum desirable SSPL and the fourth column, the more critical maximum permissible SSPL. An SSPL anywhere between these two sets of figures is designed to ensure that aided sounds do not exceed the wearer's UCL and that loud speech sounds will not be unnecessarily clipped. Had this particular person's dynamic range been small, the computer readout would have included a statement that "AGC IS RECOMMENDED".

At this point the clinician can use the generic prescription by attempting to find an electroacoustic response to approximate it from the specification sheets available. Or, the prescription can be printed out for future reference when the client returns with a hearing aid. Or, the computer program can give the clinician some options such as the following:

ENTER OPTION
1. SELECTION OF HEARING AIDS - ALL BRANDS
2. SELECTION OF HEARING AIDS - SELECTED BRANDS
3. EXIT FROM PROGRAM (1)

HOW MANY AIDS DO YOU WANT DISPLAYED? (1)

Now the computer will search through the electroacoustic characteristics of versions of hearing aids that the clinician previously entered into the program. The computer program may be written to locate the hearing aid(s) that most closely match the prescription or merely those that come within some predetermined margin of error from the prescription. In this particular example, the computer might find and show the following:

HEARING AID SPECIFICATIONS FOR ONE AID - RUN #2

MAKE: WHISTLETONE MODEL 642   TYPE: BEHIND-THE-EAR   DIR MIC: NO
BATTERY: 13   BATTERY LIFE: 220 HOURS   TEL COIL: NO   AGC: NO
AVAILABLE IN CROS: NO   AVAILABLE IN BICROS: NO   TONE CONTROL
SETTING: NORMAL   OUTPUT SETTING: MAX   EARHOOK: 1000 OHMS

	500 HZ	1000 HZ	2000 HZ	3000 HZ	4000 HZ	6000 HZ
MAXIMUM GAIN	20	34	42	39	40	−1
SSPL90	107	107	109		100	

In this example the computer located a hearing aid but needed to expand the acceptable criteria one step as noted by the notation "RUN #2". The make and model of the instrument are shown, as well as the fact that it is the requested BTE type, that this instrument does not have a directional microphone, and that it employs a No. 13 battery. The battery life (in our program for a mercury cell) is 220 hours, and there is no telephone coil or AGC option with this particular model. The electroacoustic data used by the computer to locate this version were based on a normal tone control setting, maximum output setting, and a 1000-Ω earhook, as measured in a 2-cc coupler. The computer program might well contain several other tone control, output control, and earhook variations of this particular make and model. Some computerized prescription programs also include earmold and venting information. For this particular model there was no measurable gain at 6000 Hz, as indicated by the "-1" at that frequency.

PRESCRIPTIVE STRATEGIES: OPINIONS

I have a decided bias toward prescriptive methods of hearing aid fitting, as opposed to the older comparison procedure, or, worse yet, a totally informal selection. *Advantages of prescriptions include their being readily computerized making the data manipulation more accurate than otherwise.* They add *objectivity* to the hearing aid fitting, even though one might quibble with the goal of a particular method. With little or no further effort a hard copy of the information is available to the clinician.

Prescriptions can be related to assorted make and model electroacoustic and other characteristics, making the choosing of a specific make and model easier to accomplish. However, they also minimize brand and model so that a generic prescription can be written. To my knowledge, no known weakness to prescriptive protocols has been published. Obviously, prescriptive fittings are not ideal with all hearing loss patterns, but neither would any other fitting procedure be expected to be ideal with the same patterns.

Prescriptions are easily modifiable. Thus, they can gradually be improved. As new information becomes available on the relationships between hearing loss patterns and electroacoustic information the prescriptions can be altered. They permit the researcher to look at specific parts of the prescription rather than the hearing aid fitting as a whole, hopefully resulting ultimately in the "best" prescription. That none of the prescriptive procedure has yet achieved that goal, probably none of their developers would argue.

REFERENCES

Berger KW: Prescription of Hearing Aids: A Rationale. J Audiol Soc 2:71–78, 1976
Berger KW: The Hearing Aid; Its Operation and Development (ed 3). National Hearing Aid Society, Livonia, MI, 1984
Berger KW, Gans DP, VerHoef N: Computerized hearing aid selection. Ear Nose Throat J 63:299–300, 1984
Berger, KW, Hagberg EN: Hearing aid users report on hearing aid usage. Monogr Cont Audiol 3(4), 24 pp, 1982
Berger KW, Hagberg EN, Rane RL: A reexamination of the one-half gain rule. Ear Hearing 1:223–225, 1980
Berger KW, Hagberg EN, Rane RL: Prescription of Hearing Aids (ed 4). Kent, OH, Herald Publishing House, 1984
Berger KW, Abel DB, Hagberg EN, et al: Successes and problems of hearing aid users. Hearing Aid J 35:18–20, 1982
Brooks D: Gain requirements of hearing aid users. Scand Audiol 2:199–205, 1973
Byrne D: Gain and frequency response requirements of hearing aids. National Acoustic Labs, Report 64, June 1976
Byrne D: Theoretical approaches for hearing aid selection, in Studebaker GA, Bess FH (eds): The Vanderbilt Hearing-Aid Report. Upper Darby, PA, Monographs in Contemporary Audiology, 1982

Byrne D: Hearing aid selection formulae: Same or different? Hearing Instruments 38:5–11, 1987

Byrne D, Dillon H: The National Acoustic Laboratories' (NAL) new procedure for selecting the gain and frequency response of a hearing aid. Ear Hearing 7:257–265, 1986

Byrne D, Fifield D: Evaluation of hearing aid fittings for infants. Br J Audiol 8:47–54, 1974

Byrne D, Tonisson W: Selecting the gain of hearing aids for persons with sensorineural hearing impairments. Scand Audiol 5:51–59, 1976

Carhart R: Volume control adjustment in hearing aid selection. Laryngoscope 56:510–526, 1946

Carhart R: Tests for the selection of hearing aids. Laryngoscope 56:780–794, 1946b

Carhart R, Thompson EA: The fitting of hearing aids. Am Acad Ophthalmol Otolaryngol Trans 51:354–361, 1947

Cox RM: Using LDLs to establish hearing aid limiting levels. Hearing Instruments 32:16, 18, 20, 1981

Cox RM: Using ULCL measures to find frequency/gain and SSPL90. Hearing Instruments 34:17–21, 39, 1983

Cox RM, Bisset JD: Prediction of aided preferred listening levels for hearing aid gain prescription. Ear Hearing 3:66–71, 1982

Davis H, Stevens SS, Nichols RH Jr, et al. Hearing Aids: An Experimental Study of Design Objectives. Cambridge, MA, Harvard University Press, 1947

Engebretson AM, Miller JD: A computer program for fitting a master hearing aid to the residual hearing characteristics of individual patients. J Acoust Soc 72:426–430, 1982

Engebretson AM, Popelka, GR, Morley RE, et al: A digital hearing aid and computer-based fitting procedure. Hearing Instruments 37:8–12, 14, 1986

Gans DP, VerHoef N, Berger KW: Hearing aid selection by computer. Hearing Instruments 34:17, 97–98, 1983

Hawkins DB: Variability in clinical ear probe microphone measurements. Hearing Instruments, 38:30, 32, 1987

Hawkins DB, Montgomery AA, Prosek RA, et al: Examination of two issues concerning functional gain measurements. J Speech Hearing Disorders 52:56–63, 1987

Hodgson W, Wernick JS: Canal aid versus standard custom ITE performance. Hearing Instruments 36:26, 28, 68, 1985

Humes LE: An evaluation of several rationales for selecting hearing aid gain. J Speech Hearing Disorders 51:272–281, 1986

Ickes WK: The Texas Tech method of hearing aid selection. Hearing Instruments 34:22, 24, 39, 1983

Kee WR: Use of pure tone measurement in hearing aid fittings. Audecibel 22:9–15, 1972

Keith RW, Sininger L: "New ideas"? in hearing aid fittings. Audecibel 21:9–15, 1972

Leijon A, Mangold NE, Karlsen AB: Preferred hearing aid gain and bass-cut in relation to prescriptive fitting. Scand Audiol 13:157–161, 1984

Libby ER: State-of-the-art of hearing aid selection procedures. Hearing Instruments 36:30, 34, 36, 38, 62, 1985

Libby ER: Real ear considerations in hearing aid selection. Hearing Instruments 38:14–16, 1987

Lybarger SF: Simplified Fitting System. Radioear Corp., October 1963

Lybarger SF: Selective amplification—a review and evaluation. J Am Audiol Soc 3:258–266, 1978

Lybarger SF, Teder H: 2cc coupler curves to insertion gain curves. Hearing Instruments 37:36–37, 40, 1986

Lyregaard PE: On the practical validity of POGO. Hearing Instruments 37:13–14, 16, 147, 1986

Martin MC: Hearing aid requirements in sensorineural hearing loss. Br J Audiol 7:21–24, 1973

McCandless GA: Special considerations in evaluating children and the aging for hearing aids, in Rubin M (ed): Hearing Aids. Baltimore, University Park Press, 1976, pp 171–182

McCandless GA, Miller DL: Loudness discomfort and hearing aids. Natl Hearing Aid J 7:7, 28, 32, 1972

McCandless G, Lyregaard PE: Prescription of gain/output (POGO) for hearing aids. Hearing instruments 34:16–21, 1983

Melen LA: Otometry: An emerging prosthetic discipline. Guthrie Bull 47:19–33, 1977

Nielsen HB: Hearing aid fitting based on insertion gain measurements. Audecibel 35:16–18, 1984

Pascoe DP: Frequency responses of hearing aids and their effects on the speech perception of hearing impaired subjects. Ann Otol Rhinol Laryngol 84 (Suppl 23) 1975

Pascoe DP: An approach to hearing aid selection. Hearing Instruments 29:12–16, 36, 1978

Pascoe DP: Clinical implications of nonverbal methods of hearing aid selection and fitting. Semin Speech Lang Hearing 1:217–229, 1980

Shapiro I: Prediction of most comfortable loudness levels in hearing aid evaluation. J Speech Hearing Disorders 40:323–338, 1975

Shapiro I: Hearing aid fitting by prescription. Audiology 15:163–173, 1976

Sheeley EC: Microcomputer software directory. Ear Hearing 5:371–374, 1984

Skinner M: Speech intelligibility in noise-induced hearing loss: Effects of high frequency compensation. PhD dissertation, Washington University, 1976

Skinner MW, Pascoe DP, Miller JD, et al: Measurements to determine the optimal placement of speech energy within the listener's auditory area: A basis for selecting amplification characteristics, in Studebaker GA, Bess FH (eds): The Vanderbilt Hearing-Aid Report. Upper Darby, PA, Monographs in Contemporary Audiology, 1982

Smaldino J: Comparing computer-assisted hearing aid selection software. Hearing Instruments 36:16, 18–21, 1985

Smirga DJ: Clinical experience with POGO. Hearing instruments 35:21–22, 1984

Victoreen JA: Hearing Enhancement. Springfield, IL, Charles C Thomas, 1960

Victoreen JA: Basic Principles of Otometry. Springfield, IL, Charles C Thomas, 1973

Wallenfels HG: Hearing Aids on Prescription. Springfield, IL, Charles C Thomas, 1967

Watson NA: Selective amplification. Volta Rev 41:338–340, 371, 1939

Watson NA, Knudsen VO: Selective amplification in hearing aids. J Acoust Soc Am 11:406–419, 1940

Williams DG, Webber PJ: Hearing aid selection for adults: A review. Audiol Acoust 24:2–4, 6–8, 10–12, 14–15, 1985

Appendix

HEARING AID PRESCRIPTION COMPUTER SOFTWEAR

Computer softwear tends to undergo rapid changes and new introductions. The following are the hearing aid computer programs known to us at the time this book went to press.

Central Institute For the Deaf, St. Louis, MO. "CID Selection/Evaluation Program" based CID method, plus ability to select hearing aids from the generic prescription.

College Hill Press, 4284 41st Street, San Diego, CA 92105. "Systematic Hearing Aid Prescription," by D. E. Moomaw, based on the POGO rationale.

Herald Publishing House, 647 Longmere Drive, Kent, OH 44240. The Berger prescription on disk for IBM, Apple, and in BASIC; in printed form for BASIC, FORTRAN, and Apple.

Katz Computer Software, 965 North Alvernon Way, Tucson, AZ 85711. Hearing aid selection program, unaided and aided audiometric information, and record-keeping capabilities.

Parrot Software, 190 Sandy Ridge Road, State College, PA 16801. "Select a Hearing Aid" is the Berger prescription on disk for Apple. There is also a program to search for hearing aids based on the generic prescription ("Hearing Aid Manager") by Gary J. Glascoe.

Starkey Laboratories, 6700 Washington Ave. 5., Eden Prairie, MN 55344. Available in CP/M or MS DOS with dBase II capabilities for the Starkey Matrix Program.

NOTE: Apple and IBM are registered trademarks.

Michael C. Pollack

8

Special Applications of Amplification

Over the years, there have been numerous innovations, as well as controversies, concerning the use of amplification by the hearing-impaired. These include the CROS hearing aid and its many variations, assistive listening devices, and acoustic resonators. In addition to these developments, there seems to finally be some resolution of the controversy surrounding binaural versus monaural amplification. This chapter will consider each of these four "special applications" of amplification, attempting to present all sides of the issues and to draw some conclusions. Hopefully, these discussions will stimulate thought and discussion.

MCP

MONAURAL, BINAURAL, AND PSEUDOBINAURAL AMPLIFICATION

When the literature pertaining to the nonmedical management of individuals with bilateral hearing loss is reviewed, one major area of disagreement, in the past, was whether the bilaterally hearing-impaired individual should use one hearing aid delivering sound to one ear (monaural), one hearing aid delivering sound to both ears (pseudobinaural or Y cord), or two hearing aids (binaural). While this disagreement has not yet reached final resolution, the latest data from controlled research, as well as attitudinal studies of fitters, suggest advantages of and a greater tendency toward binaural amplication.

Historically, manufacturers and traditional dispensers of hearing aids have strongly advocated binaural fittings, while audiologists have been more reluctant to

AMPLIFICATION FOR THE HEARING-IMPAIRED, THIRD EDITION   ISBN 0-8089-1886-9

do so. A great deal of formal and informal research has been performed in an attempt to demonstrate the advantage of binaural amplification. Positive case reports abound in the pages of professional publications. Yet, the disagreement continues.

Apparently, the problem is based on the fact that while users frequently report greater success with binaural than with monaural amplification, these improvements often cannot be demonstrated clinically. Audiologists are often greatly concerned with the clinical, empirical exemplification of phenomena. It may be the past lack of research evidence of the superiority of binaural fittings that often made many audiologists very cautious about recommending such instrumentation. One could interpret this reluctance as suggesting a lack of confidence in binaural test procedures.

On the other hand, the traditional dispenser often is at the other extreme, exhibiting the attitude that every individual with a bilateral loss should wear binaural hearing aids. The dispenser may base this philosophy solely on user reports of success and satisfaction and may also be influenced by manufacturer publicity claims of binaural superiority. The audiologist and the dispenser find it difficult to justify their positions to each other, especially when faced with the fact that some individuals find binaural amplification indispensable, while others are never able to properly adjust to two aids.

Rationales for Binaural Amplification

A wealth of clinical and experimental knowledge about binaural hearing has been accumulated, and many rationales for recommendations for binaural amplification are based thereon. However, the vast majority of this information was obtained with subjects whose hearing was normal. The literature concerned with binaural hearing and binaural amplification has produced varying conclusions, leading to the realization that the advantages of two hearing aids over one must be viewed as equivocal.

Wright (1959) states that the purpose of binaural amplification is to create a sound environment for the listener that is a faithful reproduction of the original acoustic event so that he can take advantage of the intensity, time, and spectrum differences of the auditory signal at each ear. These differences provide the additional cues necessary for a more reasonable approximation of the hearing experiences of the normal hearing population.

While binaural ear-level or in-the-ear (ITE) aids provide these signal differences, body aids do not. Two microphones on the chest, especially with a child, are separated by no more than 2–3 inches, while the ears are separated by 7 or 8 inches. Additionally, the head exerts a sound shadow between the ears. It is the presence of the head between the microphones that is primarily responsible for the intensity, time, and spectrum differences. Two body aids do not achieve the purpose of restoring a semblance of normal binaural auditory functioning; ear-level and ITE aids do. With the advent of powerful ear-level instrumentation, I have been recommending binaural amplification more often than in the past for both children and adults. In my experience, I have found that only in cases of the most profound hearing loss can I not find ear-level aids that will provide suitable amplification. It seems logical that hearing with two ears provides more information than hearing with one. Although speech can be intelligibly conveyed through a single neurologic channel, there are circumstances when the understanding of speech is improved considerably when it is heard through two ears. The higher level of redundancy with two-eared hearing provides advantages in sound localization and discrimination in the presence of background noise.

Another implication of binaural amplification for congenitally hard-of-hearing children relates to the fact that a prerequisite to the appropriate processing of language information is the establishment of cerebral dominance. Referring to the work of Penfield and Roberts, Lankford and Faires (1973) raise the question of the validity of monaural amplification for these children "who must rely on the processing ability of both hemispheres in order to adequately analyze and synthesize previously unlearned language." Here is another important area in need of extensive research.

Although opinion differs on the degree of improvement of speech intelligibility, there is general agreement on the advantage of binaural hearing for localization of sound (Hirsh 1950, Bergman 1957, Carhart 1958, Wright 1959). However, it is often difficult or impossible to demonstrate this clinically or experimentally. Speech discrimination scores have generally been accepted as one of the criteria in judging the superiority of binaural over monaural aids. As noted above, it is often difficult to demonstrate such discrimination improvement clinically. Here may rest the problem for the audiologist. Our test materials and procedures are not yet sensitive enough to demonstrate the known advantages of binaural hearing.

A careful examination of the studies that failed to demonstrate a binaural advantage suggests that many of them did not utilize speech intelligibility tasks rigorous enough to yield binaural results significantly better than monaural.

Clinical and Research Evidence of a Binaural Advantage

Langford (1970) summarized many of the clinical and research data, suggesting five advantages of binaural amplification—improved sound localization, increased speech discrimination in noise, greater ease of listening, better spatial balance, and improved quality.

LOCALIZATION

It has long been an accepted fact that man needs two ears for satisfactory auditory localization (Bergman 1957, Carhart 1958, Wright 1959). The rationale is that it takes analysis of input to two ears to determine effectively the distances and position in both azimuth and elevation of the sound sources. One exception is in highly reverberant rooms where differing times of arrival between direct and reflected sounds allows monaural localization with little effort.

SPEECH DISCRIMINATION

One of the most important advantages of binaural hearing is an improvement in auditory figure–ground relationships. The listener is better able to understand speech in a background noise. Koenig (1950) refers to this as a *"squelch effect,"* in which ambient background noises seem to decrease in intensity and become less disruptive. He found such noises to be more disturbing with monaural amplification than with binaural aids. This phenomenon has also been studied by Dirks and Moncur (1967), who described it as an important advantage of binaural over monaural hearing for speech intelligibility in a reverberant environment.

Gelfand and Hochberg (1973) hypothesized that the squelch effect was responsible for their finding of better speech discrimination under reverberant conditions for binaural amplification. They state that this might be due to the ability of the binaural auditory system to squelch the effects of reverberation. This was the case for both normal and sensorineural hearing-impaired subjects.

Related to the squelch effect are data reported by Tillman et al. (1963) on the head shadow effect. They found soundfield thresholds for speech to be almost 7 dB better at the ear nearer the sound source than at the far ear. In other words, the head exerts a block to the passage of sound from the near side to the far side. This is discussed in depth in the next section of this chapter, dealing with contralateral routing of signals (CROS) hearing aids. Also presented in that section are the problems related to unilateral hearing loss. It is important to keep in mind that *monaural amplification for a bilateral hearing loss creates, in essence, a unilateral hearing loss, with its related difficulties.*

There are many reports in the literature of subjective and clinical improvements in speech discrimination and intelligibility in noise with binaural systems (Harris 1965, Bergman 1957, Black and Hast 1962, Decroix and Dehaussey 1964, Heffler and Schultz 1964, Zelnick 1970b). Markle and Aber (1958) and Belzile and Markle (1959) demonstrated significantly better speech discrimination scores with binaural than with monaural aids. Cherry and Bowles (1960) found that increased speech intelligibility is related to the binaural auditory system's ability to separate sound spatially (figure–ground).

EASE OF LISTENING

Carhart (1958) indicated that "less effort is required for comfortable listening when this system (binaural) is used." Bergman (1957) and Hedgecock and Sheets (1958) related the greater ease of listening for speech to the binaural system's ability to minimize the effects of room reverberation on speech intelligibility (squelch). Langford (1970) reported that a binaural arrangement provides greater intensity to the auditory system than does a monaural aid. This allows the user to hear faint sounds with greater ease. He described situations in which binaural users turn up the gain of the remaining aid considerably if one aid is turned off. They appear to do this to maintain the signal intensity achieved with both aids on. Kodman (1961) summarized this aspect of the binaural use of hearing aids by suggesting that "another way of viewing the binaural effect is that the patient hears easier or with less effort, even though the intelligibility score is comparable, or even identical with, the monaural score" and that "binaural hearing promotes an interaural effect which is reflected in better sound balance and ease of perception."

SPATIAL BALANCE

There appears to be an increased precision in auditory orientation when some binaural listeners are confronted with a complex acoustical environment. This may result from what Huizing and Taselaar (1961) report as an interaural integration of speech presented to both ears. They suggest that under certain circumstances, distorted signals are integrated more effectively binaurally than monaurally. Dirks and Wilson (1969b) demonstrated a binaural advantage in subjects with sensori-neural hearing loss when sound sources were spatially separated so that the individual could make use of the interaural time differences.

SOUND QUALITY

Numerous case studies have yielded subjective reports from users of binaural hearing aids that sound quality is considerably better than that obtained with monaural instrumentation (Heffler and Schultz 1964, Haskins and Hardy 1960, Kodman 1961). Binaural amplification appears to provide a greater "fullness" to sound. These subjective reports are most likely the result of a summation of the four characteristics described above—better localization, improved speech intelligibility, greater ease of listening, and improved spatial balance.

On the other hand, a number of research studies have attempted unsuccessfully to demonstrate a clinical advantage for binaural aids. Hedgecock and Sheets (1958) found no statistically significant differences between monaural and binaural performance in quiet. Others who have failed to show improved speech discrimination were Wright (1959), Wright and Carhart (1960), and DiCarlo and Brown (1960). Jerger and Dirks (1961) tried to replicate the Belzile and Markle (1959) results but failed to confirm binaural superiority for speech intelligibility. Jerger et al. (1961) attempted to find objective verification for the numerous subjective reports of binaural advantage. Their results indicated that binaural systems produced little or no improvement in speech discrimination in quiet or noise.

Many reports showing an advantage for binaural amplification are based on the reports of users rather than on empirical clinical data. At the present time, the clinical measures used do not adequately reflect subjective claims of improvement. This problem was pointedly demonstrated by Dirks and Carhart (1962), who examined the reactions of subjects who used a hearing aid. Those with binaural experience expressed a strong preference for two aids. The authors noted that users for whom binaural aids were successful could not perform differentially on clinical tests. They summarized the situation by stating that no clinical test battery has been able to demonstrate the superiority of binaural aids on the basis of measurements. In other words, those who used binaural aids reported a number of subjective advantages that cannot be measured at present by clinical techniques. *The implication to be drawn from this is not that the advantages of binaural aids do not exist, but that our clinical evaluation tools are inadequate to measure them.* Another area of future research is the need to develop tests sufficiently sensitive to demonstrate the advantages of binaural aids.

A related drawback to a number of the studies that failed to show an advantage for binaural aids is that they were not designed in a manner that would adequately measure true binaural performance. Testing is often performed in quiet where good intelligibility can be achieved with one ear. In order to demonstrate binaural superiority, speech and competing signals must be presented at a signal-to-noise ratio that will be difficult for a monaural listener. Additionally, there must be some angular (azimuth) displacement between the primary and competing signal sources. Only then will it be possible to see if the binaural mode causes a release from masking or "squelch" effect.

During the past 10 years, a number of research and attitudinal studies comparing monaural and binaural hearing aid fittings have been published, overwhelmingly favoring binaural amplification (Markides 1977; Libby 1980, 1981; Scandinavian Audiology 1982; Hawkins and Yacullo 1984; Cox and Bisset 1984). Given the consistently demonstrated binaural advantages, it is surprising that audiologists continue to recommend monaural fittings for most (68 percent) of their adult patients (Curran 1985).

Mueller (1986), discussing attitudinal shifts toward binaural fittings, suggests that, in a majority of cases, "the decision to fit monaural or binaural is influenced by a belief held by either the dispenser, the referral source or the patient." While attitudes of dispensing audiologists are changing in favor of binaural, many referral sources, especially physicians, continue to demonstrate a belief that "one ear is as good as two." If a patient comes to my office, having been told by a physician or a friend who wears a hearing aid to consider only one aid, it is difficult, if not impossible, to convince that person of the advantages of a binaural fitting.

Yet, the advantages are there for most bilaterally hearing-impaired individuals. Erdman and Sedge (1986) reported on a series of preferential surveys of hearing aid users who had compared monaural and binaural fittings, including both new users and experienced binaural users. Ninety percent of both groups expressed a preference for binaural hearing aid use. Among the advantages they reported consistently, which warrant consideration of binaural amplification for most bilaterally impaired people, are (1) improved overall speech clarity, (2) better speech understanding in noise, (3) balanced hearing (stereo effect), (4) more relaxed listening, (5) natural sound quality, (6) tinnitus relief, (7) enhanced localization ability, and (8) lower volume control settings on both aids.

Arnst (1986) discusses a factor favoring binaural fittings for elderly patients, *redundancy and the central auditory aging effect.* It is well documented that hearing decreases with age and that many geriatrics exhibit speech discrimination ability that is disproportionately poor relative to the degree of their hearing loss. The degenerative changes in their auditory pathways (central as well as peripheral) results in reduced intrinsic and extrinsic redundancy of speech signals reaching the auditory cortex. These changes require the elderly patient to be more dependent on the additional redundancy cues offered by binaural stimulation. As Arnst states, "If as much binaural integrity as possible is maintained, the central auditory system's internal redundancy capacity can enhance processing of the speech signal." This is strong support for the concept of binaural fittings with geriatric patients.

Pseudobinaural Amplification

Figure 8-1 depicts an amplification mode referred to as Y cord or pseudobinaural, using one microphone, one amplifier, and two receivers. In essence, it is a monaural aid delivering sound to both ears. Available only in body aids, the Y cord arrangement is still ocassionally used with severely or profoundly hearing-impaired children.

Lybarger (1973) described four advantages of a pseudobinaural system relative to a monaural arrangement:

1. Both ears are receiving auditory stimulation
2. Somewhat better speech discrimination—although not a good as with a true binaural system
3. Lower initial cost than binaural
4. Lower operating cost through less battery consumption than binaural aids

While such hearing aid arrangements may be required for economic reasons,

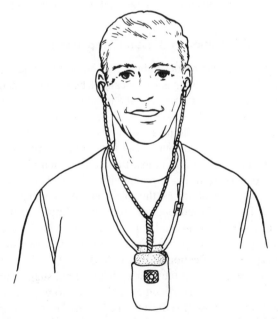

Fig. 8-1. Pseudobinaural (Y-cord) arrangement. (Adapted from Davis H, Silverman SR: Hearing and Deafness. New York, Holt, Rinehart, & Winston, 1970, p 286. With permission.)

the Y cord system provides bilateral, not binaural, hearing. The signal from one aid is split between the two ears, losing the phase, time, intensity, and spectrum cues available from a true binaural fitting. Investigative data of Wright and Carhart (1960) and Black and Hast (1962) indicate that, although both ears are stimulated, pseudobinaural aided performance is not significantly better than monaural, and is not as good as true binaural in terms of discrimination and localization. The system is only duplicating the sounds the individual is hearing with one ear. The interaural differences in phase and intensity, so necessary for localization, are absent.

Lybarger (1973) mentions the fact that not all body aids work well with a Y cord. When two receivers are used, an impedance mismatch is created that causes deterioration of the output signal. To overcome this, specially designed receivers must be used or the output impedance of the aid will be altered.

Another limitation of a Y cord is a small loss in the output reaching each ear when the signal is split (3–6 dB). Related to this problem is the realization that the balance range in output that can be obtained is limited. Although a potentiometer can be placed in the circuit, more distortion is created at high output levels. The intensity reaching each ear will be approximately the same. Therefore, a Y cord works optimally when the loss is symmetrical. If not, one ear may be under amplified or over amplified. Unfortunately, pseudobinaural aids are often recommended for young children before accurate threshold information is obtained.

Today, Y cord arrangements are less common. Generally, they are being used only when a true binaural system cannot be used due to cost or other factors.

Guidelines for Consideration of Binaural Amplification

One consistent observation throughout the literature regarding binaural amplification is that while its advantages often cannot be demonstrated clinically, user reports, after a period of experience with the two hearing aids, often strongly point to the subjective benefits. The key is an adjustment period.

A program of auditory training is often necessary for a new binaural user to take full advantage of increased sound cues for intelligibility and localization. The patient must learn to differentially adjust the gain of each aid so that the optimal summation effect occurs, resulting in potentially improved auditory perception.

The idea of adjustment raises the argument of whether or not to fit both instruments immediately. Proponents of immediate fitting argue that the user is going to eventually wear two aids and thus should start with fittings that provide the most advantageous hearing response. From the start, the user should learn to use and live with binaural amplification (Zelnick 1970a).

On the other hand, some in the hearing health field suggest that adjustment to monaural amplification is often difficult enough. Therefore, the aids should be fitted one at a time, allowing the user to adjust to one before the second is fitted. I disagree with this philosophy, based on my clinical experiences.

It has been observed that the user-adjusted gain setting of a monaural aid is generally lowered when a second instrument is introduced. With individual input to each ear, a binaural summation takes place, resulting in a lower gain setting for each instrument relative to that at which each would be adjusted monaurally. Although the binaural gain reduction is small (3–6 dB), it is obvious and consistent and could produce a more favorable sound quality.

Who should use binaural amplification? This is a question that has plagued audiologists and hearing aid dispensers. There is no pat answer—each case must be viewed individually. The guidelines presented below are based on clinical experience and common sense. They are intended only as generalized criteria.

The first consideration, naturally, must be the needs of the client. If the person is frequently confronted with situations that demand functional binaural hearing, such as business conferences, academic settings (especially in the early school years), or social settings, family gatherings or church services, binaural amplification should be given full consideration. Conversely, if the client is not confronted with these types of conditions, careful thought must be given before binaural aids are recommended. For example, if the client leads a relatively isolated lifestyle, it may be difficult to justify the gain in auditory functioning provided by a binaural system compared to the expense. This does not imply that two hearing aids should not be considered, only that the needs of the patient be paramount.

As Pascoe (1985) states, *"Hearing aids should be chosen to help restore binaural hearing. They should, in fact, be sold in pairs, just like eyeglasses."*

Clinical Evaluation of Binaural Amplification

Zelnick (1970b) begins to delineate the problem of clinical evaluation of binaural hearing aids when he states, "if the benefits of binaural hearing aids are to be demonstrated, speech stimuli and competing noise would have to be presented at such relative intensities so that the relationship between the two results in a masking effect that prevents one ear from functioning as well as both ears." If such tests are to be constructed, what competition should be used? What signal-to-noise ratio should be employed?

Other questions that need further clarification are:

1. What is the relationship between binaural amplification and such factors as recruitment and diplacusis?
2. How much benefit can be derived from binaural aids by a person with bilaterally profound hearing loss?
3. Is it possible or desirable to achieve a balance between ears through binaural amplification in a case with an asymmetrical sensorineural hearing loss?
4. How much should speech intelligibility be expected to improve in the presence of competing stimuli when binaural aids are utilized?
5. Since the better ear is generally left open in monaural fittings, and since the speech signal is frequently well above the threshold of the unaided ear, is it possible that the superior quality of the unamplified signal in one ear is of greater benefit than a second hearing aid? This may account, in part, for the

success of CROS, namely, the fact that a natural signal is being received in the frequency region where the loss is negligible.

CROS AND ITS VARIATIONS

Historically, there have been a variety of hearing loss types that have presented a confounding problem to the hearing-health team. These include patients with one ear showing normal or near-normal responses and the other ear demonstrating a severe to profound hearing loss, and patients with bilateral or unilateral high-frequency losses. In the past, a person with a high-frequency or unilateral hearing loss was considered a poor candidate for a hearing aid. Since the early 1960s this problem has been greatly alleviated through the development and modification of the CROS hearing aid. In the basic CROS design, a microphone is placed on the side of the head with the bad ear, delivering amplified sound to the better ear. A nonoccluding or open earmold is necessary with CROS to allow natural sound to reach the good ear and to reduce amplified low frequencies. Since the introduction of the original CROS aid, many variations of this design have been developed. These have widely expanded its capabilities to a point where it is possible today to provide suitable amplification for almost any type of hearing loss.

Hearing Problems Associated with Unilateral Hearing Loss

Prior to the introduction of CROS instrumentation, there were two rehabilitative avenues generally used with unilateral hearing losses that were not medically correctable: no hearing aid or a monaural instrument on the bad ear. Often, neither was very satisfactory.

There was a time when audiologists and otologists underplayed the communicative problems associated with unilateral hearing loss. They often stressed to the patient that the hearing impairment was "minimal." Rehabilitation generally consisted of a pat on the shoulder and a statement that in essence said, "You don't have any real problems—position yourself advantageously and learn to lip-read—please pay the nurse on your way out."

As coarse as this may sound, it is not without foundation. Two factors can be related to this attitude: a lack of appreciation for the many listening problems related to a unilateral hearing loss and a lack of adequate remedial procedures. After all, the unilaterally hearing-impaired patient has no difficulty on the telephone while using the good ear, does not reflect any speech and language problems, does well on soundfield hearing tests in quiet, and is under no "real" handicap because it is necessary only to "put the better ear forward." Also, because one ear is normal, most people are unaware of the hearing loss.

In reality, this individual encounters numerous communication difficulties, especially in less than ideal listening situations. These problems can be grouped into three categories.

SPEAKER ON THE SIDE OF THE IMPAIRED EAR

Tillman et al. (1963) reported on a phenomenon known as the *head shadow effect*. If speech originates on one side of the head, the signal intensity will be lower at the ear farthest from the source (far ear) than at the ear closest to the source (near ear). When measured in soundfield, with the loudspeaker at a 90° or 270° azimuth, relative to the front of the head (facing one ear directly), the near-ear speech reception threshold (SRT) will be approximately 6.4 dB better than that of the far ear. In other words, the head exerts a shadow to sound traveling around it. This effect is even greater for high frequencies (15–30 dB above 2000 Hz) than for low frequencies.

If speech is coming from the side of the bad ear (or unaided impaired ear for a monaural user), the listener is at a decided disadvantage, hearing the speech at 6.4 dB less intensity. This relatively small intensity loss can result in a substantial discrimination loss. Of course, one can turn one's head to correct this, but this is not always feasible.

The effect of the head shadow is not completely eliminated by increasing the signal intensity 6 or 7 dB. Such an increase does not compensate for the greater high-frequency shadow. If the intensity is increased by 15–30 dB, excessive low-frequency intensity results. Fletcher (1953) studied this phenomenon and concluded that the high-frequency attenuation, although relatively small, can create sufficient distortion to impose a decrease in the quality of speech, particularly for sibilant phonemes, and a resultant decrease in speech intelligibility.

If the speech is coming from the poorer ear side and noise of equal intensity originates on the side of the good ear, the unilateral hearing-loss patient experiences a great problem. In this case, the signal-to-noise ratio (S/N) at the bad ear is +6.4 dB and at the good ear is −6.4 dB, resulting from the head shadow. In other words, this individual experiences almost a 13-dB deficit relative to a normal-hearing person; the normal listener experiencing a +6.4-dB ratio at the near ear, while the unilateral listener experiences a −6.4-dB ratio at the near ear. If the conditions are reversed (speech on the good side, noise on the bad side), the unilateral listener is not at a major disadvantage relative to the normal hearer.

INCREASED DIFFICULTY HEARING IN GROUPS AND IN NOISE

One of the most common complaints of an individual with a unilateral hearing loss is difficulty in understanding speech in the presence of competing sounds. The probable cause of this complaint is the absence of the squelch effect described in the preceding section of this chapter.

AUDITORY LOCALIZATION CONFUSION

The time and intensity differences between the ears, created by the head, are virtually eliminated by a unilateral hearing loss. Without these clues it is almost impossible to adequately locate the source of a sound.

Table 8-1 summarizes the various possible combinations of the primary speech

Table 8-1
Matrix of Primary (P) and Secondary (S) Signal Locations and Effects on Unilateral
Listeners

Signal Conditions	Effects
P and S on side of good ear	No advantage or disadvantage over normal listener
P and S straight ahead	No advantage or disadvantage over normal listener
P ahead, S to either side	Disadvantage if S on side of good ear
P and S on side of bad ear	Equal head shadow—discrimination decrease due to high-frequency attenuation of speech by head shadow
P on good side, S on bad side	6.4 dB advantage due to head shadow
S on good side, P on bad side	Greatest problem—13 dB S/N difference relative to normal

(P) and secondary noise (S) signals and how the unilateral listener will function in each.

Two of the early rehabilitative approaches to unilateral hearing loss have been mentioned. The first, no hearing aid, has been described just above. The other remedial avenue involved a monaural hearing aid worn in the bad ear. This was a common approach if the poorer ear had usable residual hearing. Unfortunately, a monaural instrument for unilateral hearing loss is limited in terms of success factors.

There are a number of serious limitations to the successful use of a monaural hearing aid by an individual with unilateral hearing loss. First, there are many unilateral conductive hearing losses that can be remediated medically. If this is done after a hearing aid has been fitted, the instrument is then only temporary. Although not common today, in the past most otolaryngologists were quite reluctant to operate on a conductive ear if the opposite ear was normal. Their advice to these patients was often to position themselves advantageously and to supplement their hearing with speechreading. Second, there are people who have good speech discrimination ability in the impaired ear but who find it impossible to adjust to the combination of normal sound in the good ear and the "hollow" amplified sounds in the poorer ear. Third, there are many unilaterally hearing-impaired individuals with such poor speech discrimination ability in the bad ear that useful amplification is precluded on that side. As Harford and Musket (1964) indicated, "where the impaired ear does not offer usable residual hearing for speech, a different approach is necessary to alleviate the communicative problems of one-eared hearing."

History of CROS

Working independently of each other, Wullstein and Wigand (1962) and Harford and Barry (1965) developed similar amplification devices for unilateral hearing losses. The former researchers did not receive favorable reactions from their subjects and apparently did not pursue the matter. Harford and Barry called their instrument *CROS (contralateral routing of signals)*. The original objective was to eliminate the head shadow as a deficit. Figure 8-2 depicts the original CROS

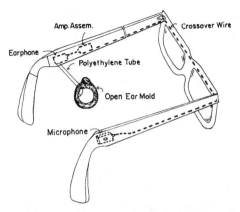

Fig. 8-2. CROS. (Reproduced from Harford E, Barry J: A rehabilitative approach to the problem of unilateral hearing impairment: The contralateral routing of signals (CROS). J Speech Hearing Disorders 30:121–138, 1965. With permission.)

arrangement in eyeglasses. A microphone is located on the eyeglass temple on the
side of the bad ear. The sounds picked up are routed through a wire to an amplifier
and receiver in the opposite temple, from where the amplified sound is delivered to
the good ear. This arrangement can be, and today most often is, incorporated into
ear-level instruments, with the signal routed either through a wire or transmitted
from microphone side to receiver side via modified amplitude-modulated (AM)
radio signals. With this configuration, sounds from the side of the bad ear are
directed to the good ear. Since this is done electronically, the effect of the head
shadow is essentially eliminated. Thus, one of the major complaints of the unilaterally hearing-impaired, difficulty hearing and understanding speech from the side of
the bad ear, is compensated for by delivering sound from that side to the better ear.

It is important that you keep in mind that the original CROS hearing aid was
intended to provide amplification for persons with no aidable hearing in one ear, and
normal or near-normal hearing in the opposite ear. Because of this intent, only
minimal gain was required to overcome the 6–7-dB head shadow. After all, since
the sound is going to a normal or near-normal ear, one would need only a minimum
of amplification. However, there are a great number of hard-of-hearing individuals
with one unaidable ear whose better ear is not normal. With these persons in mind,
many variations on the original CROS have appeared. They will be described
below.

What is meant by the term "unaidable"? Harford (1966) describes 4 conditions
under which an ear would be considered "unaidable": (1) an ear with a sensitivity
impairment beyond a point where amplified sounds can be perceived with any
appreciable degree of usefulness in terms of intelligibility; (2) an ear that manifests
a severe discrimination deficit, regardless of the degree of sensitivity loss; (3) an ear
in which the use of an earmold is contraindicated; and (4) an ear that exhibits a
markedly reduced tolerance limit and is therefore unable to utilize amplified sound.

An historic sidelight: Schaudinischky (1965) reported the development of the "audiomon" for unilateral hearing loss. This device consisted of a small microphone for sound collection in the external meatus of the bad ear that transferred the sound to a bond-conduction vibrator on the mastoid bone of the better ear. No further reports or additional data on this device have appeared.

Benefits of CROS

Experiences of clinicians, hearing aid dispensers, and CROS users have demonstrated a number of practical advantages of CROS, both anticipated and unexpected. Successful use of this hearing aid configuration has dispelled the once classic axiom that individuals with unilateral hearing loss cannot utilize amplification. Also, since the good ear receives the sound, high-gain instrumentation is not required.

The greatest and most consistent advantage reported by users is increased ease in hearing speakers from the side of the poor ear. The reason for this appears to be the elimination of the head shadow. While this benefit holds true in a relatively quiet environment, CROS appears least helpful in conditions of high ambient noise—cafeteria, social gatherings, and so on. That is, in these situations CROS may not provide a significant advantage over normal hearing. An exception to this is when the origin of the noise is on the side of the good ear and the speech is on the other side. If the S/N ratio is negative, the noise greater in intensity than the speech, CROS is of help, even under the above conditions.

Harford (1969) reported an unexpected dividend of CROS: an improvement in auditory localization ability by some individuals. Apparently some people can utilize the difference in quality between sounds entering the better ear naturally and CROS-amplified sounds to localize. If the sound is natural, the source is on the side of the good ear. If the sound is "metallic," "hollow," or "echoic," the source is on the side of the bad ear. Another factor that may account, in part, for improved localization is the time-of-arrival difference between natural and amplified sounds.

Shortly after CROS instrumentation gained popularity, the status of the better ear was found to have a direct bearing on the success that the user will have. A person with some degree of high-frequency loss in the good ear will generally experience greater success than will a person with normal hearing (Harford and Dodds 1966, Harford 1967). This phenomenon is explained on the basis of the CROS arrangement providing greater high-frequency than low-frequency amplified sound to the good ear. The presence of even a mild high-frequency loss reduces the chances of overamplification or poor subjective quality in this range. As will be explained below, the tubing delivering sound from the receiver nozzle to the ear either rests alone in the canal, with no mold, or is held in place by a plastic ring. This allows the sound from this side to enter the ear naturally. Lybarger (1967) measured the response of CROS aids with their special earmolds and demonstrated a marked decrease of response below 1500 Hz, with little or no gain below 800 Hz. Lybarger (1968) followed up on these results by writing that the "really great importance of CROS lies in its ability to give good hearing to the bilateral case where the hearing (better ear) is nearly normal in the low frequencies and drops down or off rapidly above . . . 1000 Hz." He is pointing out that as a result of the shunting of low-frequency gain, CROS can be applied to these individuals without fear of over amplifying. Low-frequency sounds reach the ear naturally. This application of CROS was not originally anticipated.

In a follow-up study of CROS users, Aufricht (1972) sent questionnaires to 60 patients. Of the 54 replies, 85 percent reported satisfaction with the instrument. These results support the findings of Harford and Dodds (1966) in which great user satisfaction was reported. On the other hand, my own experiences and those of a number of other Audiologists, lead me to question these results. Apparently, even with extensive counseling and hearing aid orientation, a considerable number of CROS users eventually abandon their aids. This was demonstrated by Smedley et al. (1974) in another study of veterans. Approximately 80 percent of their CROS subjects reported using their aids less than one-half of the time. On the basis of the criteria they employed, the authors concluded that one-half of the CROS users were not obtaining sufficient benefit to warrant continued use on any consistent basis.

Special Earmolds for CROS

The primary rationale behind CROS hearing aids is to deliver sound from the side of the good ear while, at the same time, the good ear receives sound normally from that side. If a conventional earmold was used in the good ear, sound would be prevented from entering normally. An unoccluded meatus in the better ear is an essential element of the CROS principle.

Generally, two approaches can be employed: open or free-field mold, or no mold. The open mold is essentially a plastic ring that holds the tubing from the receiver nozzle in place (see Chapter 3), for ear-level CROS instrumentation, it also provides support for the aid. Since the anchor is not essential for eyeglass aids, the open mold is often dispensed with, leaving the tubing suspended in the canal. Both of these approaches allow natural sound into the ear in addition to the amplified sound. Another important reason for leaving the canal open is the resulting damping action on the low-frequency components of sound. Since most of the intensity of speech and ambient noise is in the low frequencies, and since the typical CROS user has normal hearing below 1000 Hz, without this shunting effect, overamplification of the good ear would be a major problem. A typical CROS aid with an open mold gives little or no gain below 800 Hz and relatively uniform gain above about 1500 Hz. Figure 8-3 shows the response of the same aid with a closed and an open mold. The dramatic reduction of low frequencies with the open mold is obvious.

Various other investigations into the clinical importance of the open mold have confirmed the resulting marked decrease in low-frequency amplification and a concomitant increase in speech discrimination scores and subjective user evaluation (Lybarger 1967, 1968; Dodds and Harford 1968; Green and Ross 1968; Harford 1969; Dunlavy 1970). Lybarger (1968) summed it up by stating: "With the open

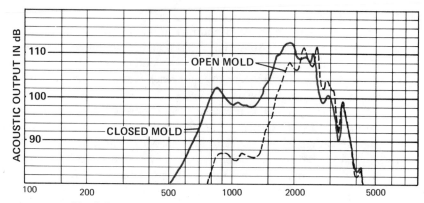

Fig. 8-3. Hearing aid response with closed and open molds.

canal arrangement, both the gain and saturation output are cut by the acoustical systems of the ear and even very loud sounds in the low frequencies would not produce an uncomfortable level through the hearing aid, as would be the case with the closed mold."

Criteria for CROS Recommendations

When considering the advisability of a CROS hearing aid, the clinician must take into account a number of factors. First, as with any fitting for a hearing aid, medical clearance should be obtained prior to a final decision. This is especially true in the case of a unilateral loss, because it may be indicative of a serious and possibly medically treatable disorder, such as chronic middle-ear pathology, Ménière's disease, or acoustic neurinoma. Second, no final decision regarding a CROS aid should be made until after a trial period of at least 30 days. It is often difficult to clinically demonstrate advantages for CROS. A trial period is essential for proper evaluation. Third, it is imperative to consider nonaudiometric factors in the selection of an appropriate hearing aid. For CROS, there are at least four areas of special consideration:

1. *What are the communication demands placed on the patient's hearing?* What are that person's communication needs? A safe rule of thumb is the greater the demand, the greater the potential benefits. Does the patient's job require frequent group conferences in which people speak to him from all directions? Is the patient commonly in social group situations?

2. *What is the status of hearing in the better ear?* As noted above, the better the hearing in this ear, the less are the chances for successful CROS use. If the good ear has a hearing loss, even if not enough to warrant an aid, the chances are greater for favorable reaction to CROS. However, the presence of normal hearing should *not* preclude a trial with CROS if it would otherwise be considered. Perhaps one of the CROS variations would be more appropriate.

3. *What is the patient's motivational level?* One who is highly motivated to improve communication ability is more likely to benefit from CROS. It can take a considerable adjustment period to successfully use CROS. Without proper motivation, as with any hearing aid, it is likely to end up in a dresser drawer. It is incumbent on the fitter to determine the motivational level and, if necessary, attempt to improve it.

4. *What is the patient's age and age at onset?* Although the age of the patient at onset of the hearing loss should not influence the decision about CROS, his present age is a factor. This is related to communication needs. A young child or a retired person may not have communication demands that would justify CROS. Ordinarily, a preschool child would not find a unilateral hearing loss enough of a handicap to justify a hearing aid. An exception, of course, would be the presence of a high-frequency loss in the better ear. When the child enters school, however, CROS should be considered.

For any one individual, the clinician may find there are other factors to be considered. These four areas are felt to be generally the most important. They have been derived from my clinical experiences as well as the experiences of others (Harford and Barry 1965; Harford and Dodds 1966, 1974; Harford 1969).

CROS Variations

As CROS instrumentation gained popularity in the mid-1960s, it became apparent that there were many hearing-impaired individuals for whom this arrangement was not satisfactory. Using great imagination and creativity, members of the hearing-health team have developed a number of variations on the original "classic CROS." These variations involve modifications of the design and applications for particular types of hearing loss. Using or eliminating the head shadow and relying on earmold modifications for frequency response alteration, these variations are allowing individuals to benefit from amplification who otherwise might not. It is now possible to meet the amplification needs of the vast majority of the hard-of-hearing population.

The first group of variations are those retaining the original CROS principle, but modifying the hearing aid/earmold coupling or the sound pickup system for the frequency response of the amplifier.

CLASSIC CROS

For review, the classic CROS, housed in either eyeglass or ear-level casings, consists of a microphone on the poorer ear side and a receiver on the better ear side. Sound picked up on the impaired side is delivered to the good ear via an open earmold. The objective of this mode is to provide the person with better hearing for speech that originates on the off (poorer) side. Classic CROS is optimally used in cases of unilateral hearing loss with a mild high frequency hearing loss in the better ear. Figure 8-2 presents a diagrammatic view of classic CROS.

HIGH CROS

Identical to classic CROS in configuration, high CROS utilizes high-frequency emphasis (HFE) instruments to further reduce low-frequency response. It is intended for bilateral high-frequency hearing losses for which classic CROS would not provide sufficient gain. High CROS utilizes the head shadow by using the natural attenuation of the head to provide more amplification of the high frequencies without feedback. An open mold is used with this modification.

MINI CROS

When it was discovered that the original CROS arrangement was not adequate for a better ear exhibiting normal responses, the mini-CROS was developed. It is the same as classic CROS except that there is no tubing from the receiver nozzle. Sound escapes directly from the nozzle, which is simply directed toward the concha. Moderate to high-gain instruments are frequently utilized because much of the amplified sound dissipates before reaching the ear. Since the microphone and receiver are separated by the head, higher output can be used without feedback problems. In other words, mini-CROS both uses and eliminates the head shadow.

FOCAL CROS

Some individuals with precipitous high frequency hearing losses cannot successfully use high CROS. Apparently they do not receive sufficient high-frequency amplification. Focal-CROS instruments are designed with a nozzle at the microphone port. A length of tubing is attached to the nozzle and extends into the meatus of the off-side ear. Thus sound is picked up in the canal, taking advantage of the resonant characteristics of the external meatus to enhance high frequencies. Some focal-CROS instruments have the microphone at the canal end of the tubing. Others retain the microphone within the aid case. With either arrangement, focal CROS reduces the need for high gain since the meatus enhances the frequencies between 2500 and 5000 Hz by 8–12 dB, resulting in less low-frequency amplification and lower distortion.

Harford and Dodds (1974) suggest two additional possible uses for focal CROS. One would be for persons working outdoors. The sound pickup may reduce annoyance from wind noise. The other is in noisy environments. The aid may reduce background noise amplification by increasing the S/N ratio through capitalizing on the acoustic attenuation offered by the pinna.

The next variations utilize two microphones delivering sound to one ear. Coincidentally, one of the first references in the literature to a special hearing aid for unilateral hearing loss employed this principle (Fowler 1960).

BICROS

Figure 8-4 illustrates the principle of BICROS, in which there is one microphone on each side sending signals to one receiver. BICROS is used in cases with one ear unaidable and the other aidable, that is, a profound loss in one ear and a moderate loss in the other. With this arrangement, sound is picked up from both

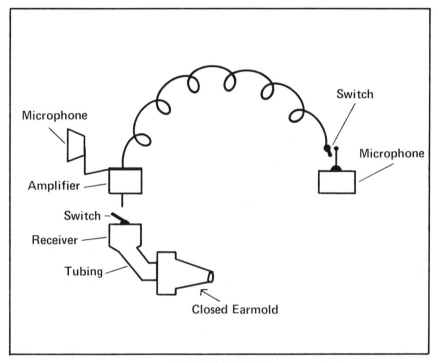

Fig. 8-4. BICROS.

sides and delivered to the better ear, in essence, giving the user two-sided hearing with one hearing aid. The off-side microphone pickup eliminates head shadow effects. A standard vented or occluding earmold is employed to allow the use of maximum gain when needed.

OPEN BICROS

This configuration is the same as BICROS except that it utilizes an open earmold or tubing alone rather than an occluding mold. It is most appropriate in cases exhibiting one unaidable ear and one ear with a high-frequency hearing loss. In this situation, an open mold is necessary to the comfort and effective amplification use derived from the resulting low-frequency damping.

MULTI-CROS

If an individual exhibits one unaidable and one aidable ear and has a wide variety of listening needs, one may consider multi-CROS. Harford and Dodds (1974) call this configuration the "epitome of flexibility." This instrument can be used as a classic CROS, BICROS, open BICROS, or conventional monaural aid. It is essentially a BICROS instrument with a separate on/off switch for each microphone. Examples of the uses that can be made of multi-CROS are: (1) in social settings or meetings where speech is originating on both sides, both microphones are on in a BICROS mode; (2) for conversation with only one person or in a noisy location, only the off-side microphone is on in a classic CROS mode; (3) if excessive ambient noise arises from the poorer side, only the on-side microphone is activated in a monaural mode; and (4) multi-CROS can also be constructed as focal CROS, mini-CROS, high CROS, or IROS (see below), depending on the needs of the individual.

Although multi-CROS is potentially very flexible, one must consider the warning of Dunlavy (1970) that "anytime you add another switch, another wire, another microphone, another receiver, or divide the instrument in any way, you are creating a potential source of trouble (breakdowns and repairs)."

The next two variations are considered by some as not true CROS modifications. However, they do employ certain CROS principles.

IROS

Ipsilateral routing of signal (IROS) instruments are monaural hearing aids using an open earmold. This term was coined by Green (1969) to differentiate it from monaural aids in which a closed mold is used. Since the aided ear is open and low frequencies are therefore damped, IROS can only be used in instances requiring relatively low gain, most often with high-frequency hearing losses. If the user has two aidable ears, binaural IROS can be employed.

The rationale for IROS is that if adequate gain can be achieved ipsilaterally without feedback, there is no reason to locate the microphone on a contralateral ear. If one carefully examines the configurations previously described, it is apparent that one of the primary reasons for placing the microphones on the off side is to take advantage of the head shadow to obtain greater gain without feedback.

CRIS-CROS

Ross (1969) points out that when two body aids are worn by an individual with severe bilateral hearing losses, these instruments do not provide true binaural hearing. The primary drawback is that the microphones are not separated by the 6–7 inches between the ears and do not have the head between them for attenuation. He suggests using two complete ear-level instruments in a double CROS or cris-CROS arrangement. In this way the user can take advantage of the head shadow to obtain maximum gain in each ear and still retain the two-eared differences.

Comments

It is my opinion that the "naming game" of CROS variations is getting out of hand. The potential number of variations on the original arrangement are probably infinite—modifying tubing or earmold, changing microphone location, altering amplification characteristics of the aid, and so on. These devices are designed to overcome some of the off-side, feedback, and response shaping problems. It would seem to be much more efficient to think in terms of two arrangements, modified as needed—CROS and BICROS.

The classic CROS can be modified in many ways: a high-frequency emphasis aid (high CROS) can be used: receiver tubing (mini-CROS) eliminated; sound pickup altered (focal CROS); a closed mold and a high-gain unit (power CROS) used; or two CROS aids can be used simultaneously (cris-cros).

BICROS can also be modified in various ways: use an open mold (open BICROS) or put in a switch to control either or both microphones (multi-CROS).

Conclusions

When one becomes familiar with the countless CROS-type hearing aids now commercially available, one realizes that great strides have been made in our ability to meet the communication needs of the hearing-impaired. The clinician can now choose amplification devices that begin to maximize communicative abilities. Although there are now CROS modifications for almost any unilateral and most bilateral hearing losses, it is inevitable that the future holds even more variations. The clinician must always be careful not to be lulled into thinking that any hearing aid solves the patients communication problems. It is a major step, but must be supplemented with other appropriate habilitative and rehabilitative measures.

ASSISTIVE LISTENING DEVICES

In recent years, a variety of products have been developed to solve one or more specific listening problems for the hearing-impaired as well as for those with normal hearing. *Assistive listening devices* (ALDs) can be an adjunct to a hearing aid, used by the hearing-impaired individual who does not use hearing aids, or used by someone with normal hearing who has special listening requirements.

For purposes of this discussion, assistive devices will be grouped into three categories: listening devices, telephone devices, and alerting/alarm devices. This discussion will not include material concerning the various hardwire and FM auditory training systems currently on the market or material regarding group and auditorium listening systems. Suffice it to say that most of the listening systems that are described below are also available in larger models designed for classrooms, theaters, or churches.

Listening Devices

Essentially, listening devices are designed to deliver sound directly to the listener, who has direct control over the intensity of the sound through a personal receiver. These devices help to overcome the common problems of background noise, distance, and reverberation. While hearing aids are designed to assist the hearing-impaired individual in almost all listening environments, listening devices are designed to help in only one or just a few situations and are designed for short-term use, while hearing aids are designed for full-time use.

TV LISTENING SYSTEMS

One of the most common problems encountered by individuals with hearing impairment, from relatively mild to profound, is difficulty in hearing and understanding sound from the television. If hearing-impaired individuals turn the volume on the television high enough to be comfortable for them, regardless of whether they are wearing hearing aids, other people in the home and, possibly, neighbors complain about the loudness of the sound.

Three styles of audio systems and one video system have been developed to assist the hearing-impaired with these difficulties. They include infrared carrier wave products, electromagnetic induction loop systems, hardwire amplification devices, and closed-caption decoders.

Infrared carrier systems. Infrared light waves are just beyond the red end of the visible spectrum and are invisible to humans. This concept is utilized in a number of TV systems currently on the market. A microphone picks up the sound from the loudspeaker of the television and transmits it to an infrared converter, usually placed on top of the television set. The converter changes the electrical energy to light energy and transmits it on an infrared carrier beam. The listener wears a receiver containing an infrared light-sensing "eye." The light energy is then converted to sound energy, the intensity of which is regulated by a volume control on the receiver. The user wears lightweight earphones.

In this way, hearing-impaired individuals can maintain control over the loudness they receive, while the volume on the TV is set to a level comfortable for others. While the sound quality is excellent with these systems, there are certain limitations to their use. The "eye" of the receiver must be in a direct line with the emitting elements of the transmitter. Fortunately, all the individual infrared systems are either sufficiently lightweight to be rotated to directly face the receiver unit or have multiangle emitting elements.

The ease of use of such systems makes them readily adaptable for use in larger environments, such as auditoriums (requiring multiple transmitters to cover the large area), noisy areas such as large meetings or cocktail lounges, where certain individuals may want to listen to a radio or television broadcast, and courtrooms.

Electromagnetic induction loop TV systems. These systems utilize the same principle as classroom loop-amplification systems. They allow for physical mobility of the user, which some other systems do not permit. The only requirements are that the user must have a hearing aid with a functional "telephone" switch and stay within the area of the loop. With this system, a microphone picks up sound from the TV or radio loudspeaker and transmits it to an amplifier/transducer that is connected to a coil loop placed around the perimeter of the room. The transducer converts the electrical energy from the microphone into electromagnetic waves. This electromagnetic energy is transmitted through the wire loop and picked up by the induction coil in the hearing aid. The user then has direct control over the intensity of the received signal via the volume control of the hearing aid. Loop systems are susceptible to outside electrical interference and do not always maintain a uniform signal over a given area. One of the primary advantages of this, as well as infrared and hardwire systems, is the maintenance of a good signal-to-noise ratio for the listener. Another factor that must be evaluated when considering the use of a loop system is the efficiency to the telecoil in the hearing aid. Use of a high-gain hearing aid does not ensure high gain with the use of the telecoil. Additionally, it is dangerous to assume that the frequency response of the telecoil will be the same as that of the hearing aid. It would be necessary for the hearing aid user to have a demonstration of such a system in a dispenser's office before purchasing it.

Hardwire amplifier systems. Chronologically among the earliest assistive systems used by the hearing-impaired, hardwire systems, as the name implies, utilize a direct wire connection between the microphone, amplifier, and receiver, either direct audio input to a hearing aid or external earphones worn by the user. While this type of system lends itself very well to multiple inputs and multiple receivers, there are the obvious disadvantages of the hardwiring. Such systems are used less frequently today than in the past and are commonly being replaced by frequency modulated (FM) and infrared systems.

Closed-caption decoders. Many television programs today are accompanied by "subtitle" presentation of the words being spoken along the bottom of the TV screen. This captioning is invisible on a standard television set unless a special closed caption decoder is employed. This type of system is most advantageous for the severely and profoundly hearing-impaired individual who cannot enjoy the sound from television even with a hearing aid or any of the above-described assistive systems. This system allows the individual to "see" the dialogue while still enjoying the other visual aspects of the television program.

PERSONAL LISTENING DEVICES

Many hearing-impaired individuals have difficulty in conversational situations, even when using hearing aids, because of the severity of their loss, high levels of background noise, or both. Individual listening devices generally consist of a microphone, amplifier, and earphone receiver. Because they are larger than a typical hearing aid, most personal listening systems have a broader frequency response and greater gain capability than do most hearing aids. Additionally, because the microphone of the system can be positioned close to the sound source, the signal-to-noise ratio can be significantly improved. Many of the personal systems are also usable with a neck loop induction coil that is utilized with the telecoil of the hearing aid.

Telephone Assistive Devices

In addition to loud bell ringers and light signalers for use with the telephone, which are discussed below, a variety of telephone amplifiers are currently on the market. There are three categories of these types of devices, volume control in the telephone handset, add-on amplifiers for use with modular telephones, and portable amplifiers that are attached to the receiver of any telephone. All of these can be of significant benefit to the hearing-impaired and normal hearing population who have difficulty understanding conversation on the telephone.

Another type of assistive device for use with the telephone is the *telecommunications device for the deaf (TDD)*, computerized systems that utilize a typed message for transmission and reception via the telephone, and LED display for the typed message and/or a printer. Both the sender and the receiver of the telephonic communication must have the TDD devices. The telephone handsets are placed in the TDD unit by both the sender and the receiver. The sender types the message, which is converted to electronic impulses and transmitted over telephone lines and converted to the visual display at the receiving end. They are designed for the profoundly hearing-impaired. Most telephone companies are allowing special long-distance rates for registered TDD users. Also, many public service companies, as well as a number of private businesses, have some type of TDD communication system available for their deaf customers.

Alerting/Alarm Devices

Advances in electronic technology have allowed for the development of a number of alerting and/or alarm devices for the hearing-impaired. The alerting/alarm signals utilize the visual, tactile, or auditory sensory modalities. In other words, the signal can be a flashing light, a loud horn or bell, or a vibratory stimulus. The alerting/alarm devices are designed for a multiplicity of uses, including alerting an individual when the phone or doorbell rings, an alarm clock sounds, a smoke detector goes off, or a baby cries.

The various systems allow for a variety of signals to be used, as described above. For example, the phone or doorbell ringing can cause a light to flash or a loud horn to sound. An alarm clock sounding can cause a bright light to flash or a pillow or bed vibrator to be activated. Many of them are also available with personal vibrating units that are activated as a signal that a baby is crying, a phone or doorbell is ringing, or the smoke detector is sounding. For the hearing-impaired, these alerting/alarm devices can be extremely useful, even life-saving. For those with normal hearing, these alerting devices can be useful in knowing when the baby is crying or the phone is ringing in another room in the house. Additionally, the flashing light and loud horn alerting systems have also been utilized in various work environments where either ambient noise levels are too high to allow a phone ring to be heard or where the sound from a ringing phone would be detrimental, that is, a television or radio studio.

Needs of the Marketplace

Assistive listening devices are finally coming of age. They are a much-needed adjunct to conventional hearing aids for the hearing-impaired. Hearing aids do not yet meet all the needs of the hearing-impaired population. Assistive devices allow these individuals to lead a more active life and participate in activities they enjoy.

However, most of the population are not aware of assistive devices. It is incumbent on all members of the hearing health team to acquaint the public with these systems. Display and demonstration centers in office waiting rooms are an excellent means of conveying information to the public. Additionally, public service programs and multimedia advertising will assist in getting the message across.

Appendices at the end of this chapter present sources of information about ALDs and their manufacturers and distributors.

ACOUSTIC RESONATORS

At one time or another everyone has cupped a hand behind their ear in order to hear better. The effect of this action is to make speech a little easier to hear. Figure 8-5 displays probe microphone open-ear resonance curves, with and without a hand cupped behind the ear. As can be seen, the effect of cupping the ear is to lower the resonant frequency and increase the amplitude at the lower peak frequency by about 11 dB.

This phenomenon has been utilized for centuries to assist the hearing-impaired. As Berger describes in chapter 1, ear trumpets, speaking tubes, and ear inserts served as sound collectors to make better use of natural ear resonance amplification. These devices are based on the principle of the Helmholtz resonator, developed in

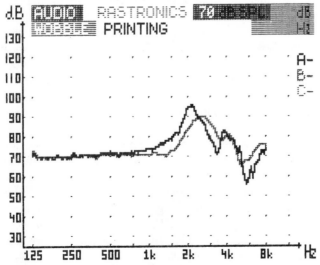

Fig. 8-5. Open-ear resonance curves measured with probe microphone. (A) ear cupped; (B) normal resonance.

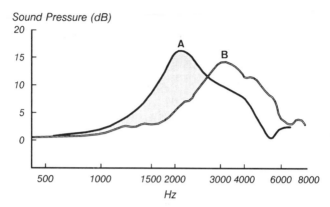

Fig. 8-6. Shift in ear resonance peak and amplitude caused by an acoustic resonator: (A) effect of resonator; (B) normal resonance. (Courtesy of Innovative Hearing Corp.)

the mid-1800s, demonstrating that all cavities have a resonant frequency at which the walls vibrate sympathetically, increasing amplitude (Gerber 1974).

In the past few years, new products have been introduced that are small adaptations of the Helmholtz acoustic resonance principle. At the time of this writing, there are two such devices on the market: the Innovaid 600, manufactured by Innovative Hearing Corporation, and the Earlens, developed by Sound Acoustic Systems, Inc. Both are nonelectronic ITE hearing devices that work on the principles of sound collection and acoustic resonance.

The Innovaid 600 is a custom unit, made from an impression of the ear, and tuned, within the range of about 1800–2000 Hz, while the Earlens is a stock product, available in three sizes.

The average external ear and canal resonate at about 2800 Hz, naturally amplifying sound in this range by 10–15 dB (see Chapter 2). The acoustic resonators have the effect of lowering the resonant frequency to the range of 1000–2000 Hz, shifting the natural 10–15 dB of amplification to the lower-frequency range. Both brands of resonators also cause an insertion loss above 3000 Hz. Figure 8-6 shows both the shift in resonance and insertion loss, measured in a Zwislocki coupler attached to a KEMAR ear.

Both types of acoustic resonators are intended only for individuals with a *mild hearing loss* who might not yet be ready for electronic amplification, whether psychologically or as a result of the degree of loss, but who need some assistance hearing in certain situations. According to Lampert (1986), the ideal candidate for an acoustic resonator is one demonstrating *a sensorineural loss of no more than 25–40 dB in the range from 1000 to 2000 Hz, with even better hearing in the lower frequencies.* Figure 8-7 depicts the audiogram of a person who would be considered a good candidate for an acoustic resonator.

Subjectively, the benefit of a resonator is usually very subtle. Most users of resonators report *little or no increase in the subjective loudness of sound, but a*

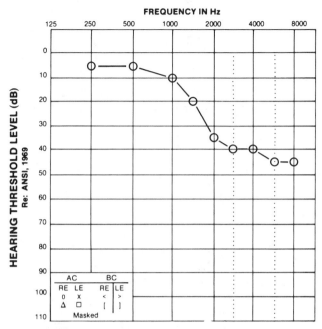

Fig. 8-7. Audiogram of a typical resonator candidate.

distinctly increased clarity of speech. In other words, speech is not perceived as louder, but noticeably more distinct—easier to understand. This is a very important concept to be stressed when counseling potential users about a resonator.

Holden (1984) reported on two research studies with 112 Innovaid 600 users. Table 8-2 presents average functional gain data for warble tone thresholds. As can be seen, between 1500 and 2000 Hz there was a gain of 9.1 to 12.4 dB, with a peak average gain at 1750 Hz. The same study revealed that 75 percent of the subjects demonstrated improved speech discrimination in noise (4–36 percent at S/N = 0).

TABLE 8-2
Average Functional Gain for Warble Tones
with the Innovaid 600*

Frequency (Hz)	Functional Gain (dB)
1000	3.0
1500	9.6
1750	12.4
2000	9.1
2500	0.3

Adapted from Holden KA: Evaluation of the Non-electronic Innovaid 600 Hearing Device and Its Effectiveness in Hearing Improvement. Innovative Hearing Corporation Report, 1984

As was noted above, the Innovaid is a custom unit, while the Earlens is a stock device available in three sizes. The Innovaid 600 is, to a limited extent, tuned during the manufacturing process. Varying the size of the cavity and the sizes of the peripheral and medial sound openings allows tuning of the acrylic Innovaid bubble within the range between 1800 Hz and slightly above 2000 Hz. Thus it can, to some extent, be designed for the needs of the user. Additionally, if worn binaurally, the two units can be tuned to slightly different frequencies, resulting in a wider summated resonance peak. This tuning capability seems to be an advantage of a custom resonator over a stock unit.

In my experience, acoustic resonators have a very limited, but definite, applicability. They are potentially useful for individuals with a mild loss and high motivation. There are certain advantages of resonators over conventional hearing aids for someone with such a loss: (1) the amplification is more natural, eliminating electronic distortion problems; (2) because resonators are not electronic, there are no feedback difficulties; (3) there is no electronic circuit noise that often bothers hearing aid users who have a mild loss; (4) they can be easily inserted and removed for use when needed; and (5) they can be readily cleaned in water and are not subject to breakdown from moisture, as are electronic aids.

There are also disadvantages to the use of resonators. First, successful electronic hearing aid users generally do not function well with resonators because they do not experience any increase in loudness. Second, resonators do not offer much assistance when used in the presence of high levels of ambient noise. This is apparently due to the high-frequency insertion loss. Third, they cannot usually be used successfully in the wind because even the slight breeze caused by walking outdoors can be focused through the sound port and be very noisy. One patient I fitted with binaural resonators, with a strong caveat not to wear them outside, rejected them after experiencing high wind noise and resulting headaches while playing golf on two occasions. Fourth, because they are made of lightweight plastic, they are subject to breakage. Fifth, they are of limited value for use with the telephone. Sixth, resonators are of value only in a limited number of situations, such as watching TV, in small groups and theater, or church. Seventh, it has been my experience that if a patient is not successful in using a resonator, it is difficult to them convert them to using electronic aids.

Appropriate counseling is critical when fitting resonators. It is very important that the patient have realistic expectations of the benefits and limitations related to their use. Also, the user must acknowledge their communication problems and be motivated to do something about them. If both of these conditions do not exist, prognosis for success is very limited.

Acoustic resonators are not intended to be a replacement for electronic hearing aids, but as a complement to them. Some people with a mild hearing loss either cannot or will not use hearing aids. For many of these people, resonators can be an interim form of assistance until their hearing loss increases to the point where they can use or will accept conventional aids. Resonators fill a need for a segment of the hearing-impaired population, if fit judiciously and with proper counseling.

REFERENCES

Monaural/Binaural/Pseudobinaural Hearing Aids

Arnst DJ: Binaural amplification in cases with central auditory deficit. Hearing J, 39:27-29, 1986

Belzile M, Markle DM: A clinical comparison of monaural and binaural hearing aids worn by patients with conductive or perceptive deafness. Laryngoscope 69:1317-1323, 1959

Bergman M: Binaural hearing. Arch Otolaryngol 66:572-578, 1957

Black JW, Hast MH: Speech reception with altering signal. J Speech Hearing Res 5:70-75, 1962

Carhart R: The usefulness of the binaural hearing aid. J Speech Hearing Disorders 23:41-51, 1958

Cherry EC, Bowles J: Contributions to a study of the cocktail party problem. J Acoust Soc Am 32:884, 1960

Cox RM, Bisset JD: Relationship between two measures of aided binaural advantage. J Speech Hearing Disorders 49:399-408, 1984

Curran JR: ITE aids for children: Survey of attitudes and practices of audiologists. Hearing Instruments 36:20-25, 1985

Davis H, Silverman SR: Hearing and Deafness. New York, Holt, Rinehart, & Winston, 1970, p 286

Decroix G, Dehaussey J: Binaural hearing and intelligibility. J Auditory Res 4:115-134, 1964

DiCarlo LM, Brown WJ: The effectiveness of binaural hearing aids for adults with hearing impairments. J Auditory Res 1:35-76, 1960

Dirks D, Carhart R: A survey of reactions from users of binaural and monaural hearing aids. J Speech Hearing Disorders 27:311-322, 1962

Dirks D, Wilson R: The effect of spatially separated sound sources on speech intelligibility. J Speech Hearing Res 12:5-38, 1969a

Dirks D, Wilson R: Binaural hearing of speech for aided and unaided conditions. J Speech Hearing Res 12:650-664, 1969b

Dirks D, Moncur JP: Interaural intensity and time differences in anechoic and reverberant rooms. J Speech Hearing Res 10:177-185, 1967

Erdman SA, Sedge RK: Preferences for binaural amplification. Hearing J 39:33-36, 1986

Fletcher H: Speech and Hearing in Communication. Princeton, NJ, D Van Nostrand, 1953

Gelfand SA, Hochberg I: Binaural and monaural speech discrimination under reverberation. Annual Meeting of the Acoustical Society of America, 1973

Harris JD: Monaural and binaural speech intelligibility and the stereophonic effect based upon temporal cues. Laryngoscope 75:428-446, 1965

Haskins H, Hardy W: Clinical studies in stereophonic hearing. Laryngoscope 70:1427-1432, 1960

Hawkins DB, Yacullo W: The signal-to-noise ratio advantage of binaural hearing aids and directional microphones under different levels of reverberation. J Speech Hearing Disorders 49:278-286, 1984

Hedgecock LD, Sheets BV: A comparison of monaural and binaural hearing aids for listening to speech. Arch Otolaryngol 68:624-629, 1958

Heffler AJ, Schultz MD: Some implications of binaural signal selection for hearing aid evaluation. J Speech Hearing Res 7:279-289, 1964

Hirsh IJ: Binaural hearing aids—a review of some experiments. J Speech Hearing Disorders 15:114–123, 1950

Huizing HC, Taselaar M: Experiments on binaural hearing. Acta Otolaryngologica 53:151–154, 1961

Jerger J, Dirks D: Binaural hearing aids, and enigma. J Acoust Soc Am 33:537–538, 1961

Jerger J, Carhart R, Dirks D: Binaural hearing aids and speech intelligibility. J Speech Hearing Res 4:137–148, 1961

Kodman F: Successful binaural hearing aid users. Arch Otolaryngol 73:302–304, 1961

Koenig W: Subjective effects in binaural hearing. J Acoust Soc Am 22:61–62, 1950

Langford BG: Why binaural? Audecibel 19:151–158, 1970

Lankford S, Faires W: Objective evaluation of monaural versus binaural amplification for congenitally hard of hearing children. Paper presented at Meeting of the American Speech Hearing Association, Detroit, 1973

Libby ER: Binaural Hearing and Amplification, Vols. I and II. Chicago, Zenetron, 1980

Libby ER: Binaural amplification. Ear Hearing 2:183–233, 1981

Lybarger SF: Advantages and limitations of the "Y" cord. Hearing Aid J 26:6, 34, 1973

Markides A: Binaural Hearing Aids. London, Academic Press, 1977

Markle DM, Aber WA: Clinical evaluation of monaural and binaural hearing aids. Arch Otolaryngol 67:606–608, 1958

Mueller HG: Binaural amplification: Attitudinal factors. Hearing J 39:7–10, 1986

Pascoe DP: Hearing aid evaluation, in Katz J (ed): Handbook of Clinical Audiology (ed 3). Baltimore, Williams & Wilkins, 1985, pp 527–549

Scandinavian Audiology: Binaural effects in normal and impaired hearing. Supplement 15, 1982

Tillman T, Kasten R, Horner J: The effect of the head shadow on the reception of speech. Paper presented at Convention of the American Speech and Hearing Association, Chicago, 1963

Wright HN, Carhart R: The efficiency of binaural listening among the hearing-impaired. Arch Otolaryngol 72:789–797, 1960

Wright HN: Binaural hearing and the hearing-impaired. Arch Otolaryngol 70:485–494, 1959

Zelnick E: Options in the fitting of binaural hearing aids. Nat Hearing Aid J 23:89–37, 1970a

Zelnick E: Comparison of speech perception utilizing monotic and dichotic modes of listening. J Auditory Res 10:87–97, 1970b

CROS and Its Variations

Aufricht H: A follow-up study of the CROS hearing aid. J Speech Hearing Disorders 37:113–117, 1972

Bergman M: Binaural hearing. Arch Otolaryngol 66:572–578, 1957

Dodds E, Harford E: Modified earpieces and CROS for high frequency hearing losses. J Speech Hearing Res 11:204–218, 1968

Dunlavy AR: CROS: The new miracle worker. Audecibel 29:141–148, 1970

Fowler EP: Bilateral hearing aids for monaural total deafness: A suggestions for better hearing. Arch Otolaryngol 72:57–58, 1960

Green DS: Nonoccluding earmolds with CROS and IROS hearing aids. Arch Otolaryngol 89:512–522, 1969

Green DS, Ross M: The effect of a conventional versus a nonoccluding (CROS-type) earmold upon the frequency response of a hearing aid. J Speech Hearing Res 11:638–647, 1968

Harford E: Bilateral CROS. Arch Otolaryngol 84:426–432, 1966

Harford E: Recent developments in the use of ear-level hearing aids. Maico Audiological Library Series 5(3), 1967

Harford E: Is a hearing aid ever justified in a unilateral hearing loss? Otol Clin N Am 153–173, 1969

Harford E, Barry J: A rehabilitative approach to the problem of unilateral hearing impairment: The contralateral routing of signals (CROS). J Speech Hearing Disorders 30:121–138, 1965

Harford E, Dodds E: The clinical application of CROS. Arch Otolaryngol 83:455–464, 1966

Harford E, Dodds E: Versions of the CROS hearing aid. Arch Otolaryngol 100:50–58, 1974

Harford E, Musket C: Binaural hearing with one hearing aid. J Speech Hearing Disorders 29:133–146, 1964

Lybarger SF: Earmold acoustics. Audecibel 16:9–20, 1967

Lybarger SF: Some comments on CROS. Nat Hearing Aid J 21:8, 1968

Ross M: Changing concepts in hearing aid candidacy. Maico Audiological Library Series 7(10), 1969

Schaudinischky LH: New hearing aid for the monaurally deaf restoring binaural hearing. Arch Otolaryngol 60:461–466, 1965

Smedley TC, von Khaelsberg J, Clement JR: Success and failure patterns among CROS and BICROS users. Paper presented at Meeting of the American Speech and Hearing Association, Las Vegas, 1974

Tillman T, Kasten R, Horner J: The effect of the head shadow on the reception of speech. Paper presented at Meeting of the American Speech and Hearing Association, Chicago, 1963

Wullstein HL, Wigand ME: A hearing aid for single ear deafness and its requirements. Acta Otolaringologica 54:136–142, 1962

Acoustic Resonators

Gerber SE: Introductory Hearing Science. Philadelphia, Saunders, 1974

Holden KA: Evaluation of the Non-electronic Innovaid 600 Hearing Device and Its Effectiveness in Hearing Improvement. Innovative Hearing Corporation report, 1984

Lampert JL: The acoustic resonator: Selecting candidates. Hearing Instruments 37:40–43, 1986

Appendix A

Sources of Information about Assistive Listening Devices

Council on Assistive Devices and Listening Systems (COADLS)
P.O. Box 32227
Washington, DC 20007

Consumers Organization for the Hearing-Impaired (COHI)
P.O. Box 8188
Silver Spring, MD 20907

National Association for Hearing and Speech Action (NAHSA)
10801 Rockville Pike
Rockville, MD 20852

The Organization for the Use of the Telephone (OUT)
P.O. Box 175
Owings Mills, MD 21117

Self Help for Hard-of-Hearing People, Inc. (SHHH)
4848 Battery Lane, Suite 100
Bethesda, MD 20814

The Washington Area Group for the Hard-of Hearing (WAG-HOH)
P.O. Box 6283
Silver Spring, MD 20906

Appendix B

Manufacturers and Distributors of Assistive Listening Devices

Products Key

1. Personal amplifiers
2. Infrared TV listening system
3. Induction-loop TV listening system
4. Hardwire TV listening system
5. Visual alerting devices

6. Auditory alerting devices
7. Tactile alerting devices
8. TDD/TTY
9. Telephone amplifiers
10. Telecaption decoders

American Communication Corp. 5,8
180 Roberts Street
East Hartford, CT 06108
(203) 289-3491

Audex 1,2
713 N. 4th Street
P.O. Box 3263
Longview, TX 75606
(214) 753-7058

Audiobionics Inc. 8
9817 Valley View Road
Eden Prairie, MN 55344
(612) 941-5464

Hearing Aid Center, Kalamazoo 1
P.O. Box 3055
Kalamazoo, MI 49003
(616) 381-6930

Hal Hen Company Inc. 1,3,4,5,7,9,10
P.O. Box 6077
Long Island City, NY 11106
(718) 392-6020

Heidico, Inc. 5,6,7,8,9,10
444 S. Montezuma Street
Prescott, AZ 86301
(602) 445-9554

Julian A. McDermott Corp. 5
1639 Stephen Street
Ridgewood, NY 11385
(718) 456-3606

Krown Research, Inc. 8
6300 Arizona Circle
Los Angles, CA 90045
(213) 641-4306

Metavox, Inc. 1
8375 Leesburg Pike, #421
Vienna, VA 21180
(703) 759-2995

Nady Systems, Inc. 2
1145 65th Street
Oakland, CA 94608
(415) 652-2411

National Captioning Institute 10
5203 Leesburg Pike
Falls Church, VA 22041
(703) 998-2471

National Hearing Aid Distrib., Inc.
1,4,9
145 Tremont Street
Boston, MA 02111
(800) 343-2266

National Technical Systems 5
26525 Golden Valley Road
Saugus, CA 91350
(805) 251-6622

Nationwide Flashing Signal Systems,
Inc. 5,7
8120 Fenton Stree
Silver Spring, MD 20910
(301) 589-6671

Oticon Corporation 3
29 Schoolhouse Road
Somerset, NJ 08873
(800) 526-3921

Oval Window Audio 3
306 Congress Street
Portland, ME 04101
(207) 775-7292

Phone-TTY Incorporated, Inc. 5,7,8
202 Lerington Avenue
Hackensack, NJ 07601
(201) 489-7889

Phonic Ear, Inc. 1,9
250 Camino Alto
Mill Valley, CA 94941
(800) 227-0735

Precision Controls, Inc. 5,7,8
14 Doty Rd.
Wanaque, NJ 07420
(201) 835-5000

Quest Electronics 7
510 S. Worthington St.
Oconomowoe, WI 53066
(414) 567-9157

Rastronics USA, Inc. 1,3,5,6,7,9
1125 Globe Ave.
Mountainside, NJ 07092
(201) 654-6034

Sonic Alert, Inc. 5,6,7
209 Voorheis Street
Pontiac, MI 48043
(313) 858-8957

Siemens Hearing Instruments, Inc.
2,7,9
685 Liberty Ave.
Union, NJ 07083
(800) 631-7965

Ultratec, Inc. 5,8
6442 Normandy Lane
Madison, WI 53719
(608) 273-0707

Unex Corporation 2
5 Liberty Way
Westford, MA 01886
(617) 692-3000

Westclox Div., General Time Corp. 5
520 Guthridge Court
Norcross, GA 30092
(404) 447-5300

Wheelock, Inc. 5,6
273 Branchport Avenue
Long Branch, NJ 07740
(201) 222-6880

Williams Sound Corp. 1,3,4
6844 Washington Ave. South
Eden Prairie, MN 55344
(612) 941-2896

Daniel L. Bode

9

Speech Signals and Hearing Aids

One of the most common misconceptions held by the general public is that hearing aids can restore hearing to normal. Anyone who believes this and begins to wear an aid is suddenly made aware that this is not the case. This appears to be the number one reason why so many hearing aids end up in a dresser drawer. In another chapter of this book, Derek Sanders points out the importance of providing the hearing aid user with realistic expectations. Understanding why hearing aids do not generally restore normal auditory functioning and being able to explain this to your patients is a major step in realizing these expectations.

In this chapter, Dan Bode undertakes the task of explaining many of the questions often asked by lay persons and members of the hearing health team. Relating basic principles of speech acoustics and noise interactions to hearing aid hardware and physiological dysfunction in the ear, Dan describes some of the complex relationships between speech signals and hearing aids.

MCP

This chapter is an overview of the major interactions among speech signals, noise, hearing aids, and impaired listeners. The topic is complicated by many variables associated with (1) speech acoustics, (2) noise spectra, (3) electroacoustics of hearing aids, (4) complex speech—noise interactions, (5) earmold acoustics, and (6) variability among sensorineural listeners in degree and configuration of hearing impairment.

Any one of these topics could be the sole focus of this chapter. Of necessity, discussion in this chapter is general rather than particular. The cited references will

AMPLIFICATION FOR THE HEARING-IMPAIRED, THIRD EDITION

aid the interested reader who wishes to pursue further the specifics of a topic that is briefly described here.

Two issues are addressed regarding persons with sensorineural hearing impairment: (1) why hearing aids typically do *not* restore hearing to normal and (2) why we are not able to prescribe hearing aids at present. The review moves from speech acoustics to speech—noise interactions, then to sources and types of distortion along the path from talker to listener, and finally, to a discussion of the two questions posed above. Throughout the review, practical limitations of current clinical knowledge are emphasized.

CHARACTERISTICS OF SPEECH SIGNALS

Complexities of Speech

Speech acoustics are complicated because of the instant-to-instant interactions of sound pressure, frequency, phase, and duration. Sound pressure levels (SPL) for soft, conversational, and loud speech at a distance of 1 m are approximately 50, 65, and 80 dB, respectively. These average values typically describe overall measures of low-frequency vowel components. Consonants, which are generally more important for speech perception, may have average levels about 20 dB less than these values (House et al. 1965, Pickett 1980). However, the acoustic cues for consonant perception cannot be easily considered independent of the vowel environment. Many important cues are contained within vowel–consonant and consonant–vowel transitions as a consequence of coarticulation during production (Liberman et al. 1967).

In the frequency domain, speech contains components that are important for speech perception covering a range from about 100 Hz to at least 5000–6000 Hz. However, it is impossible to say which frequency components are most important to a listener because of at least three considerations: the type of listener, the type of listening task, and the objectives of an audiologist in a given situation, such as diagnostic testing, hearing aid evaluation, auditory training, prediction of an individual's performance and needs in work, academic or social environments. One must consider the entire frequency range from 100 to 6000 Hz as potentially important, depending on unique considerations. For example, in working with a child who is learning speech and language, we may wish to emphasize low frequencies (100–1000 Hz) so that the child might benefit from prosodic cues (pitch, duration, loudness), whereas under other listening conditions (e.g., noise backgrounds, consonant perception training) emphasis of high frequencies may be the desired goal.

Durational characteristics of speech further complicate our topic. Vowels and some consonants may have durations at average talking rates of approximately 100–200 msec, while many consonants (plosives in particular) may be as short as 40–50 msec (Liberman et al. 1967). Normal listeners can easily make use of these cues, despite the fact that hearing sensitivity decreases substantially as the duration of a signal is reduced. Temporal integration and other time-oriented characteristics of auditory perception *may* be dramatically worsened for some sensorineural listeners (Gengel 1972).

During high-level output at the receiver stage, hearing aid transducers may not be able to follow short-duration signals without considerable distortion. That is, the aid may add transient distortion both by altering the speech signal and by continued response after the original signal ceases, possibly masking the next phoneme. (See Chapter 2 for a description and discussion of transient distortion.)

Many of the acoustic components in speech occur simultaneously (in parallel) as a result of coarticulation of phonemes. The acoustic results of primary interest here are the transient features of plosives (p, b, t, d, k, g, ch, dz). These phonemes represent about 25 percent of the consonants in spoken English and thus are very important for speech perception. Not only do some impaired listeners have difficulty hearing these cues even through high-fidelity earphones, but output transducers of hearing aids may not be able to reproduce these transients without distortion.

Since transient speech sounds have rapidly changing sound pressures, frequencies, and durations, it is a challenge to understand how normal listeners perceive these cues. It is even more intriguing to know how hearing aids and impaired listeners interact to process these complex and subtle features of speech, especially when these cues are competing with environmental noises and with speech from other talkers during everyday listening. Contextual restraints and redundancy cues in connected speech probably account for many of these abilities (Sanders 1982).

Speech Perception

A fairly recent development has been the increasing awareness that criterion speech discrimination scores can be subjected to analytic study. That is, rather than only assessing performance on the basis of percentage correct perception of monosyllables, efforts have been made to determine the types of errors and confusions that impaired listeners make under aided and unaided conditions (Picard 1974). Given that we could know the types of errors a listener makes and the acoustic characteristics of the phonemes involved in the errors, we might then be in a better position to prescribe amplification.

Considerable research is needed since the topic is more complex than believed, and relevant acoustic cues for speech perception by normal listeners still is enigmatic. A variety of speech materials and analysis systems are available for research and clinical use, but normative data regarding perception of specific material have not been established for clinical use. Until more is known of these complexities, and until we have demonstrated reliable and valid assessment procedures, educated and insightful clinical evaluations remain the pragmatic approach.

One major obstacle is that we do not understand the normal speech perception processes, let alone those of hearing-impaired listeners with or without hearing aids. For analysis and/or instructional purposes we reduce the total communication system into components for convenience and ease of study. However, consideration of the total communication process seems essential if we are to understand the relevant effects of components. The need exists for operational theories of speech perception processes, especially speech perception by listeners with hearing impairment. Major attempts have been made in terms of normal processing (Stevens and House 1970, Liberman et al. 1967), and hypotheses have been offered regarding impaired reception (Carhart 1967, Boothroyd 1968). A continuing and constructive interchange among audiologists, psychologists, speech scientists, and other disciplines interested in speech perception is needed (Elkins 1984).

Intelligibility versus Prosodic Cues

Efforts are often directed toward making speech more intelligible for hearing-impaired listeners. Of additional value to human communication are the prosodic cues present in conversational speech (Liberman 1972). Pitch, duration, loudness, and juncture are important cues for language perception since subtle meanings are often conveyed through the prosody factors. For example, the two following sentences emphasize the importance of juncture cues:

1. The sons raise meat.
2. The sun's rays meet.

Given that contextual cues are not present, these types of sentences can be easily confused, but potentially more so for the impaired listener who cannot detect these subtle cues. A dramatic challenge is the severely or profoundly hearing-impaired child whose hearing loss occurred prior to the development of language. In the absence of auditory stimulation, the question arises as to whether the child can develop appropriate oral language skills. If the child does not hear prosodic cues, appropriate features are often missing in the speech of these children.

This topic becomes complicated by other existing questions. One question has been the masking effect of low frequency vowel sounds on higher frequency consonants. (Danaher et al. 1973; Danaher and Pickett 1975). Amplified vowels may reduce the impaired listener's ability to identify second transitions and other consonant cues. The paradox then becomes: Do we provide such individuals with hearing aids that emphasize low frequencies (for prosodic cues), high frequencies (for intelligibility cues), or some combination thereof?

Two practical approaches are possible in the absence of definitive clinical research. One is to select an aid that has a suitable filter control capability so that highs and lows can be independently controlled depending on the listener's needs. Another approach is to select two aids, one delivering low-frequency cues to one ear and one delivering high-frequency cues to the other. A listener could summate the two types of signals and have prosodic and intelligibility cues simultaneously or independently, depending on the particular listening situation.

The importance of prosodic cues to quality judgments and to hearing aid acceptance by a listener needs further study. Speech intelligibility may be sought at the expense of selecting aids that are comfortable in varying listening conditions and have acceptable quality for the listener. Whether these subjective benefits are amenable to positive change via auditory training procedures (and/or experience in listening during trial periods) has been subjected to preliminary appraisal (Bode and Oyer 1970).

CHARACTERISTICS OF NOISE

Just as speech signals have varying sound pressures, frequencies, and durations, noise contributes its own moment-to-moment fluctuations, complicating the task of an impaired listener attempting to use a hearing aid.

Many problems with hearing aids and their selection would be reduced if they were to be used only in "quiet" situations. Indeed, measurements of hearing aid performance are studied in quiet listening conditions only. Impaired listeners have most of their reported difficulties understanding speech in noise, and it is to alleviate these problems that they seek personal amplification.

Environmental noises in those conditions where a hearing aid is needed vary in both spectrum and duration. Frequency components are typically confined to the low frequencies (below 1000–1500 Hz), with progressively lesser amounts in the higher frequencies. The low-frequency range is where many impaired listeners have the most residual hearing. Hearing aids amplify both the desired speech signals and any environmental noises having components between the effective high- and low-frequency cutoffs of the hearing aid.

Hearing aid users often face the situation wherein whatever speech-to-noise ratio (S/N) exists at the face of a microphone also exists in their ear canals at higher levels, for *both* the speech and the noise. Aids with frequency distortion and peak clipping may worsen the existing S/N (Bode and Kasten 1971). Worsened S/N ratios may explain a major portion of the problems experienced by hearing aid users. Hearing aid use may be further compounded by alterations in speech-to-noise ratios *within the listener* due to distortions resulting from his own unique hearing impairment.

Because of these interactions, and to add face validity to test procedures, audiologists have long recognized the importance of using noise or competing speech background during hearing aid evaluations (Tillman and Olsen 1973, Goetzinger 1978, Tillman et al. 1970). Many practical objectives may be achieved by such testing. First, the speech understanding task is made more difficult than in "quiet," thus sensitizing the task to subtle differences. Second, face validity is added to the protocol in that more realistic listening environments are simulated. Third, if a particular hearing aid has greater distortion than others being evaluated, the resulting speech-to-noise ratio could be worsened with a concomitant reduction in the criterion speech understanding score. Fourth, given a differential interaction between aids and an individual listener's unique speech–noise processing abilities, the consequences can be realistically assessed by testing in noise. For these reasons, those engaged in hearing aid research and clinical evaluation of aids are increasingly making use of some form of background competition.

Agreement has not been reached regarding the type of noise, overall levels, and speech-to-noise ratios to use for research or clinical purposes (Konkle and Rintelmann 1983). The types of "noise" have included: (1) white noise (equal spectrum level at all frequencies within the passband of the earphone or loudspeaker), (2) sawtooth noise (a low-frequency fundamental with odd harmonics), (3) "speech" noise (equal spectrum levels at all frequencies up to about 1000 Hz and then 6–12 dB/octave decrease in levels above 1000 Hz, i.e., a spectrum simulating the long-term average for real speech), (4) recordings of one or more talkers producing speech, (5) cafeteria and/or traffic noises (to achieve some face validity and also to add moment-to-moment fluctuations in levels and durations), and (6) white noise that is modulated and/or interrupted.

Given the variety of possible noise backgrounds, the differences of opinions among professionals regarding *the* best noise(s) to use, and the various noise–speech interactions reported in the literature, it is not surprising that controversy surrounds this topic.

Currently, individual researchers and clinicians must make well-considered but tentative decisions, such as (1) *this* specific noise will be used for *this* specific purpose, (2) levels will be calibrated so that speech-to-noise ratios that exist during testing will be known, (3) normal listeners will be tested first in order to establish and maintain normative limits, (4) reconsideration of these decisions will be made at reasonable intervals, and (5) efforts to standardize testing conditions among clinics will be supported.

SPEECH–NOISE INTERACTIONS

Critical Ratios and Effective Masking

The "critical ratio" in decibels, and the "critical band" in hertz (Scharf 1970) have been of substantial practical and theoretical value to audiologists. Knowing, for example, the critical ratio associated with each audiometric frequency and the spectrum level (or level per cycle) of a given noise, one is able to predict average pure tone thresholds for normal and many impaired listeners in this noise.

The formula for critical ratio is:

$$(a) CR(dB) = T(N) - LPC$$

where T(N) is the established threshold in noise of the signal and LPC is the level per cycle, or spectrum level, of the wideband noise. It then follows that:

$$(b)\ T(N) = LPC + CR(dB) = EL\ (effective\ Level)$$

The calculation of spectrum level is:

$$(c)\ LPC = OL(N) - 10 \log BW$$

where OL(N) is the measured overall SPL of the noise and BW is the bandwidth of this same noise.

For example, given an OL(N) of 80 dB SPL and a "conventional" audiometric earphone having an approximate bandwidth of 10,000 Hz, and by substituting in formula (c) above, we obtain a LPC of 40 dB. Then, given a CR(dB) of about 30 dB for speech material (50 percent response level) we are able to use formula (b) above and predict a T(N) for this example of 70 dB. Most normal listeners and many impaired listeners (given that they do not have a threshold for speech in quiet of greater than this level) would be expected to demonstrate a 50 percent speech threshold of about 70 dB SPL, that is, at a -10 S/N.

Understanding the above concepts, and having the appropriate CR(dB) values for speech and for pure tones, the audiologist can calculate and calibrate the testing system so that the T(N) or "effective level" of the noise is known, whether for masking the nontest ear or for determining the levels to employ during a hearing aid evaluation procedure.

Both the effective level (EL) and the T(N) of the preceding example is 70 dB SPL. The definition of effective masking level (EML) takes into account the threshold in quiet, T(Q), in the following formula:

$$(d) EML = -T(Q) = T(N) - T(Q)$$

This formula expresses a basic definition of psychoacoustic masking: *the shift in threshold of audibility of a signal in the presence of another sound.*

The concepts and calculations given above can aid in understanding what is happening during many clinical test procedures. They are also helpful in comparing normal and impaired performance in "simple" listening conditions, that is, speech materials in broadband, equal energy per cycle noise.

Normal and Impaired Perception in Noise

The CR(dB) concepts developed in the previous section should be viewed primarily as capable of predicting performance of normal listeners. However, many impaired listeners *probably* will perform close to the normal levels in noise. This is why some audiologists and psychoacousticians refer to noise as the "great equalizer." That is, although the EML will differ among listeners because T(Q) varies, the EL of noise will be similar for most listeners.

Research is needed before we can understand and predict the impaired listener's behavior in simple noise environments. Although impaired listeners can differ dramatically from "normal" in quiet conditions, the separation between populations seems to be quantitatively much less during listening in noise environments (Bode 1978). For example, an impaired listener might show a 40 dB deviation from a normal listener during tests in "quiet" but less than a 5-dB difference in noise. We are not saying that the hearing-impaired listeners would not have a substantial handicap relative to their normal-hearing peers. Rather, we are saying that the *quantitative* difference in noise appears to be much smaller than usually assumed. Thus there is a continuing need for reliable and valid speech tests in noise, such as procedures using adaptive tests (Bode and Carhart 1973, 1974, 1975).

Binaural Unmasking

An interesting phenomenon that has excited students of human hearing is called binaural unmasking, masking level differences (MLDs), or release from masking. Reviews of binaural hearing and MLDs provide background and summary information (Green and Henning 1969, Levitt and Voroba 1974).

Basically, an MLD is obtained whenever a phase, time, and/or level difference between either signal (S) or noise (N) exists between the two ears during dichotic stimulation with both the signal and the noise. One of the simplest binaural conditions is conventionally designated N_0S_0, wherein both noise and signal are each *identical* at two ears; that is, all noise components in the ear are *exactly the same* in all respects as the noise in the contralateral ear and the signal is exactly the same in each ear. This general condition is called *diotic stimulation,* as opposed to *dichotic listening,* which exists when there is *any difference* in signal or noise presented to the two ears.

Typically the N_0S_0 condition is used as a reference in the systematic study of changes that occur in listener performance as time, intensity, and/or spectral differences are introduced between ears. A dramatic improvement in thresholds can be obtained if specific conditions exist at the two ears. It has been found consistently that N_0S_π *or* $N_\pi S_0$ conditions result in the greatest improvement, that is, a "release from masking" in signal detection. The subscript π means that the signal *or* noise is out of phase *between* the ears by 180 degrees; intensity levels between ears are the same for the signal and for the noise. The improvement in detection thresholds (the MLD), relative to the N_0S_0 condition, can be as much as 15–20 dB for low frequencies (around 250–500 Hz) and 3–4 dB for higher frequencies (1500–2000 Hz upward) with intermediate changes between these regions.

Most of the research with MLDs has been done with pure tone signals, but some investigations have used speech stimuli (Levitt and Rabiner 1967; Carhart et al. 1967, 1968a; Carhart et al. 1968b). Here the findings have shown about a 6–8-dB improvement in intelligibility thresholds for spondee words (low-frequency cues) and about 3 dB for monosyllabic words (high-frequency cues) when either N_0S_π or $N_\pi S_0$ conditions are compared to the N_0S_0 condition.

Laboratory studies have generated interest in applying these data to the study of impaired hearing under specific conditions of binaural listening (Schoeny and Carhart 1971, Briskey, 1978). Better understanding of normal and impaired binaural hearing in noise, maximal benefits of various binaural conditions, and realistic goals for binaural hearing aid fittings will be valuable rewards for the student of audiology and ultimately for hearing-impaired listeners (Hawkins and Yacullo 1984, Cox and Bisset 1984).

SOURCES OF DISTORTION

Many types of distortion can exist between talker and listener, with distortion referring to *any change* in an original speech signal in its path from a talker's mouth to eventual analysis by a listener. Linguistic distortion within either the talker or listener (or both) is not considered in the present context. In addition to noise variability discussed earlier, there are major sources of distortion, as described in the following paragraphs.

Talker Variability

A talker's production of speech can distort the resulting acoustic signal either through inadequate or inappropriate generation and propagation of the acoustic signal. Distortion at the source (including visual cues) can increase the difficulty of an impaired listener's perception of the intended message.

Reverberation

In many listening environments, speech can be distorted by damping and/or introduction of energy not present in the original signal. An example is any hard-walled, reverberant condition in which the original speech is complicated by the addition of reflected frequencies. Typical classrooms, hallways, and other structures with high reflecting surfaces can add serious distortion to a transmitted speech signal (Ross 1972, Nabelek and Mason 1981).

Talker-Microphone Distance

A problem facing a hearing aid user is the often uncontrollable distance between the talker and the hearing aid microphone(s). In general, as this distance increases, the overall level of the speech decreases, with high-frequency components showing the greatest potential decrement. This is due to the ease with which high-frequency sounds are reflected back toward the source by obstacles in the environment. Further, *given that environmental noise often remains relatively constant in level, while the level of the speech decreases as a function of distance, the S/N ratio at the microphone can progressively worsen* (Niemoller 1978).

Directional and Head Shadow Effects

Depending on talker and microphone location, differences in spectral components at the microphone can occur. For example, if a talker is directly to the *right* of the listener (90° azimuth) and the microphone is on the *left* side of the listener's head, several changes in spectrum can exist: (1) there can be about a 0.8 msec time difference between the two sides of the head; (2) speech at the aided side can be about 6.5 dB less intense than on the unaided side; and (3) as a result of head reflection and diffraction effects, component high frequencies can be attenuated more at the aided than at the unaided side. Interest in binaural hearing aids, and in the various contralateral routing of signal (CROS) aids, has resulted in efforts to eliminate or reduce and, in some instances, utilize these effects [see Chapter 8; also Harford and Dodds (1974)]. Effects of the pinna also have been investigated, with evidence suggesting that the pinna is important for localization of front-to-back and elevation (Freedman and Fisher 1968). Microphone placement in the ear canal could enhance these cues and high-frequency signals.

Hearing Aid Distortion

A considerable amount of time has been expended in the study of the effects of hearing aid electroacoustic distortions on speech perception (see Chapter 2). Frequency response, bandwidth, harmonic and intermodulation products, and transient response have been studied with equivocal results, probably because of the traditional difficulty of isolating one "cause" while controlling effects of other sources of distortion [see Bode and Kasten (1971); also Chapter 2)].

Coupling Between Aid and Ear

How the aid is coupled to the ear canal of a listener can have dramatic effects on the performance of the hearing aid and the listener (Killion 1981). Open, closed, vented, tubular earmolds and use of inserts have been studied in recent years. Studies have indicated (1) the importance of knowing what negative and positive effects result from specific types of coupling, and (2) the inadequacies of typical coupler measurements of a hearing aid's characteristics in predicting what energies actually exist in a listener's canal (see Chapter 3).

Listener Variables

An impaired listener's unique difficulties in processing speech continues to warrant study (Preminger and Wiley 1985). Reduced sensitivity at different frequencies can distort an incoming speech signal by frequency filtering. Further, depending on the location and specific pathology, impaired discrimination among phonemes at comfortable levels above threshold can reflect a combination of other sources of distortion, such as bilateral asymmetries in sensitivity, aural harmonics, inefficient spectral analysis within the cochlea, abnormal masking effects, loudness recruitment, impaired temporal integration, and processing deficiencies in the central nervous system.

Complex Interactions of Distortion

Briefly stated, given all the above *possible* sources of distortion, it is impressive that so many impaired listeners do so well with hearing aids. The expectation is that they should not have satisfactory experiences. *We typically are placing low-fidelity amplification on ears (which can further distort the speech signal) and then expecting the listener to show substantially improved performance!*

Those listeners who are successful with hearing aids seem to have minimal distortion in the pathway from talker to listener, and those who are unsuccessful have greater total distortion. Sometimes the solution is relatively easy; often it is not. Given the complexity of the topic, and the associated difficulties of impaired listeners, one need not apologize for the absence of simple solutions.

PRESCRIBING AIDS AND PREDICTING PERFORMANCE

Prescription of a remedial procedure implies that prediction of probable outcome is possible (Marshall and Bacon 1981). In general, the state of the art in hearing aid evaluations is such that we are not able to predict speech perception performance; thus, given that we have unaided measures with a particular listener, we are not able to prescribe a specific set of hearing aid characteristics that invariably will predict speech recognition scores for this listener. In chapter 7, Berger addresses contemporary approaches that have improved prescriptive accuracy to a major extent.

We have examined data from routine clinical hearing aid evaluations to assess possible predictive interactions among conventional tests (Bode et al. 1972, Dodds and Bode 1972). Results were obtained from representative and similarly conducted evaluations with 68 clients seen in the Northwestern University Hearing Clinic. Intercorrelations among 26 aided and unaided tests were analyzed by computer, with the primary objective of identifying factors that influence test performance of hearing-impaired listeners. All persons had been tested in "quiet" and against "competing messages" both unaided and aided.

In viewing the results, five factors appeared to account for test performance: (1) aided monosyllabic discrimination, (2) test ear sensitivity, (3) nontest ear sensitivity, (4) interear high-frequency response, and (5) aided speech reception threshold (SRT).

One of the intriguing results, in addition to the identification of the five factors, was the statistical independence of these factors. Knowledge of the clients' performance on those tests involving one factor did not provide predictive information regarding their performance on tests associated with any of the other factors. Most importantly, knowledge of either (1) unaided sensitivity in the test ear, (2) unaided sensitivity in the nontest ear, or (3) the unaided high-frequency response in either ear did not allow prediction of how the listeners functioned with hearing aids. This conclusion applied regardless of whether we were attempting to predict aided speech reception threshold or aided monosyllabic discrimination (either in quiet or in competing speech conditions).

Further, since *aided* speech reception threshold and aided monosyllabic discrimination appeared to be independent factors influencing test performance, predictions from one type of test result to the other were not feasible. That is, knowledge of a client's speech reception threshold with a hearing aid did not provide reliable information regarding that person's speech discrimination score with this hearing aid, either in quiet or in the competing speech conditions. Granted, knowledge of aided SRT and of the intensity level of speech stimuli impinging on the aid allows specification of the sensation level of the speech, but this knowledge does not enable us to predict discrimination of speech materials. The monosyllabic discrimination factor apparently underlies many types of monosyllabic speech tests (Carhart and Tillman 1972).

Competing message testing in our studies provided realistic information regarding the impaired listeners' performance with hearing aids, information that was neither obtained nor predicted by discrimination testing in quiet. This conclusion was related to the fact that the mean difference between best and worst aided performance in quiet was only 6 percent while competing message testing showed an average 15 percent difference between conditions. Clinical decisions regarding which hearing aid to recommend, of course, are enhanced when the differences among aids are maximized.

These perspectives perhaps have been considered during traditional hearing aid evaluations. The results provide validational support for these considerations and highlight the practical importance of attempts to explain and predict performance of clients on a variety of tests. Further refinement of measures of each factor should considerably increase our ability to estimate and/or predict the performance of impaired listeners with hearing aids.

The search for underlying factors that account for, or explain, test results with clients is a continuing need, one that has been only minimally explored. The potential for reducing a large variety of test results to a few factors that explain listener performance is one of the objectives. Achievement of this goal might reduce the number of constructs needed to understand the complex auditory behaviors encountered in clinical testing situations and in everyday life.

CONCLUSION

I have attempted to suggest answers to the two issues mentioned at the outset: why hearing aids typically do not restore hearing to normal and why we are unable to prescribe hearing aids with a reasonable degree of confidence.

The solution to the first issue is that *one cannot expect hearing aids to interact with damaged, distorting hearing mechanisms in such a way that the listener with sensorineural impairment will function similarly to one's normal hearing peer.* The practical goals, given present status of hearing aids and the limits of our knowledge, are rather to reduce or overcome the speech sensitivity impairment as much as possible, to provide maximum understanding of speech delivered in "noise" to the hearing aid, to provide prosodic cues when possible, and to achieve all of this with maximal comfort and minimal adjustment on the part of the listener. This entire book is addressed to current procedures and issues involved in accomplishing these goals.

The answer to the second question, regarding prescription of hearing aids, has been only partially suggested here. However, the issues discussed here and throughout this book should convince the reader that although the question is simple, the answers are not. Given the wide variation in complexities of speech signals, in the pathway and noise interactions existing in everyday life, in the electroacoustic characteristics of hearing aids, in the idiosyncratic nature of various sensorineural pathologies, and in the generally unknown features and dimensions of speech perception, we can be sure that much remains to be accomplished. A variety of activity is currently underway, including applied research, sophisticated clinical testing, relevant legislative and professional action, and cooperative standardization efforts. These efforts, as well as the increase in the number of individuals attacking present problems, serve to encourage those who seek to understand the interactions among speech signals and hearing aids and to implement means wherein the deleterious effects of these interactions can be minimized.

REFERENCES

Bode DL: Adaptive speech testing applied to hearing impaired listeners. Annual Convention, American Speech and Hearing Association, 1978

Bode DL, Oyer HJ: Auditory training and speech discrimination. J Speech Hearing Res 13:839-855, 1970

Bode DL, Kasten RN: Hearing aid distortion and consonant identification. J Speech Hearing Res 14:323-331, 1971

Bode DL, Dodds E, Carhart R: A factor analysis of competing message testing in hearing aid evaluations. J Acoust Soc Am 52:184(A), 1972

Bode DL, Carhart R: Measurement of articulation functions using adaptive test procedures, in IEEE Transactions on Audio and Electroacoustics, AU-21, 1973, pp 196-201

Bode DL, Carhart R: Stability and accuracy of adaptive tests of speech discrimination. J Acoust Soc Am 56:963-970, 1974

Bode DL, Carhart R: Estimating CNC discrimination with spondee words. J Acoust Soc Am 56:1216-1218, 1975

Boothroyd A: Statistical theory of the speech discrimination score. J Acoust Soc Am 43:362-367, 1968

Briskey RJ: Binaural hearing aids and new innovations, in Katz J. (ed): Handbook of Clinical Audiology (ed 2). Baltimore, Williams & Wilkins, 1978, pp 501-507

Carhart R: Factors affecting discrimination for monosyllabic words in background noise. Paper presented at the Annual Convention of the American Speech and Hearing Association, 1967

Carhart R, Tillman TW, Johnson KR: Release of masking for speech through interaural time delay. J Acoust Soc Am 42:124-138, 1967

Carhart R, Tillman TW, Johnson KR: Effects of interaural time delays on masking by two competing signals. J Acoust Soc Am 43:1223-1230, 1968a

Carhart R, Tillman TW, Dallos PJ: Unmasking for pure tones and spondees: Interaural phase and time disparities. J Speech Hearing Res 11:722-734, 1968b

Carhart R, Tillman TW: Individual consistency of hearing for speech across diverse listening conditions. J Speech Hearing Res 15:105-113, 1972

Cox RM, Bisset JD: Relationship between two measures of aided binaural advantage. J Speech Hearing Disorders 49:399–408, 1984

Danaher EM, Osberger MJ, Pickett JM: Discrimination of formant frequency transitions in synthetic vowels. J Speech Hearing Res 16:439–451, 1973

Danaher EM, Pickett JM: Some masking effects produced by low-frequency vowel formants in persons with sensorineural hearing loss. J Speech Hearing Res 18:261–271, 1975

Dodds E, Bode DL: Evaluation of clinical hearing aid selection procedures. ASHA 14:473, 1972

Elkins E (ed): Speech Recognition by the Hearing Impaired. ASHA Reports 14. American Speech-Language-Hearing Association, Rockville, MD, 1984

Freedman SJ, Fisher HG: The role of the pinna in auditory localization, in Freedman SJ (ed): The Neuropsychology of Spatially Oriented Behavior. Homewood, IL, Dorsey Press, 1968, pp 135–152

Gengel R: Auditory temporal integration at relatively high masked threshold levels. J Acoust Soc Am 51:1849–1851, 1972

Goetzinger CP: Word discrimination testing, in Katz J (ed): Handbook of Clinical Audiology (ed 2). Baltimore, Williams & Wilkins, 1978, pp 149–148

Green DM, Henning GB: Audition. Ann Rev Psychol 20:105–128, 1969

Harford E, Dodds E: Versions of the CROS hearing aid. Arch Otolaryngol 100:50–57, 1974

Hawkins DB, Yacullo WS: Signal-to-noise ratio of binaural hearing aids. J Speech Hearing Disorders 49:278–286, 1984

House AS, Williams CE, Hecker MHL, et al: Articulation testing methods: Consonantal differentiation with a closed-response set. J Acoust Soc Am 37:158–166, 1965

Killion MC: Earmold options for wideband hearing aids. J Speech Hearing Disorders 46:10–20, 1981

Konkle DF, Rintelmann WF (eds): Principles of Speech Audiometry. Baltimore, University Park Press, 1983

Levitt H, Rabiner LR: Binaural release from masking for speech and gain in intelligibility. J Acoust Soc Am 42:601–608, 1967

Levitt H, Voroba B: Binaural hearing, in Gerber SE (ed): Introductory Hearing Science. Philadelphia, Saunders, 1974, pp 187–206

Liberman AM, Cooper FS, Shankweiler DP, et al: Perception of the speech code. Psychol Rev 74:431–461, 1967

Liberman P: Speech Acoustics and Perception. Indianapolis, Bobbs-Merrill, 1972

Marshall L, Bacon SP: Prediction of speech discrimination scores from audiometric data. Ear Hearing 2:148–155, 1981

Nabelek AK, Mason D: Effect of noise and reverberation on binaural and monaural word identification. J Speech Hearing Res 24:375–382, 1981

Niemoeller AF: Hearing aids, in Davis H, Silverman SR (eds): Hearing and Deafness. New York, Holt, Rinehart and Winston, 1978, pp 293–337

Picard M: Effects of selective amplification upon consonant intelligibility in normal and sensorineural listeners. Unpublished doctoral dissertation, University of Illinois, 1974

Pickett JM: The Sounds of Speech Communication. Baltimore, University Park Press, 1980

Preminger J, Wiley TL: Frequency selectivity and consonant intelligibility in sensorineural hearing loss. J Speech Hearing Res 28:197–206, 1985

Ross M: Classroom acoustics and speech intelligibility, in Katz J (ed): Handbook of Clinical Audiology. Baltimore, Williams & Wilkins, 1972, pp 756–771

Sanders D: Aural Rehabilitation (ed 2). Englewood Cliffs, NJ, Prentice-Hall, 1982

Scharf B: Critical bands, in Tobias JV (ed): Foundations of Modern Auditory Theory, Vol 1.
New York, Academic Press, 1970, pp 159–202
Schoeny ZG, Carhart R: Effects of unilateral Ménières disease on masking-level differences.
J Acoust Soc Am 50:1143–1149, 1971
Stevens KM, House AS: Speech perception, in Tobias JV (ed): Foundations of Modern
Auditory Theory, Vol 2. New York, Academic Press, 1970, pp 3–62
Tillman TW, Carhart R, Olsen WO: Hearing aid efficiency in a competing speech situation.
J Speech Hearing Res 13:789–811, 1970
Tillman T, Olsen WO: Speech audiometry, in Jerger J (ed): Modern Developments in
Audiology. New York, Academic Press, 1973, pp 37–74

Derek A. Sanders

10

Hearing Aid Orientation and Counseling

It is a rare hearing aid user who can put on a new instrument and use it optimally without rather extensive counseling and orientation. This involves much more than simply showing the individual where the controls are and how to put the aid on and take it off. It includes discussions of the proper manner in which to adjust to the new and often abrasive sound of the aid, and of identification and remediation of the tangential psychological aspects of hearing loss.

This chapter systematically considers the various factors involved in assisting a hearing-impaired person derive maximum benefits from a hearing aid. Each of the basic steps in hearing aid management is presented and discussed in a realistic manner. Derek Sanders also explores the personal adjustments the candidate for a hearing aid must be assisted to make in order to use the aid successfully. Derek's discussion of what a counselor should be and what that role involves is based on many years of experience. The approach described is humanistic in that it deals with the individual rather than the hearing impairment. The combination of a reality orientation and a real sensitivity to the often subconscious feelings of the hearing aid candidate makes this chapter a valuable resource for the reader.

MCP

ACCEPTING THE COUNSELING ROLE

One of the most difficult aspects of writing a chapter on counseling is the recognition that many audiologists and speech pathologists are uncomfortable with

AMPLIFICATION FOR THE HEARING-IMPAIRED, THIRD EDITION   ISBN 0-8089-1886-9

the idea that counseling is a necessary part of our professional responsibility. Even when we do acknowledge this aspect of our role, we feel that we lack both the training and confidence to fulfill it. We are not even sure of the nature and extent of the counseling support we should provide to our clients and their families (Luterman 1984). Our most worrisome concern is that, unwittingly, we may harm our client psychologically, that we will give the wrong advice or say the wrong thing. We often are equally worried that we will not know what to say, that we will make fools of ourselves, or that we will be embarrassed by our client's emotional response, be it anger or tears. These apprehensions are perfectly understandable, and, within the perspective from which they arise, justified. They are certainly concerns that must be addressed and resolved before you can feel comfortable about accepting your role as counselor.

That goal cannot be achieved by reading a single chapter in a text. It is also unlikely, however, that you will enter a course of professional training to achieve competence in counseling. You are indeed faced with a dilemma, for although you may not feel competent to provide counseling, the need for it on the part of your client is always there. Most adults fitted with a hearing aid will make an adequate although not necessarily an optimal adjustment even without your guidance. Some will have considerable difficulty doing so, while a few will fail to come to terms either with their hearing handicap or with the aid. They become dissatisfied, disgruntled hearing aid users, or simply give up, attributing their dissatisfaction to everything except their need for counseling.

The needs of the parents of young and school age children fitted with amplification, particularly during the teenage years, are even greater. Unfortunately, we tend either to simply present "lectures" to parents and "lessons" to school children, or we decide that it should be the teacher or psychologist who should provide the service (Luterman 1984). The temptation simply to avoid this issue of counseling, therefore, is great and often is succumbed to. This was recently evidenced by the experience of a student in one of my undergraduate courses. She came to me after class saying that our discussion of hearing impairment in the course was very relevant for her, since she had just that week been fitted with an in-the-ear (ITE) hearing aid. She asked if she could talk with me about her hearing loss and about the hearing aid. The audiologist in the Speech and Hearing Center in her town had given her only the briefest information about the aid. She knew nothing about her hearing loss or her measured performance with and without the aid. She also had many feelings to express about feeling handicapped at age 20. The audiologist had no doubt performed well in terms of this young woman's amplification requirements but had failed to recognize her need for information and psychological support. *The advent of the ITE and the canal fitting seems to have resulted in even less concern for the adjustment needs of the client.* I assume that the audiologist feels that *if the handicap is not made visible by the stigma symbol of a hearing aid, the feelings of being different will not arise.*

The need for at least some degree of psychological support becomes hard to dispute if you believe that the decision to purchase a hearing aid necessitates facing the reality of being hearing-impaired. Such an admission, even to oneself, initially gives rise to feelings of reduced self-worth. One is no longer one's normal self, no longer the same as one's peers, one is deviant. We categorize people with impaired hearing, we refer to them as "the hearing impaired," "the deaf," or "the communicatively disordered." This process of categorization, of labeling, has been extensively discussed in the literature of deviancy (Goffman 1963). It has been shown that simply being identified as "different" is alone enough to evoke a range of predictable feelings and reactions, *even when the actual difference does not exist* (Freedman and Doob 1968). Imagine yourself, then, suddenly reclassified from the "normal" category, with all its implications of health and well-being, into the unknown category of "hearing impaired." With the label comes all the negative connotations of age, of being less than fully aware of what is going on. A whole repertoire of jokes exists illustrating so-called humor of not hearing. Similarly, imagine learning that your young child has just been labeled by an audiologist or an otologist as "not normal," for that is what the label "hard of hearing" or "deaf" means to parents and, unfortunately, to society.

We have a responsibility, therefore, to adopt a model of hearing aid fitting that goes beyond the provision of technological expertise. We must address the emotional needs of the person along with the acoustic needs. The new hearing aid user, and that person's family, need to know about the hearing deficit and about the hearing aid, but they also need to work through the feelings associated with all that a hearing aid and the need for it means to them and to significant other persons. My goal in this chapter is to discuss the major components of a model intended to assist you in establishing a counseling relationship with your client. I do not expect you to feel confident about counseling when you have read this. However, I hope to motivate you to address the adjustment needs of your client as part of an effective hearing aid fitting service. I hope you will feel more comfortable about assuming this role and will feel receptive to the counseling education your clients can provide you through your relationship with them.

THE NATURE OF THE TASK

To a great extent our apprehensions about our counseling role and our reluctance to accept it arises from our definition of the term. The term *counselor* is commonly, and correctly, used to identify a professional who has completed a formal course of study and training that equips that person to deal with emotional and adjustment problems of clients. However, the word *counsel*, from which *counselor* derives, is a generic term. The Webster New World Dictionary defines it as "a mutual exchange of ideas, opinions, etc., discussion and deliberation, advice resulting from such discussion." Thus there exist today financial investment counselors, real estate counselors, retirment counselors, and so on. I use the term *counseling* in this generic sense. We must accept responsibility for counseling about the adjustment that having a hearing impairment and using a hearing aid necessitates. We must provide counsel to parents who learn that their child is deaf. Our task is to provide information to our clients, to exchange ideas with them, and to discuss and deliberate about the problems they perceive and the feelings they are experiencing.

Therefore, the task before you is most appropriately viewed as developing a cooperative problem-solving relationship. You bring to it your knowledge and experience about hearing impairment; clients bring theirs. Remember, however, that no matter how extensive your experience has been, unless you are yourself wearing a hearing aid(s) you only *know about* the effects of a hearing problem, you do *know* what it is like to be hearing handicapped. When I tell this to my clients, I communicate my need for their input into the task of choosing an appropriate hearing aid fitting, and learning what to expect from it. I make it clear that there is really no such group as "the hearing-impaired." A hearing impairment has a different impact on each individual. It creates special problems for each person, problems influenced by the type of communication demands made upon them, the listening environments they have to function in, and the social activities in which they participate. I explain that the effect of the hearing deficit will be greatly influenced by their feelings about it, their understanding of what is happening, and their fears for the future. Likewise, their perceptions of the attitudes and reactions of their immediate family and of their friends, employers and colleagues, to their communication difficulties and their needs will contribute further to the overall success in the effective use of amplification. To the extent that hearing-impaired people can modify these attitudes favorably, they will be able to function with less apprehension. Thus, to be effective, the solutions we seek with the client must be solutions to very individual problems, those that the particular client you are working with is encountering.

This approach allows you to communicate acceptance of the validity of the client's difficulties and anxieties and your personal interest in assisting in the client's efforts to reduce them. You need to empathize with the client, to attempt to perceive the problem from that person's point of view. *Success is achieved when your understanding of the client's problems and needs and the perceptions the client has of them are in accord.* Counseling seeks to bring two perceptual worlds together so that two individuals, you and your client, can work cooperatively, seeking to resolve a well-defined problem. This challenge often is hard for the audiologist or speech language therapist to accept, for it necessitates rejecting the security of the authoritarian role of a specialist who best knows what is needed. *Rather than impose solutions, your value lies in your ability to assist the client to identify and define problems and to adopt acceptable and effective ways of reducing them. Your role is to facilitate the process, not to determine it.*

UNDERSTANDING THE PROBLEM

As audiologists, teachers of the deaf, or hearing therapists, we are particularly concerned with the effects of the hearing deficit on a person's ability to communicate. Yet, as Ramsdell (1970) points out, this is not, as one might expect, the area of greatest impact of the hearing impairment. Ramsdell maintains that the most serious effects of impaired hearing, particularly a rapid loss of hearing, lie in the resultant reduction or loss of a "feeling of relationship with the world," which is maintained largely through auditory contact. This primitive hearing function, which permits the ongoing monitoring of events of daily living, provides the auditory background that gives a person the feeling of being a participant in the surrounding changing world. Reactions to these changes occur at a preconscious level: "The constant reaction establishes in us states of feeling that are the foundation for our conscious experiences, a foundation which gives us the conviction that the world in which we live is also alive and moving" (Ramsdell 1970, p. 438). It is this primitive monitoring that serves as the coupler between the pattern of activity of our own personal system and that of the environment as a whole.

It is important, therefore, that you be sensitive to the impact that a reduction in the efficiency of this coupling may be expected to have on the hearing-impaired person. The severity of its effects will be greatest in cases of sudden or rapid hearing loss. In such cases, it may induce severe depression, which is cause for referral for psychiatric guidance. However, most of the people with whom you work will have experienced a progressive loss of hearing over a number of years, rather than a sudden loss. The progressive effects are insidious and, therefore, hard to recognize. Even the person who experiences a sudden onset of deafness will probably be fully aware of the reason for the overwhelming depression that follows, which, Ramsdell points out, occurs even when a person is facing practical difficulties in a realistic way. It is reasonable to assume, therefore, that with slowly deteriorating hearing one will be unaware of the origins of one's feelings of progressive detachment and insecurity, one's inner loneliness felt even when one is with one's family. This feeling is deeper, less tangible, than those that can be explained by the problems of speech communication. As a counselor, you need to assist the hearing-impaired person to explore these vague feelings of insecurity. You can provide a framework for this process by discussing the role hearing plays in keeping an individual aware, at a preconscious level, of being a part of things. It helps for the client to understand the importance of this preconscious awareness of one's environment and the disturbing effect that its reduction or loss can give rise to. Explaining the role sound plays in localizing and identifying events around us and permitting us to behave appropriately will further help the client to realize the legitimacy of feelings of insecurity and anxiety. Lack of understanding of such feelings often causes serious concern for the hearing-impaired person who does not identify the cause. Ramsdell states: "Knowing the cause of depression does not remove it but fortunately the mere understanding of the reason for a feeling state does much psychologically to relieve its intensity" (p. 439).

The problem frequently is compounded by the fact that hearing-impaired people often feel that their inability to cope is a weakness. They are ashamed to admit to difficulties they are experiencing and the anxieties that beset them. Sometimes they may even repress their conscious concerns. Parents of deaf children frequently experience feelings of guilt and inadequacy. As a counselor, you must be aware of the likelihood that your client may be experiencing these feelings and be alert to the defensive behavior that results from them (Sandlin 1974).

CLIENT REACTIONS TO THE HEARING HANDICAP

In an article on the psychologic reactions to hearing loss, Rousey (1971) identified the most common patterns of defensive maneuvers an individual, including a hearing-impaired person, may use when under stress. These include regression, repression, reaction formation, isolation, undoing, projection, turning against self, and sublimation. He stresses the role objective anxiety plays in provoking one or more of these defensive reactions. Objective anxiety arises from anticipation of being punished or penalized for the state of one's behavior. Clients' perceptions of how others treat persons with handicapping conditions will therefore have considerable bearing on their pattern of adaptive behavior (Freedman and Doob 1968). Their objective anxiety may result in modified self-perception sufficiently unacceptable as to cause them to deny the severity of their hearing handicap.

They may project the problems they are having onto others, accounting for their difficulty in hearing correctly by accusing others of mumbling, of deliberately excluding them from conversations, or they may blame the room acoustics. When such projections can no longer be supported, a person will often begin to withdraw from threatening situations, such as quit a job, avoid group meetings, decline responsibilities that involve group discussions, withdraw from training programs, cease to attend plays or movies, or decline invitations to dinner parties. These defense reactions are frequently accompanied by self-deprecation. Since such adaptive behavior, negative though it may seem, is necessary to maintain the identity of the person, and since the real cause is either not recognized or not admitted, one's self-esteem begins to lower to make it compatible with one's behavior. This forced shrinking of one's lifestyle may seriously shrink one's self-image. This progressive erosion of the normal lifestyle of the client, and usually of the spouse, is the ultimate and most serious effect of impaired hearing.

When the cause of the difficulties is consciously identified as the loss of adequate hearing, the most common reaction, according to Rousey (1971), is one of mourning, a natural concomitant of loss. This, he points out, is related to Ramsdell's idea of separation of the individual from the world around him, a world that seems "dead," giving rise to depression or an all-pervading sense of sadness.

Rousey also explains that the loss of hearing frequently gives rise to a feeling of pain and mortification. He discusses mortification in terms of its two closely related derivatives, shame and self-esteem. He quotes Fenishel's description of shame as "constant fear of being criticized, ostracized or punished." Rousey (1971,

p. 386) goes on to state, "It is probably certain that patients who express a conviction of shame over the need to wear a hearing aid or their hearing loss are struggling with some of these issues." These feelings are closely related to self-esteem.

THE SIGNIFICANCE OF CONSIDERING THE USE OF A HEARING AID

Unlike much consumer behavior of today, the decision to buy a hearing aid almost never constitutes impulse buying. The client in your office finally has had to accept the unpalatable fact of, at least in some important situations, being no longer able to function as a normal-hearing person. The realization of this fact explains the consultation this client has sought. It does not necessarily mean, however, that the person has adjusted to the need or has come to terms with its implications. For many clients the need to accept the reality of a hearing loss, for having to face up to the need for help and the need for a hearing aid, may constitute a real threat to their self-image. To acknowledge this hearing loss, particularly by wearing a hearing aid, is a definite act requiring acceptance of the fact that one is less than completely normal. This may be too great a step for a person to take without sympathetic support. Yet, the individual realizes that failure to do so will mean living with what has become an unacceptable problem. Rousey draws our attention to the fact that the fear engendered by the threat to one's self-esteem may be handled by the development of varying degrees of arrogant behavior. This may be directed at anyone associated with the client's difficulties, whether a member of the family or a helping specialist, such as yourself. As a counselor, aware of such possible reactions, you will be less confounded by your client's apparently conflicting behaviors of support seeking and rejection of helper.

It is unjustifiable to assume that the presence of a client in your clinic necessarily indicates willingness to use a hearing aid. Clients often seek consultation only to satisfy the persistent entreaties of a spouse or other close friend or relation. The person may be silently adamant about not wearing a hearing aid. Some even go so far as to purchase the aid, only to reject it as soon as they feel they have satisfactorily demonstrated that they cannot tolerate it. They frequently reject the aid because "it advertises my hearing loss." Parents of a young, deaf child may neglect to have their child wear the aid when they take the child shopping, on a trip to the park, or to a community event because "I don't want people to know my child isn't normal." Freedman and Doob (1968), in a fascinating study of how a deviancy or stigma affects the behavior of people, indicate that if the problem is not known to others, people will attempt to conceal it, which often leads to avoidance of social contacts, so that life style shrinks, as described earlier. There is little point in proceeding with a hearing aid selection process until a client, or the parents of a child, are positively motivated toward its use. Shore (1972) states, "If the parents of a deaf child reject the use of an aid their child will do the same. Therefore, it is necessary that the consultant learn how the parents feel about amplification. It is possible that in some cases it may take as many as three or more sessions to modify the thinking of parents who are anti-hearing aids."

THE PROCESS LEADING TO CONSULTATION

Usually your client will have passed through a number of years during which the insidious effects of a slow, progressive deterioration of hearing have gone unnoticed. The reduction in acoustic information at first is compensated for unconsciously by greater use of the redundance naturally occurring in communication interaction. This, however, of necessity requires increased demands on cognitive functions, closer attention to the speaker, and greater listening effort, all of which can be very tiring. Gradually comes the realization that something is wrong and life is much harder than it used to be. Even at this point, many people genuinely may fail to realize that the problem originates with themselves.

The individual with a borderline hearing handicap is not the only one who commonly misperceives the nature of the problem. The spouse, son, daughter, or other relatives, often attribute the occasional misunderstandings to inattention, moodiness, lack of interest, or preoccupation with some activity. This explanation of the communication breakdown may even give rise to hard feelings, complaints, and recriminations. Interpretations of family members, or even persons in the work setting, are reinforced by the observation that hearing-impaired individuals do, indeed, understand most of the time, and can get what was missed "if they pay attention." What is not realized is that such keen attention cannot be sustained over time, or under certain listening conditions. This period is often one during which annoyance and frustration have colored communciation relationships in the family because of a lack of awareness of the cause of what is happening.

When the hearing aid candidate is an older person, the inattentive behavior, difficulty with easy monitoring of casual conversation, and poor memory of what was said (but only partially heard), often are quite unjustly attributed to problems of aging. For some, the hearing loss may exacerbate true problems of aging to the point at which the person can no longer cope with life outside a nursing home.

By the time your client is in your office the realization that hearing is a significant problem has occurred. The communication demands in the person's life, young or old, now exceed the ability to meet them. No redundancy remains to compensate for lost acoustic information in important situations. Often, before acknowledging the hearing deficit, your client denied having a problem, hoped it was a temporary difficulty, and deferred seeking help. This client may even have been deterred from seeking help by a physician, even an otologist, who insisted that the loss was not severe enough to warrant use of an aid. A physician whom I fitted with binaural aids confessed to always having told his patients that they should put off getting a hearing aid as long as possible, viewing it as an undesirable last resort. Acknowledgment of the problem is often made difficult because the spouse has insisted for a long time that this client's partner was "going deaf," a very frightening prospect for your client. Indeed, the decision to "see about an aid" is often made under pressure from family members. Just having to admit that one had been wrong is, itself, often difficult, facing the implications of the confession is often much harder. I must be cautious, however, not to overdramatize the course of events. Nor must I too readily generalize these observations to all clients. Many will seek your help with a positive attitude. They have faced the reality of the problem and are ready, often anxious, to do something about it. A client even may admit to having no negative feelings about wearing a hearing aid, their only concern being that it may not help. *Identifying the client's needs is an essential part of counseling.*

The achievement of the goal of an optimal hearing aid fitting, therefore, is heavily dependent on your sensitivity to the particular stage of problem resolution your client has reached. You need to know how positive the person feels toward the purchase of a hearing aid(s), for success in the use of amplification is predicated on coming to terms with the need for it. It is perfectly possible to assess, fit, and dispense a hearing aid(s) to a client without any reference to the psychological adjustment involved. However, to do so is merely to fit hearing aids to ears, ignoring the obvious fact that the hearing aid must fit the person. It eventually must be accommodated by the individual's self-image just as much as by that individual's auditory system.

The basis of understanding the problem, therefore, lies in realization that a change in our ability to continue to cope with the demands made on us, whether that change be externally or internally induced, poses a threat to our psychologic stability. We may react to this threat in a number of ways, each of which has been discussed. Only when one has adjusted to the change in a manner that does not shrink lifestyle and self-image can maximal adaptation be said to have occurred. It is a counselor's role to assist the client to achieve this goal. The success with which a client is able to maintain a normal lifestyle, or with which a child successfully meets the emotional social and psychological challenges of development, will be the true measure of the effectiveness of a counseling program. Creating an emotional climate conducive to such growth in a hearing-impaired person and that person's immediate family is your first task.

BUILDING A TRUST RELATIONSHIP

The willingness and ability of a client to explore feelings and experiences as they relate to the hearing handicap requires a trust relationship. For this to occur, the counselor must communicate a sincere interest, concern, and respect for the individual. Clients must perceive you to be genuinely accepting of the reality and importance of the difficulties they are experiencing and must believe that you understand, or are genuinely attempting to understand, the problems. We communicate these attitudes through our actions, words, and gestures. Try to be very conscious of your client from the first encounter, look for genuine opportunities to convey respect and concern. I always greet clients in the waiting room even before seeing them in the consultation room. If I am running a little late I tell them about how long it will be before I can see them. When I see a client I have kept waiting, I apologize, often explaining why I am running late. I ask a husband, wife, mother, other relative, or friend accompanying the client to come into the consulting office with the client, explaining that although only the client has a hearing problem, the family and close friends experience a communication problem, which is one of the things we hope to change.

You communicate acceptance of your clients by listening attentively to what they tell you, by nodding to indicate that you understand. It helps to begin the interview by expressing interest in the history of your clients' difficulty, inquiring how long they have known about it, what persuaded them to inquire about a hearing aid at this time, and how they feel about doing so.

By identifying with the client you are able to communicate understanding by such comments as "that must be very frustrating" or "you probably feel very inadequate when that happens." I point out that although I do not know what it is really like to have a hearing problem, I do know, from others I have worked with, that it creates feelings of insecurity in difficult communication situations and often leads to embarrassment and a feeling of inadequacy.

Tyler (1969) says that *the essential components of an effective counselor are attitudes rather than skills.* An attitude that defines the process of hearing aid selection and fitting as one that requires the input of the client and the family from the beginning is likely to foster the client's trust in your professional expertise. Remember, however, that your behavior must be genuine. *A lack of sincerity is quickly detected by a client and will result in a barrier between you and that person.*

IDENTIFYING FEELINGS

We discussed earlier the probable experiences a person has had as a result of an unidentified progressive hearing impairment. I make a point of identifying these feelings that the hearing-impaired individual and the family members experience when communication breakdown occurs, with the intention of legitimizing them, making them understandable, and normalizing them for both parties. I endeavor to help them acknowledge the feelings and to examine the cause of them. By relating the feelings to particular situations or events, they become more susceptible to modification. *Problem situations often respond to management strategies, raw feelings do not.* I identify those feelings commonly experienced by persons with impaired hearing.

Apprehension

Apprehension arises from knowledge that there is a high probability that in a given situation one will not understand. It is a well-justified feeling based on not having control in a communication situation. It is related to *fear of embarrassment*, of making a fool of oneself. Both feelings usually respond to strategies and techniques that increase one's control of the communication situation. For example, advise the listener that you have a problem hearing and may not always catch what has been said; make sure that you position yourself where you can see and hear best; ensure that you ask for a repetition or clarification of information when you lose track of a a conversation, or ask a question that will focus the main topic for you. You can reduce the chance of embarrassment only if you remain an active participant in the communication situation.

Fear that the Problems You are Encountering are Related to the Aging Process or to a Psychological Inability to Cope

This fear is not an unreasonable one if you fail to realize how complex the effects of a reduction in acoustic information really are. I point out the effort involved in listening, the constant demand to fill in bits of the message not received, the difficulty in remembering what was not heard fully and thus was poorly recorded in memory. Understanding how large a problem a person has been managing to cope with does much to reassure that person that these fears have been attributed to the wrong cause.

Concern About Personality Change

A number of clients confess to being anxious about changes they feel are occurring in their personality. They refer to feeling depressed, to having lost the zest for life, to being hyperirritable, to having a constant feeling of unease. These feelings relate back to Rousey and to Ramsdell's explanation of the psychological ramifications of impaired hearing discussed earlier. Again, I point out that *what they are experiencing is the effect of their attempts to cope with changes they really did not understand.* To the extent that our moods and behaviors reflect what is going on inside us, personality does change with circumstances, but it is not one's basic personality that has changed. Given an acceptable level of restoration of listening ease, one can be confident that the client will see the surrounding world more optimistically.

Tension and Stress

The final feelings that I identify for the client are those of tension and stress, which result from the burden of always having to work hard at communicating, always with the added stress of the emotions I have discussed here. An effective hearing aid fitting will make a noticeable difference in how exhausting the client feels life has become.

The Family's Feelings

I have found it helpful to discuss the feelings experienced by the family members. It is not easy always to be patient and understanding when a person you live with can only understand what you say under certain listening conditions. When my wife suffered a hearing impairment for a period of 5 weeks, I found, to my embarrassment, that I was soon saying "Oh, never mind" when she asked me to repeat something she had not fully heard. I realized how superficial much of what I say is; it really did not warrant repeating. I felt awful about it, but yet I found it a constant effort to remember not to talk from another room, when the dishwasher was running, or when she was not looking at me. The volume of the television set bothered me even though I knew it was necessary. I learned, then, that a hearing impairment also creates stress for family members. I now mention this to parents, expressing the fact that I understand how the spouse or children may feel. I accept that as people with normal hearing, we are not always as sympathetic or accommodating as we really would like to be toward those we love. I make a point of the fact that I expect the hearing aid to afford benefit to the hearing members of the family, too, that they will be as much a judge of its effectiveness as the person who wears it. Indeed, on a postfitting visit, it is often the family members who are enthusiastic about the benefits the hearing aid provides.

Reviewing the Subtler Effects of Hearing Impairment

Your ability to show your awareness of the many subtle effects of hearing impairment will contribute greatly to the achievement of rapport with your client. The individual with the problem, of course, often is aware of these effects, but may not have attributed them to the hearing impairment. The person frequently has noticed changes in feelings, emotional behavior, attitudes, and interest in life, and has worried about them. The person may not have mentioned these concerns even to the family. When changes in mood or behavior have been commented on negatively by family members, the person often has felt the complaint or comment was justified. This situation adds guilt to the complex of emotions to be dealt with. I wish to assure you that I am not talking about an occasional individual with unusual problems. Usually we do not learn how others feel because we give them no opportunity to tell us. We conclude that most of the clients we meet are dealing with their hearing handicap well, that all they need is a hearing aid and everything will be taken care of. The naiveté of this assumption is enormous. How many times have you been asked "How are you today?" to which you have replied "fine" or "I'm okay" when in truth you are really troubled inside? It is reasonable to assume that a person who daily has to surmount the handicap imposed by the hearing impairment will experience negative feelings. It is equally reasonable to realize that these in turn will affect self-image and behavior. Thus I try to communicate to my client that I assume living with a hearing impairment is not an easy task. I explain that I have learned from others who have hearing impairments that it can be a very stressful experience both for the hearing-impaired person and for the members of the family. I mention that others have expressed concern about the restrictions on their lifestyle they have had to accept and the problems this has created for other family members. Those of us who hear normally fail to understand that it is not enjoyable to go to a movie or theater when you understand only half of what is said. We do not realize the apprehension caused by fear of not understanding what someone says to you at a dinner party or reception, at a club meeting or a picnic. We have no idea of the constant fear of making a fool of oneself by giving an inappropriate response, to say nothing of having missed or misunderstood a call in a card game. These apprehensions arise from the communication problems that occur in social situations. Hearing-impaired persons frequently deal with these problems by avoiding them. They socialize less, decline invitations where there will be more than just a few people, do not attend church anymore because they cannot hear the preacher. "It's years since I went to a play or a concert. I used to enjoy them, but what's the use when you can't hear" is a commonly heard complaint.

Equally serious are the games the hearing impaired person plays at work to avoid people knowing about the hearing impairment. One chief architect in the company he owned said "I'm sure the people who work for me think I'm a bear, but with my hearing problem I have to be aggressive or I'm lost." So at work, where it is difficult to withdraw from situations, a repertoire of subterfuges is often evolved for protection and survival. The price, however, is high, one of constant apprehension.

Even at home the hearing-impaired person functions under varying degrees of stress. The inability to hear as well as other members of the family often causes frustration and friction in communication situations. Not being able to easily follow conversation at the dinner table, being unable to communicate easily in the car, not understanding one's grandchildren, are all very real problems that must be adapted to. The family adapts as best it can. Unfortunately, this usually involves a degree of withdrawal on the part of all parties. The hearing members tend to say "never mind" when not understood, and to slowly and unconsciously exclude the hearing-impaired person from conversations. The hearing-impaired person begins not to make the considerable effort needed to follow conversation and either withdraws psychologically, or physically leaves the group.

The essential point here is that *these are all normal, rational reactions to what is an abnormal situation.* It is important to stress to the clients and their families the reasonableness of what has occurred. It is an enormous relief to see as perfectly reasonable reactions or behaviors one has come to consider aberrant, and finally to understand why they are happening. I like to discuss with my clients and their families some of the effects I know hearing impairment has on cognitive processes, that is, the way the brain processes speech. I point out to them that when I am in a conversation or listening to a play or lecture, I receive far more information in the speech signal than I need, because I have normal hearing. I remind them that we can follow the gist of what is said when only half the information is present. Because of the luxury of excess information, the normal-hearing person has several advantages that are lost when hearing impairment occurs. With more information than we need, we can afford to pay less attention to the actual details of the speech message. We devote our attention to the content, to what is meant by what is said rather than what actually was said. Similarly, the excess redundancy means that when the message content becomes more complex or less familiar, or when poor acoustic conditions (noise and reverberation) make listening more difficult, we make use of the extra information available in the speech signal. We process the information more carefully to continue to maintain good comprhension. Hearing-impaired persons enjoy no such luxury. If they are "getting by" in a situation in which the difficulty increases, they have no reserve of information to draw on and soon will be lost. The point is that they have to use so much brain power to reason out what was said, that they have little or no time to consider the implications of what was meant. Listening becomes hard work instead of pleasure. Unfortunately, the observation that they have difficulty in concentrating, in following what is being said, often is attributed to the gradual loss of one's facilities with age; a concern heightened by the recent publicity concerning Alzheimer's disease. This incorrect assumption, unfortunately, is reinforced by the fact that when one no longer can follow the conversation, one's mind wanders to more rewarding activities, and one does in fact no longer pay attention. It is unreasonable to expect a person to do so when so little reward is obtained. Now the scenario gets worse. It is quite understandable that you have difficulty remembering conversational detail you were unable to catch, or even parts of conversations you had stopped paying attention to. Suddenly you are addressed, a question is asked, a comment called for, but you cannot remember what was said because you did not hear it. So hearing impairment indirectly takes its toll on memory, for how can you remember what you do not adequately hear? *We are not dealing simply with difficulty in hearing, but with the far more complex effects that reduced hearing has on how a normal person's whole processing system is disrupted by reduced auditory information.*

It may seem that the counseling process described above is too involved and too time-consuming to be accommodated in the time allowed for a hearing aid fitting. In fact, it is a time saver. Much of what I do is planned development of my relationship with the client; it is interactional conversation with a purpose. *I find that the time invested for this purpose before the actual fitting contributes greatly to successful use of the hearing aid.* It cuts down on the number of clients who experience adjustment problems. Each client's needs are different. I have tried to increase your sensitivity to what those needs frequently include. I am confident that you will monitor them as they related to a particular client and will find that you learn which topics require discussion, while recognizing those aspects of adjustment with which the client feels comfortable.

INFORMATION COUNSELING

Much of the anxiety that arises from an identified disability often exceeds what you as a specialist consider justified. It has been difficult for me to understand that the level of anxiety experienced by a person is not predictable from the type or severity of the disability. A person with a moderate hearing problem may experience far greater distress over the diagnosis than another person whose hearing difficulty is severe. A parent of a child with a cleft palate may exhibit fewer adjustment problems than another parent whose child has a minor hearing difficulty. These variations in the degree of anxiety a person or family feels about a problem usually arise from differences in the makeup of the persons involved. However, the level of anxiety usually is significantly raised by lack of information concerning the problem, its real significance, and the prognosis for improvement. *Therefore, informational guidance seeks to provide hearing-impaired people with a clear understanding of the type of hearing problem they have, the effects such problems are known to have on performance, and how those effects vary under different conditions.* A client should be advised of alternative ways of reducing the effects of the hearing deficit, what each alternative involves, and the prognosis for achieving significant improvement. Informational counseling describes the objective realities of the situation. This contrasts with personal adjustment counseling, which is concerned with helping the client to achieve a perception of the situation that is conducive to problem-solving.

You have the theoretical and technical knowledge necessary for the selection and fitting of the most appropriate hearing aid(s). It is important that the client realize that the hearing aid is as much a custom selected and adjusted device as are the lenses in a person's glasses. Unlike glasses, however, it does not correct the problem. It is a tool by which communication can be improved, it is an *aid to hearing*.

The client must understand the need for it, what it may or may not achieve, and how to use it. Equally important, your client must want to use it, feel confident about being able to use it effectively, and feel positive about using it. Finally, both of you must have a clear understanding of the ultimate adjustment goal toward which you are to work. It may be that after a successful hearing aid selection, orientation, counseling, and the trial use, the client will achieve the established goals alone. Sometimes, however, even with the appropriate tool, the task takes longer and requires greater resources.

Explaining the Hearing Impairment

In some states, medical clearance is required before a hearing aid can be fitted; such clearance always is advisable. However, medical consultation does not mean that clients clearly understand what the physician told them about the impairment. It is wise, therefore, to begin by explaining why a referral has been made for a hearing aid trial. Since most clients have sensorineural impairments, you should reinforce their understanding that these are not medically reversible hearing problems since they involve damage to the sense organ and/or nerve of hearing. When there is a conductive loss or conductive component, you should explain that at present the specialist does not feel medication or corrective surgery will solve the problem or contribute further to the improvement of hearing. This point should be made because some persons, particularly the parents of hearing-impaired children, have the impression that a hearing aid is a corrective device and that after a period of use it will no longer be necessary to wear it. A question frequently asked is: "Will he not become dependent on the aid?" This question is evidence of the same type of faulty reasoning. The answer is, of course, "We hope so," that is to say, we hope that amplification will permit a level of communicative behavior that otherwise would not be possible. The dependency is on the higher level of functioning that the aid makes possible—a very worthy goal to strive for.

Audiometric Test Results

It is always reassuring to know that a specialist whom you are consulting really does understand your problem. Explaining what the audiogram and speech audiometry results mean and making predictions about the effects of the impairment on the individual's ability to hear, will usually win quite a lot of confidence. To do this, I begin by explaining what the audiogram is and what it tells me. Even when this has been done before, it is helpful to remind the client what we are dealing with. Avoid all technical terms unless you give the lay equivalent. Begin by explaining that the figures at the top of the chart represent the pitches, or "frequencies," of the tones they heard. The higher the pitch, the higher the numbers. For instance, I explain that by "using tones of pure pitch we can determine whether the ear detects all pitches equally well or whether some are more difficult to hear than others. The pitches that play the greatest part in speech comprehension are 500 to 4000. The numbers down the side of the chart represent how strong the tone is, the right ear results being shown by circles, the left by crosses." Given this information, the client is ready to read the audiogram. "Normal sensitivity lies in the area 0–20 dB, or units of loudness"; you draw a line across the 20-dB level. You and the client then consider whether either ear has normal sensitivity for any pitches, examine whether the two ears follow approximately the same pattern across the audiogram, or whether one has better hearing than the other. You both discuss the pattern of the loss of sensitivity for the different pitch ranges. It may be relatively equal for all pitches or you may observe that the loss becomes greater as the pitch gets higher. You label this pattern for the client, for example, as a "relatively flat loss," "a gradually sloping loss as the pitch rises," or a "steep ski slope loss beginning in the middle pitch range." You might use this information when you describe the effects of audiogram shape on speech intelligibility.

The client always wishes to know how severe the hearing loss is. The otologist has often given percentage loss figures. These really do not prove very helpful in terms of an appreciation of the functional significance of the problem. A client is often most satisfied when the audiologist explains that to understand the degree of loss it is necessary to consider three pitch ranges. These are as follows: the low range (125–250 Hz), where the voice energy lies; the middle range (500–2000 Hz), where most of the information lies; and the high-pitch range (3000–8000 Hz), where a few high tone consonants such as sh, s, f, etc. lie. You could categorize the *level* of impairment as (1) mild (20–35 dB), (2) moderate (40–55 dB), (3) moderately severe (60–75 dB), severe (80–90 dB), or profound (95+ dB). You then look at the audiogram in the three pitch ranges to find, for example, that the client has only a very *mild* problem hearing voice in the low range, but that in the important middle pitch range, which contains so much speech sound information, the impairment is moderately severe, while hearing loss for the high tone is severe, that in fact sounds in this range are not audible at all. You might then summarize by saying "so you have a hearing loss which is mild for low voice tones, moderately severe for most of speech, and severe for high pitched sounds." Clients with steep high-frequency losses with an abrupt decrease in thresholds above 1500 or 2000 Hz need a different explanation. They need to understand that normal hearing provides a cushion of extra information that we draw on when listening conditions become poor or the listening task difficult; for example, when noise levels compete with speech, when there are high reverberation times, when there are multiple speakers, when a person has a foreign dialect, or when the details of the message are critical or complex. A hearing loss above 1500 or 2000 Hz creates a significant handicap under these conditions because the normal cushion of information has been greatly reduced and the reserves are not available to supplement the reduced information available in poor listening conditions.

Speech Discrimination Results

After you and the client have looked at the audiogram together, you might explain that the chart is interesting now, not for the hearing that has been lost, but for the hearing that remains. You both want to know how much you can expect from that hearing when you reach it by amplifying the sound. This, you explain, is what the discrimination test results give an approximation of. They show how much the distortion of a damaged organ of hearing, "the cochlea," affects the clarity of speech when it is loud enough. You explain that just to follow the gist of a conversation, one needs to hear half of all the speech signal. Comfortable listening under favorable conditions requires 70–80 percent information. You both then examine the scores the client obtained—for example, 88 percent in the right ear, and 76 percent in the left suggesting better clarity in the right ear, which borders on normal discrimination potential.

To help the client better understand why they have difficulty understanding everything, even when it is loud enough, you could explain sensorineural impairment as an unwanted filter that takes out some important information from speech sounds. I find the analogy of baking a cake to be helpful. Each cake requires a recipe for its production; each recipe is specific to a specific type cake; and each calls for a specific combination of ingredients in prescribed quantities. If ingredients are omitted or the quantities not accurately measured, the quality of the cake will deteriorate, perhaps even to the point where the cake is inedible. Speech perception is the same. Each individual speech sound has a recipe. To be clearly perceived all the ingredients must be present in the correct proportions. A sensorineural hearing impairment reduces the strength of the ingredients, but seldom does so equally. Some ingredients are removed completely, some reduced in loudness. The result is distortion. The sound may be audible but unclear or perhaps unrecognizable. Two sounds, dependent for their recognition on high-frequency (pitch) ingredients, may be audible but indistinguishable when a severe hearing loss in the high tone range removes these components. "So, you often hear but cannot make out what has been said. That is the problem we are going to try to overcome with a hearing aid(s)."

You might communicate to the client at this point the extent to which you predict amplification will help. This should always be stated positively—"You are an excellent candidate for a hearing aid, Mrs. Collins" or in another case, "Even though a hearing aid is not going to solve all your hearing problems, it's going to make things easier."

Amplification Need Profile

Having stressed adjustment needs so strongly, I can now address the more practical issue of the specific situations and communication activities in which amplification must provide help.

I work part of my week in a private agency devoted exclusively to providing appropriate hearing aid fitting, counseling, and rehabilitation for hearing-impaired persons. In such a setting, service must be paid for in full. This contrasts markedly with the way clinics, supported in part by community funding or by universities, can operate. As a result, I have a conservative approach to the method of need profiling. However, a few clients may require an intensive profile. For this reason, I include approaches suitable to both situations in my discussion.

The informal need profile constitutes an analysis of the particular communication demands that the client encounters but cannot comfortably satisfy. The point of such an analysis is that it should be highly individualized. It should constitute a data base that you, the client, and the immediate members of the client's family can use to (1) identify problem communication situations, (2) assess the *functional* benefits the hearing aid(s) provides in real life environments, (3) identify situations that remain problems even with amplification, and (4) assess the effectiveness of communication strategies targeted at situations that continue to present difficulty.

For most clients, you will be able to obtain the information for the communication profile in informal discussion. It is most useful to include in this discussion the spouse, close family members, or any other person in close relationship with the client. They can often be more objective than the client about the communication difficulties experienced at home and in social situations. Together you should identify the particular situations that present communication problems. You might ask first about *difficulties at home,* then about those that are experienced *at work,* and finally about problems *in social or recreational activities.* You could make a written note of each situation in which difficulty is experienced, for it is from this information that you and the client will determine your goals and expectations for amplification.

Once the problem situations are identified, it is advisable to analyze each situation. You could ask the client to try to think of particular situations that illustrate the difficulty and to answer the following questions:

1. Where were you when the problem arose?
2. What, briefly, was the situation?
3. How many people were you with?
4. What was the nature of the communication?
5. Were you an active participant?
6. What were the room acoustics like?
7. Was there a lot of noise?
8. How far were you from the speaker?
9. How much difficulty did you experience?

I wish again to stress that I obtain this information through discussion with the client and whomever accompanies that client. As you work together to develop the communication profile you are also developing a cooperative working relationship. Fitting a hearing aid requires team work. You are the leader of a team, not a dictator who knows what is best for your client, who tells the client how to feel and behave. *Your role is to guide the client in the search for the most appropriate approach.*

For each of the three environments, home, place of employment, and social situations, it is a good idea to write out a set of goals that you and your client seek to achieve. The hearing aid alone may not allow you both to fully achieve each goal, although it usually moves you closer to each. For example, your goals for the home environment may include:

1. To be able to communicate easily in a face-to-face situation in the living room without/with the help of watching the speaker
2. To be able to participate comfortably in conversation in the living room when two to four guests are present with/without watching the speaker
3. To be able to follow dinner table conversation easily
4. To hear the television well at a normal level of loudness

Socially the goals might be:

1. To be able to join in conversations at dinner parties
2. To be able to follow the sermon in church
3. To be able to take up bridge again
4. To enjoy attending a play
5. To be able to follow a talk at the gardening club

While at work, the goals may be a significant improvement in the ability to:

1. Understand what the customer has asked me without having to ask them to repeat what they said
2. To have significantly less difficulty following the discussion in staff meetings

3. To be able to follow more easily the instructional videotapes in the training course that is giving me trouble
4. To understand with significantly less difficulty conversations at the table in the cafeteria.

Obtaining the information necessary to identify specific problem situations and establishing appropriate goals based on those problems is not very time-consuming. It is valuable in that it evidences your concern for individualized relevance in your approach to your clients' problems. It shows your clients that you are addressing their difficulties in a highly individualized manner.

Under some circumstances, it may be helpful, and economically justifiable, to conduct an in-depth analysis of communication difficulties. With an ever-increasing emphasis on cost-effectiveness, even in funded agencies, it is necessary to carefully consider the necessity for administering a lengthy communication profile before deciding to do so. Several scales have been developed to provide comprehensive information.

High et al. (1964) first developed and tested the hearing handicap scale, designed to assess the effect of hearing loss on the subject's performance in ordinary hearing situations arising in an urban environment. They used two tests of 20 questions each related mainly to speech communication and to a lesser extent to audition of background noise and warning signals. The response was specified in terms of the frequency with which difficulty was encountered in each situation. The limitations of this tool, as have been pointed out by Giolas (1970), lie in the rather narrow homogeneous nature of the items. A number of important aspects, particularly vocational status and attitude toward the handicap, are not included.

Giolas in his 1970 article appeals for further investigation into tools that explore the effects of hearing loss upon everyday functions. In discussing this need he states:

> While it is reasonable to assume that a loss in sound reception will effect some handicap, the nature of the handicap in the everyday life situation is unknown. This is pointed out by repeated encounters in the clinical setting with individuals demonstrating quite similar audiograms and quite dissimilar functional behavioral problems. Still another way to look at the ineffectiveness of threshold measures as indicators of special handicap is to recognize the implications of a stable audiogram. Even after successful aural rehabilitation where there is obvious improvement in communication skills, the audiogram is not expected to improve. This points out once again that the status of a given handicap cannot be meaningully assessed from threshold measures.*

Such a scale, as suggested by Giolas, was designed and developed by Noble and Atherley (1970). Their instrument, the Hearing Measurement Scale for Disability, includes 42 scoring items weighted to give a measure of disability. The ques-

*Reproduced from Giolas TG: The measurement of hearing handicap. Maico Audiol Libr Serv 8:6, 1970. With permission.

tions used cover areas of speech and hearing ability in different situations, acuity for nonspeech sounds, localization, speech distortion, effects of tinnitus, and personal opinion about the effects of the hearing deficit.

In follow-up publications, Atherley and Noble (1971) and Noble (1972) discussed the effectiveness of the tool as tested with specific populations. They describe it as a workable device that can provide useful clinical information about individual hearing-impaired persons or about groups of persons with a hearing deficit.

The dispenser may wish to use one of the already tested scales or seek the flexibility of developing variants of these for his own use. Remember, in developing the scale, attempts are to be made to both identify the types of communication situations in which problems occur and the degree of difficulty.

The scales I suggest in Appendixes A–D at the end of this chapter illustrate the type of approach that may be taken. Notice that after each question the person is asked to identify the frequency with which the situation is encountered. Each answer is rated on a scale ranging from +2 to −2; the frequency of occurrence is rated 1–3. This permits an average rating to be computed for degree of difficulty in communication situations in a specific environment. By multiplying the value of the answer by the value of a question, for example, "I experience a fair amount of difficulty" (value −1) by the frequency of occurrence of the situation, for example, "very often" (value 3), a weighted value (−3) is obtained. The same difficulty experienced only seldom reduces the weighted value in this example to −1. The absolute value ($a \times b$) indicates the level of importance that the communication situation has for the client.

Developing Realistic Expectations for Amplification

Once the profile has been developed, it is necessary to address directly the question of what the hearing aid is likely to be able to contribute to the task of reducing communication difficulty in the situations identified. *The most appropriate time to discuss realistic expectations for achieving benefit from the aid is after aided testing has been completed, but before the client leaves for the trial period.* Using the unaided/aided test results I again emphasize that the main contribution of the aid is to make more auditory information available. I point out that the organ of hearing remains damaged and that the hearing aid cannot restore normal hearing. Its effectiveness must be judged on how close it comes to meeting justifiable expectations. These concern the improvement amplification is predicted to make in the person's ability to function in everyday situations.

It is most important, therefore, that the client have realistic expectations for what those benefits are likely to be. *Too often disappointment arises because the client was not informed about the capabilities and limitations of the aid.*

When a young child is being fitted for amplification, the need for counseling parents in terms of what to expect is, if anything, more critical than when an adult is involved. Ross (Chapter 6) discusses this need and makes specific reference to the writings of McConnell (1968) and Luterman (1971). In addition, I refer the reader to an article by Horton and McConnell (1970). For an in-depth treatment of the hearing-impaired child's use of sensory information, I would suggest Stark (1974).

The aim of this discussion is to forestall the disappointment that arises from expecting too much. Writing about the disappointment frequently expressed by new hearing aid users, Niemeyer (1974) states:

> As long as he carries on a conversation with a single person, in a quiet room that is, as long as he uses the hearing aid under similar acoustic conditions as those prevailing at the time of selecting the hearing aid on the basis of the speech audiometric results, his understanding is good and this already means an important step forward to him; the interpretation of succeeding sound events, diachronous hearing, does not present any insuperable hurdles to him. However, when he wants to participate in group conversations, or when conversations take place in a noisy environment, his understanding falls off considerably; synchronous hearing, the perception of acoustic events simultaneously presenting and the isolation of the speech signal from the noise is poor. This particular handicap already distresses most of the patients with internal ear deafness even before they use a hearing aid and the situation is even, accentuated by amplification through the aid. The hearing handicapped individual who places his hopes in the technical hearing prosthesis again feels shut out and unable to share fully in group conversations.*

Honest counsel concerning expectations will do much to engender the attitude and expectations appropriate to the trial period with the hearing aid.

Correcting False Assumptions

The lack of understanding of what a hearing aid can and cannot do that I encounter, even among hearing aid users, continues to surprise me. Perhaps they have been given this information and have forgotten it, perhaps they were never told. Clients often tell me "no one ever explained that to me before." I make this observation to emphasize the importance of educating one's clients, of enabling them to learn about the hearing aid(s) potential, limits, function, and care. Certainly most potential users of hearing aids have incorrect concepts of what a hearing aid can do. They and their families frequently assume that the hearing aid will actually restore normal hearing.

Perhaps the most common incorrect assumption made by the potential hearing aid user is that in some way the hearing aid is selective and only amplifies speech. This concept may not be specifically expressed, but the reaction of clients to the noise of amplified nonspeech sounds is evidence that their expectations do not coincide with reality. This aspect of amplification must be discussed quite carefully to avoid hasty rejection of the aid. Also, arrangements must be made to minimize

*Reproduced from Niemeyer W: Psychological aspects of hearing-aid fitting. J Audiol Tech 12:3, 1973. Maico Audiol Libr Serv 10:5, 1972. With permission.

the effects of environmental noise in early experiences with the aid. The problem of adjustment to noises in the world, even to one's own voice if it has not been at normal loudness for several years, is one of perceptual patterning. It is not infrequent for persons who have had their hearing restored to near normal by a stapedectomy operation to experience a difficult period of adjustment. Occasionally, a person will admit to wishing that the surgery had not been performed.

Von Senden (1960) reported similar reactions by his subjects to the restoration of sight following cataract removal. The problem arises from the discrepancy between the established perception of the auditory or visual world, and the sudden change in the information received after surgery or amplification. This discrepancy may be sufficiently disturbing as to threaten the client's stability, a situation not dissimilar to the effect of a sudden onset of deafness. It is the overwhelming feeling of being unable to cope with the changed situation that threatens and causes a person to reject that situation rather than adapt to it. This situation can and should be prevented by counseling the hearing aid candidate.

The nature of the situation should be explained, emphasizing that the person not only has been shut off from normal speech perception for a long time but also has been effectively cushioned against the constant noise background that once was heard everyday with increasing loudness. People learn to identify the components of this noise so that they are able to accept it as normal despite its unpleasantness. To a degree, they become only partially aware of it. *When a person has grown accustomed to relative quiet, sudden exposure to environmental sounds at near-normal levels of loudness can be a very negative experience and will take time for that person to adjust, because the process involves subconscious reassessment of the relative loudness of common sounds.* By being aware that this is to be expected, the audiologist may gain the client's agreement not to make a hasty decision to reject amplification. Hearing aid evaluation and informational counseling attempts to help clients to increase their objectivity in assessing the value of a hearing aid. It also helps to keep their observations and their feelings in two clearly identified categories.

At this point the client usually is anxious to see an aid, to know what types are available, or to see an earmold, even a battery. You might explain, "We will go into the details of the aid when we do the fitting. My concern now is to explain what I want the aid to do." To achieve this, you could return to the audiogram. You should remind the client that the hearing loss has two aspects: loss of loudness and unevenness of sensitivity to different pitches. The hearing aid, you point out, can provide as much power as needed. To a great extent, the hearing aid, together with the technology of the earmold when a postauricular aid is worn, will shape the amplified sound. This gives different emphasis to the different pitches as needed by the client. This way we not only put back loudness, but also information. It should be stressed, again, that there are limits. Only so much loudness will be acceptable, and the ear is not normal, so there will always remain an element of distortion. "You will never hear as well as when your hearing was unimpaired," you might explain. "My goal is to make you able to communicate more normally." You need to get across the fact that *no hearing aid can correct a sensorineural hearing deficit as glasses correct a muscular visual defect*. No system of amplification can compensate for the loss of function of some components of the sense organ of hearing. *What an aid does is to allow the use of what remains*. It is an "aid" to hearing, not a restorative device.

Be honest about what you believe a client is justified in expecting from the hearing aid. If an aid can reasonably be expected to bring communication performance to within normal level in all but the most difficult listening situations, then the hearing aid candidate's demands may justifiably be set high. If, on the other hand, poor maximum discrimination determines that amplification can do little more than increase the ability to follow conversation in the most favorable listening conditions, and even then, mainly because of the increased ease with which the person can interpret visible speech cues against the background of increased auditory information, the expectations for improvement must be more conservative.

Choosing the Appropriate Type of Hearing Aid

It is our responsibility as audiologists to determine which type of hearing aid(s) and which model and setting will be best suited to the client's needs. Indeed, our assessment of the potential benefits to be derived from amplification should be based on an optimal fitting. Sometimes, however, despite careful counseling, the client has a preference for a particular type of hearing aid. For example, a client may insist on a canal fitting or an ITE fitting or, similarly, may decline even to try binaural hearing aids, insisting that just the single aid will probably suffice. The client simply may not wish to spend the money on a second aid.

Even among audiologists there exist different philosphies and guidelines concerning fittings. Each of us must function according to what we believe to be in the best interests of the client. We are obligated to identify for the client what the best fitting would be and to explain why we believe anything less than that would represent a compromise. If, despite our best efforts, the client insists on an alternative fitting, you will have no choice but to accede to these wishes graciously unless you feel that to proceed with such a fitting would be unethical. A decision to decline to make less than an optimal fitting is made difficult by the realization that undoubtedly, somewhere, the client will obtain such an aid.

The fact is that it is sometimes necessary to temper our ideals with pragmatism. If clients are adamant about their choice, even after careful counseling, you may decide that the second-best fitting will be better than no fitting. The final decision to purchase an aid, even to try one, does after all rest with the client. A recent example with which I am familiar is a lawyer who insisted on purchasing two canal aids. He did so despite advice to the contrary. Even though it was explained that his hearing loss is borderline for that category of aid, and that his history of slow deterioration in hearing thresholds suggest that the aids may prove inadequate in a year or two, he still purchased them. It was two canal aids or no aids. He was prepared to take the financial risk and to hear less successfully than we feel he could with a different binaural fitting.

Our role is to inform, advise, and to guide. We cannot impose our wishes on the client even in his or her best interests.

The Role of the Amplified Signal in Communications

For those children and adults for whom normal auditory performance is not possible to achieve by amplification, it will be necessary to explain, in as simple a manner as possible, that communication is a total process that is made easier because it takes place within a context. Within the auditory channel, the constraints of language limit how the speaker may put together speech sounds, words, sentences, and phrases. The meaning content exerts further constraints, which operate on the visible aspects of speech. Added to this are the cues provided by the speaker's dress and gestures and the immediate environment so that the situation is one in which the listener, unconsciously familiar with these factors, can afford to miss part of the acoustic signal yet still be able to perceive the message. Counseling, therefore, should place the hearing aid within the larger context of the total communication event. The hearing aid user should not assume either that all the information must be perceived through the aid if speech is to be understood, or that if the aid provides less than complete comprehension, it is not worth using. With auditory and visual communication, it may well be possible to close the communication gap. This type of information also will be of value to the adult user of a hearing aid, particularly when less than complete benefit from amplification is possible. It will help the user to understand that the successful use of amplification is not to be assessed as complete understanding of speech in most situations but rather as the degree of improvement it permits in overall communicative behavior. Honest counsel will do much to engender the attitude and expectations appropriate to the trial period with the hearing aid.

Instructing Your Client in the Operation and Care of the Hearing Aid

Such instruction used to require quite a lot of counseling time when body-worn aids were the only type of hearing aid available. The increasing use of canal aids, common use of ITE models, and otherwise almost universal fitting of postauricular hearing aids has simplified the controls and hearing aid user. You need to remember, however, that many of your clients are elderly, many have reduced tactile and motor coordination ability, and most are somewhat apprehensive about wearing the aid(s). It is important to decide how much information about the aid a given person needs and can absorb, how often it needs to be gone over, and how best to present what you wish them to know. Remember, an alert woman of 93 years of age, such as a woman I recently fitted with a hearing aid, may absorb the instruction more easily than a very tense anxious man half her age. Again, each person's needs are special. It is particularly helpful at this time to have a family member or good friend present.

This enables an observer to see how the aid is to be worn and taken care of. It makes going over the instruction booklet together easier after the client gets home, since two persons were present when the same information and procedures were explained and demonstrated in the office. If the aid to be fitted is a postauricular model, you could first try the earmold to ensure a comfortable fit, at the same time measuring and cutting the tubing. You might then explain that you first want the individual to learn to inset and remove the mold easily, showing the two important parts to pay attention to when fitting the mold in the ear: the canal projection and the helix area. Then you could show how to hold the mold while inserting it and slowly and carefully, hooking the helix area under the skin flap, snugging the mold home by gently pressing on the concha ring. Sometimes you may wish to demonstrate this while inserting a mold into your own ear, or you might insert the mold into your client's ear while the client holds a mirror to watch. You may be surprised by how apprehensive and tense many clients become about their ability to perform this task. Again, it is important to identify these feelings as quite normal. Stress that there is no hurry, that it may take a few attempts to figure it out, but that once they get it right it will all seem quite easy. Try to appeal to the client to be patient and not to struggle with the task: "If you have to struggle, then you need to change how you are putting the mold in the ear." While the client is attempting to insert the mold, you may gently guide a hand. You might also reward patience verbally, "That's a very patient approach, Mr. James, take your time, you'll get it in a minute." When the mold eventually is inserted, you could commend the client, "Excellent. May we do that just once more so you really get the feel for it?" When a client shows frustration you could interrupt the process, identifying the frustration early. "Let me show you once more" or "Let me guide your hand" or even "You are finding this very frustrating, let's take a break to look at the hearing aid. We'll come back to the mold in a moment. I promise you, you will get the hang of it."

Once the mold can be inserted and removed satisfactorily, you could explain the particular controls on the aid being tried, showing how the battery is correctly inserted and how to turn the aid on. Particular care should be taken to explain the role of the T (telephone) switch. Clients must know that they will not hear people or sounds in the environment when the control is set to T. You should point out that this is the first thing to suspect if the aid appears not to be working, or to produce only a hum. Explain that for normal use, the switch must be set to M (or an appropriate letter code for microphone). At this point it might be wise to explain that just before they leave for the trial period, you will demonstrate how to use the aid to talk on the phone both on the M and on the T setting. You could also explain the use of the volume control including the "off" switch if it is not part of the volume control. Once these controls have been explained, have the client turn the aid to "on," turn volume to full, while cupping the aid in the hands close to the ear. If the client can hear the resultant feedback, this check should always be made before putting on the aid. You should also ask the client to set the input controls, first to M, then to T, then to O.

The client is now ready to try the aid. For the postauricular, you might tell them not to worry about the hearing aid until the mold is comfortably in the ear, to simply let the aid hang by the tubing. Then show the client how to hook the aid behind the ear. Finally, verbally guide the client in an exploration of the hearing aid, first finding the on switch and then gradually increasing the volume to comfort level. The significant point I wish to make is that in hearing aid orientation the client's feelings are important to successful acceptance and use of the aid. Some clients will have no problems inserting the mold, fitting the aid behind the ear, and finding and operating the controls. They exhibit a comfortable positive attitude. Some, however, even with your counsel, support, and encouragement, remain apprehensive. The apprehension generates a sense of insecurity, inadequacy, even self-helplessness.

Some clients will remark, "Oh, I'll never learn to do this" even before they have actually tried. Others may claim the mold is not the correct one, that it does not fit. They may express how clumsy they feel, even how stupid because they are experiencing difficulty. You need to acknowledge and accept the expression or manifestation of these feelings. Point out that it is not unusual for it to take time to learn how to insert the mold, to find and operate the controls. Acknowledge the real limitations of mildly arthritic fingers, of reduced sensation in the fingertips. Share with the client that you, too, have experienced such feelings in new situations, that you do not expect them to master the task immediately. *You must counteract and reduce the negative feelings. You must prevent the client from struggling with the task.*

At this point in the discussion, you will probably acknowledge the importance of providing adequate informational and support counseling *before* the fitting of the hearing aid. The amount of support needed will vary from minimal to maximal. You will need to be the judge for each client. In a genuinely cooperative problem-solving relationship such judgment should not be difficult.

The use of the ITE and canal type aids is much easier for the client. However, the same considerate instruction and support should be provided. The feelings about the aid may be just as strong, but the manipulation problems, presuming the aid is appropriate for the client's finger dexterity and sensitivity, will be minimal.

Explanations for special fittings (e.g., binaural, CROS, BICROS) should be made with special care. The client should really understand the basic principle of the system and how to operate it.

Before the client leaves, you should explain and demonstrate how to use the aid on the telephone. With the postauricular aid, you should demonstrate this on both the M and T settings. Explain how to avoid feedback with all three types of aids. It is essential that the client try the telephone in your office, even if listening on an intercom or to a recorded time and temperature, weather, or movie listing.

Working with Parents of the Young Hearing-Impaired Child

In the case of young children, parents should be given this information. Downs (1971) outlined and discussed methods for maintaining three cardinal principles, which she lists as (1) keeping the hearing aid on the child, (2) keeping the hearing aid functioning on the child, and (3) using the hearing aid as an amplification device to aid hearing. Downs identifies such practical problems as an earmold and receiver that will not stay in an infant's ear, a problem that may be solved by connecting them by a small tube molded to the ear so as to permit the receiver to be positioned behind it, or perhaps by placing the aid on the back of the child, thus keeping the cord away from the child's hands. For the child who keeps pulling the aid out, she recommends carefully rechecking the selected volume level, lest it be too high, and ensuring that the mold is comfortable. If these points check out negatively, then the child will need to be trained (Downs 1966). Downs discusses the problem of feedback pointing out the need for frequent new molds for growing children and emphasizing the need for frequent analysis of the performance of the hearing aid. Care and maintenance information must be simply, carefully, and—if necessary— repeatedly explained and demonstrated to parents. However, never underestimate the ability of school-age hearing-impaired children to become sophisticated hearing aid users. Paulos (1961) convincingly demonstrated the effectiveness of a program specifically designed to educate these youngsters in the nature of their hearing difficulty and in the role of amplification. It is the child's hearing problem; the child has to wear the aid; the child knows what it is like. I, therefore, treat children with the same respect as I do adults, for with such an approach, children usually manage to impress me with their competence. This experience can be an important step in personal adjustment counseling.

In addition to understanding the hearing aid, the audiologist will need to explain how to care for it. The most important aspects of care involve the following instructions:

1. Handle the aid gently; it is an expensive instrument. Avoid placing it where it will get hot, such as on a radiator or in the glove compartment of the car. Keep the aid dry and do not clean it with anything other than an almost dry cloth. Make quite sure that food and dust are not trapped on the microphone grill of a body aid.
2. Open the battery compartment when the aid is not in use. The battery will continue to drain even if the volume control switch is off.
3. Ensure that the terminals of the battery socket and the battery contacts are noncorroded and clean. They may be gently roughened with the small end of an emery board used for shaping fingernails. The prongs of the cord should be kept bright in the same manner. Should corrosion occur, it may be removed by using a damp cloth sprinkled lightly with baking soda.
4. Always carry spare batteries. Zinc-air cell batteries are preferable to mercury because they have approximately twice the lifespan and do not require refrigeration for long-term storage. If you use a battery tester, do so sparingly, for it, too, consumes battery power.
5. Wipe the earmold or plastic shell casing for the ITE and canal aids regularly with a tissue. Remove wax carefully from the canal opening of the mold or aid,

using an opened paper clip for the mold and the special tool provided with the ITE and canal models.

6. If the hearing aid gets wet, immediate action may preserve it by (a) removing the batteries at once, (b) draining all water from it, or (c) drying it with absorbent cloth, and placing it in a warm—*but not hot*—place. The low heat of a hair drier could be used. A jar containing silica gel or a dry pack pouch available from your hearing aid dealer will provide an excellent dry climate for the aid when it is not in use.

Checking the Hearing Aid and Identifying Problems

When first fitted with a hearing aid, a person often finds that the sounds heard are different from those expected. This is a result of the combined filtering effect of that person's hearing impairment and the frequency characteristics of the aid. Adult hearing aid users will become accustomed to how speech and environmental noises sound through the hearing aid. This provides a norm against which a subjective judgment can be made as to whether the aid is functioning as expected. For young children, parents must make this decision. They should make a point of frequently listening to speech and noise through the child's aid in order to develop an auditory image of how it sounds when functioning well. They should routinely listen to the aid each day to check its function before putting it on the child.

From time to time, things will go wrong with the hearing aid. These malfunctions should be detected immediately in order that the hearing aid user not be deprived of amplification for longer than is absolutely necessary. When an aid is believed not to be functioning properly, the user or the parents of a child should be able to run simple checks to eliminate some basic causes before making a trip to the hearing aid dealer.

The following checks should be made routinely, either by the user, or on his behalf by a person with good hearing.

THE BATTERY

Open the battery case and remove the battery. Using a simple battery tester, which every hearing aid user should have, test to ensure that the battery is at the required voltage. Even a new battery should be tested before use. Discard or store old batteries in a box clearly marked "used batteries." Check that the terminals of the battery and the contact points of the aid are bright. If they are not, they can be cleaned with a pencil eraser or with a fine emery board. Insert the battery, making sure that the + and − signs on the battery match those marked on the hearing aid.

If the aid does not function at all, the prime suspect is a dead battery. Replacement of the battery in this case will render the aid functional again. Intermittent function of the aid may arise from a faulty connection between the battery and the contacts. When this is the case, it is often observed that tapping the aid lightly will cause it to function briefly, only to have it go off again very soon. Cleaning the terminals and connections often will correct this.

Sometimes a hearing aid user is concerned that the battery appears not to last very long. This is not an unusual complaint after purchase of a more powerful aid, which places a heavier drain on the battery than did the previous hearing aid. A hearing aid wearer should be advised of how many hours a battery should be expected to last. Once having begun to use the aid regularly, the user or parents of a child should be encouraged to keep a log of the number of hours the aid is on each day. After 2 or 3 weeks, they will know the weekly average in-use hours that can then be compared to the expected battery life.

THE EARMOLD, TUBING, AND CONNECTIONS

The earmold should be kept free of wax. If the mold becomes completely blocked, the aid will appear not to function. When an aid is reported "dead" after checking for a dead battery, check for a wax plug in the mold. If it is dirty, clean it carefully as described above. Check the tubing, which on ear-level devices connects the mold to the hearing aid. This tube must be unobstructed to allow the sound to travel from the aid to the ear. If moisture forms and condenses in the tube, the passage of sound will be blocked. Similarly, if when the aid is inserted, the tube becomes kinked, the sound will be prevented from reaching the ear. Care must be taken to avoid this occurring when inserting the mold. Someone can be asked to check the tubing, or it may be possible for the user to check for himself by using a mirror. Sometimes kinking will occur if the tube is too long. In this case the hearing aid dispenser should be consulted. Stiff, discolored, or cracked tubing should be replaced. In some cases, it may be advisable for the hearing aid user to have extra tubes available as replacements and that someone be able to change a tube if the client is not able to do this. This is necessary only when it is difficult for the client to get to the hearing aid dispenser.

Finally, check that the connections between the tubing, the earmold, and the aid are clean and unobstructed. If the connection on the hearing aid is blocked, consult the hearing aid dispenser.

THE CONTROLS

Improper setting of the controls is not an infrequent cause of apparent malfunction. Particular attention should be paid to the on/off switch, which must be in the on position for use, and to the M/T switch. When used normally, the aid must be switched to M for environmental microphone. When switched to the T (telephone) circuit position, the environmental microphone will not operate. The telephone circuit enables the client to listen to a telephone conversation without distraction from amplified environmental sounds. The T setting is appropriate only for telephone use.

The tone control should be on the setting recommended by the dispenser. Expressed dissatisfaction with the quality of the sound of the aid may arise from the tone control inadvertently having been moved from the usual setting, thus changing the characteristics of the amplified sound.

It is difficult for a non-hearing aid user to listen to a hearing aid without a plastic hearing aid stethoscope (available from Hal Hen Products). This allows the mold and tubing to be reproved from a postauricular aid and the ear hook opening to be pushed into the rubber cup at the end of the stethoscope. The canal opening on canal and ITE aids likewise can be pushed into the cup to enable you to listen to the aid.

Turn the volume control on and rotate it up and down, listening for scratchiness or dead spots. The loudness of the sound should grow smoothly as the volume control is turned more fully on. A sudden jump in loudness, or lack of control over loudness, indicates that the volume control is defective. The volume control should be neither exceptionally loose nor very stiff. Rotating the volume control gently up and down a half dozen times occasionally will overcome scratchiness caused by dirt. Intermittent function of the aid may originate in a faulty volume control. Similarly, check the "on/off" switch, turning it back and forth to check for loose contacts.

Check tone controls, listening for appropriate changes in pitch and quality of the sound. Check the telephone switch to ensure that speech over the telephone is amplified on the T setting while environmental sounds are not. If the sound is weak on the T setting, replacement of the telecoil may be necessary.

BODY AID CORD AND RECEIVER BUTTON

Check for breaks in the cord of a body aid by rolling it back and forth between finger and thumb while listening for "cut-outs." A faulty cord may result in intermittent sound or absence of sound. If in doubt, replace the cord. The firmness of the connections between the cord and the aid, and the cord and receiver button, should be checked. Terminal prongs should be straight and clean.

The receiver button should be inspected for cracks or chips in the plastic case. These are indicative of trauma to the receiver and often identify hidden damage to the internal components. It is advisable to have an extra receiver button as standby. The snap connection between the receiver and the earmold should be tight. A plastic washer should be used to ensure maximum seal.

FEEDBACK

Feedback, which is caused by the amplification of sound leakage from the aid, will be recognized by its characteristic squeal or whistle. This most often results from an ill-fitting earmold. To check for the cause, remove the hearing aid and close the opening in the canal of the receiver by pressing your thumb against it. Now turn the aid on full. If the whistle no longer occurs, the fault is undoubtedly in the poor fit of the mold when placed in the ear. This can be confirmed if the feedback whistle can be stopped by pressing the mold more tightly into the ear when wearing the aid. In a body-worn aid, the mold should be disconnected from the receiver and the open nozzle of the receiver covered with your thumb to check whether the whistle can be stopped. If feedback cannot be stopped when you block the sound outlet from your aid with your thumb, the aid should be returned to the dealer.

Whistling will sometimes occur in postauricular aids if the wearer stands with an ear close to a reflective surface or if a hand is close to the aid while adjusting it. This is normal and is not a cause for concern. Under no other circumstance should feedback be tolerated. Most importantly, it should never be controlled by reducing the gain below the optimal amount required by the client.

User Adjustment to the Hearing Aid

Most new hearing aid users will begin to make an immediate adjustment to amplification. Indeed, the usual response is one of surprised pleasure at all the sounds now audible. Providing the specifications of the hearing aid settings are appropriate, most clients will leave the office wearing the hearing aid and will continue to do so consistently. A few will choose to be selective about when they wear it. This is commendable when appropriate. A very small number of clients will experience adjustment problems. These may be anticipated by you when there are legitimate psychoacoustic factors, such as recruitment, to account for the initial problem. Sometimes even after careful counseling the client remains apprehensive about using the hearing aid on trial. In such cases, a conservative approach to wearing the aid is advisable. Using the profile of hearing difficulties, I recommend that you identify those acoustical and communication environments in which the most favorable response to the hearing aid may be expected. These should constitute the initial experiences in hearing aid use. They should occur among people with whom the person feels comfortable and who, perhaps because of counsel, are sensitive to the feelings of apprehension and embarrassment the hearing aid user may experience. These kinds of environments will provide favorable acoustic experiences and will minimize *psychological reactions to wearing the aid.* Referring to this consideration of the client's feelings about his aid, Newby (1964) says: "Thus even the beginning hearing aid user should be successful with the aid, at home with members of his family."

The schedule of use planned for the client should be as individualized as other management procedures. Care should be taken not to unwittingly expose your clients to more listening situations than they can immediately adjust to. In Niemeyer's words (1974), "the hearing aid novice must patiently acquire his skill in dealing with the confusion of varying and rapidly changing acoustic impressions. In the initial stages he needs encouragement, guidance, and instruction to enable him to master an adaptation and training program of increasingly difficult steps." Schedules should be designed to control two parameters: (1) the environment in which the aid is worn, and (2) the duration of its use. The aim is to increase both.

As I have already stated, initial experiences with the aid are best made at home, where the noise level is low and reverberation is minimized by curtains, carpets, and upholstered furniture. Recommendations should be made that the aid be tried initially for two or three periods of about an hour each day, until the user feels comfortable with it. Since a perceptual adjustment will be involved, the person should experiment with different settings of the volume control, not simply to determine the appropriate level, but to develop some concept of how the volume control affects the loudness of sounds. Clients should be advised to see how their own voices sound to them when they speak at soft, normal, and loud levels. Reading out loud or conversing with a cooperative family member will help them to become accustomed to their "new" voice. Listening to the voices of children or grandchildren, whose natural levels of pitch are quite a lot higher than adult voices, may bring a lot of pleasure, provided the children are not shouting or all talking at once. The radio and television should be listened to when adjusted to comfortable loudness by a person with normal hearing. The volume control of the hearing aid may need to be adjusted for this activity.

The hearing aid user should gradually expand both listening time and the range of things listened to. Using the "home profile," the user should begin to explore using the hearing aid in situations that previously presented difficulty. The person can be helped to rank those situations by using the overall item rating score (degree of difficulty × frequency). Have the client keep brief notes of difficulties and successes.

A person who feels fairly comfortable using the aid around the home can begin to try wearing it in similar situations when visiting friends or relatives. The schedule should then be expanded to incorporate activities that can be planned by reference to the profile sheets for business, social, or school environments.

During this period, hearing aid counseling should continue, preferably as part of a comprehensive program of management of the person's communication problems. Auditory and visual communication training sessions, speech improvement, and adjustment counseling should be part of the support program based on the client's needs.

After 2 or 3 months, adjustment to the aid will hopefully be demonstrated by the client's growing dependency on it as an aid to living the kind of life the hearing problem had previously encroached upon. It is hoped that the aid will become as natural to this client as eyeglasses are to those who cannot function without them. This will be an appropriate time at which to reassess communicative performance, using the profile development charts. Comparison of scores, item by item or section by section, will reveal whether, in the considered judgment of the client, improvement has resulted from using the hearing aid. It will also identify situations in which further investigation and training may be fruitful. Wherever possible, it helps to have the same questions answered by the husband, wife, parent, boyfriend or girlfriend of the client. This parallel pre- and postamplification evaluation by someone close to the client aids in objectifying the perceived effects of the hearing aid on actual communication performance.

Downs (1966) outlined a program to aid parents in establishing hearing aid use by their young child. She suggests that in many cases, counseling the parents to help them accept the child's hearing loss may be the first step. I will discuss this more in the final section on personal adjustment counseling. Downs (1966) advocates the firm approach: "we tell him what is going to be done, and we do it."

Starting early in the morning, Downs recommends showing the child the aid while pointing to the clock (e.g., 9:00 A.M.), indicating a 5-minute time span during which the aid will be worn. Using physical constraint if necessary, gently insert the mold with the hearing aid turned off. If the child accepts it without protest, occupy the child for 5 minutes in a pleasurable manner. A child who rejects the mold should be constrained for the 5-minute duration and be talked to reassuringly. It is recommended that this be repeated 4 times a day until the mold is accepted. At the next session, Down advises that the parent turn the aid on one-quarter volume and speak softly and soothingly into the aid. The aid may then be inserted into the harness, while the child is occupied pleasantly for 5 minutes. A child who objects should be held firmly for that period.

The next stage (second week) extends the time to 15 minutes and expands the environment by walks around the house to help the child to relate the sounds he hears to the objects or events that make them. I have discussed the importance of this procedure in a discussion of a chapter on auditory and visual training in another text (Sanders 1982).

The third stage (third week), as described by Downs, increases the time the aid is worn to four 30-minute sessions in which the mother draws attention to the sounds her daily home activities generate.

The fourth week extends the time to 45 minutes, with the aid set at the volume setting recommended by the teacher of the deaf or the audiologist. By the sixth to eighth week, the aid hopefully will be worn most of the day. However, Downs recommends three exceptions: (1) three 10-minute breaks each day, (2) nap time, and (3) rough play.

A program such as that outlined by Downs depends on the support and guidance of parent counsel. Hearing-impaired children, even those with severe losses, should be under the constant supervision of an audiologist or a teacher of the deaf. In most cases, these children will need an intensive training program in which effective use of amplification is a major goal.

The period of adjustment to the use of a hearing aid is, for both child and adult, one that demands both a perceptual and a psychological adaptation. Adjustment to the aid is a vital component of a larger psychologic reality of being a hearing-impaired person. I would like, therefore, to remind the audiologist that, although for purposes of continuity I have discussed informational and personal adjustment counseling separately, in reality they will need to be treated as interwoven components of the orientation and counseling process.

To this point, my discussion has been concerned mainly with informational counseling. To complete this chapter, the nature of the adjustment counseling task with which you will be involved must be examined.

PERSONAL ADJUSTMENT COUNSELING

The Counselor's Role

The most common view of a counselor is that of a person with the necessary training and experience to permit that person to diagnose a problem, to determine what is needed to effect a solution, and to direct the client in a manner aimed at achieving the changes believed necessary. The problem with such a definition is that the burden of responsibility for success or failure lies with the counselor. Furthermore, the solutions arrived at are based upon the counselor's perception of the problem, which may only vaguely approximate the client's concept of the difficulties.

Brammer (1979), in examining the process and skills involved in the helping relationship, asks for whose benefit the helping process exists. We all recognize the need our client has for our help, but Brammer urges us to consider the fact that we, too, need growth and development. Unfortunately, as a counselor, the respect that comes with being an "expert" and the power inherent in being perceived by others in this role may be found to be very rewarding. Great satisfaction may be derived from the knowledge that a client needs you and may even be dependent on you.

Each of us must ask ourselves to what extent our attitudes, behaviors, and methods in the helping relationship are motivated by our own needs for self-enhancement or emotional gratification (Brammer 1979). "Why do I feel such an urge to help?" These feelings are quite natural, and not confined to beginning counselors. To experience them should not cause you to experience guilt. However, you should recognize them, acknowledge them, and realize that they are self-gratifying no matter how well you rationalize them. As such, they will not aid the counseling process. Such feelings on the part of a counselor may in fact hinder the growth process, since you are seeking to have your clients achieve independence, not dependency, and to learn how to define and solve their own difficulties, not to have solutions provided for them.

Tyler (1969) feels that success in helping others is as much a result of the kind of person you are as it is on what you actually do. Thus, learning to be a successful counselor primarily involves discovering how to make better use of the sensitivities you possess already. Combs, et al. (1971) in their work concluded that the overriding factor in differentiating effective from ineffective counselors is not the knowledge the counselors have or the methods they use, but how they view themselves. These authors identified five self perceptions that greatly contribute to success in counseling:

1. *Identification* with humankind; the perception of oneself a part of the human scene rather than divorced from it.
2. *Adequacy*; a feeling of knowing how to cope with one's own stresses and problems, of being in control of one's life.
3. *Trustworthiness*; a sense of confidence in oneself as dependable, reliable, and a sense of confidence in one's model for dealing with life.
4. *Being wanted*; feeling liked, accepted, respected by others; being able to evoke a warm response from others.
5. *Self-worth*; knowing oneself as a person worthy of others positive regard; seeing oneself as having integrity, honesty, and as having contribution to make.

Numerous authors have listed the traits that they consider important to successful counseling (Rogers 1951, Kodman 1966, Tyler 1969, Combs et al. 1971, Hansen et al. 1982, Luterman 1984, Gargiulo 1985). All agree that accurate empathy, unconditional positive regard for the person we are seeking to help, and genuineness, are probably the most important traits.

ACCURATE EMPATHY

Accurate empathy involves listening very carefully to the clients' problems and feelings about their problems in order to obtain as clear a picture as possible of how the situation looks and feels to him. Rogers (1951) states:

> It is the counselor's aim to perceive as accurately as possible all of the perceptual field as it is being experienced by the client, with the same figure and ground relationships, to the full degree that the client is willing to communicate that perceptual field; and thus having perceived this internal frame of reference of the other as completely as possible, to indicate to the client the extent to which he is seeing through the client's eyes.*

Thus empathy is necessary if you are to be able to absorb the emotionally laden, poorly defined problem expressed by your clients and reflect it back to them with an objective focus that may permit them to see their difficulty in a new light or, as Rogers (1951) says, "with a new quality," facilitating his search for a solution.

For example, a client may express the feeling: "I don't think I could wear an aid; I mean—I'd feel funny about it." An empathic helper might clarify the statement by saying: "You feel the aid would in some way be degrading; that others would think less of you," encouraging the client to clarify this feeling with: "Well yes, I mean it's like admitting to having a weakness."

Thus empathy helps guide your clients to explore their feelings. The process involves your mirroring clients' feelings yet at the same time clarifying and focusing these feelings for them. Brammer (1979) says that we can achieve empathy by listening, by striving to understand the client's perception of his/her problem and his/her world.

UNCONDITIONAL POSITIVE REGARD

This involves accepting the client as he is. To quote Rogers (1951) again:

> The primary point of importance here is the attitude held by the counselor toward the worth and the significance of the individual. How do we look upon others? Do we see each person as having worth and dignity in his own right? If we do hold this point of view at the verbal level, to what extent is it operationally evident at the behavioral level? Do we tend to treat individuals as persons of worth or do we subtly devaluate them by our attitudes and behavior? Is our philosophy one in which respect for the individual is uppermost? Do we respect his capacity and right to self direction, or do we basically believe that his life would be best guided by us?†

---

*Reproduced from Rogers C: Client-Centered Therapy. Boston, Houghton Mifflin, 1951. With permission.
†Ibid.

GENUINENESS

This arises from the empathy with and respect for a client, which permits you to feel at ease in the counseling situation, to feel unbeaten, and thus able to act in a manner congruent with your true self. It means not putting on the mask of professionalism. Genuineness is evidenced by rejection of the impressive jargon of a profession, by a relaxed, friendly manner, by an ability to accept suggestions from the client and even criticism if appropriate. "The personality of the helper must play a vital part in any helping relationship. It is the helper's use of himself which makes the interaction whatever it is to become. If a helper's self is to have such a significance, it must be involved in the dialogue" (Combs et al. 1971, p. 57).

These three conditions of accurate empathy, unconditional positive regard, and genuineness have been shown to correlate with a high degree of counselor effectiveness (Kodman 1966).

The Problem

I have already considered this problem in some detail under the heading "Understanding the Problem" and have discussed the conflict that often arises between the need to seek assistance and the acceptance of the hearing loss that act involves. The feeling of being shut off from the world, which Ramsdell (1970) explained, and the loneliness, sadness, and depression often arising from that feeling, were discussed. I pointed out that hearing-impaired people often feel ashamed of their inability to cope and judge their inadequacy as a weakness. Ramsdell's description of the hearing-impaired person's feelings of threat to self-esteem and the arrogant behavior that may be used as a way of handling this threat have been considered. I suggested that the idea of wearing a hearing aid brings these feelings into focus, since it requires not only acknowledgment of one's hearing difficulty, but a willingness to let others know about it.

Parents of hearing-impaired children face all of these problems, plus the acute feelings of responsibility that give rise to guilt. "What did I do to deserve this?" "If I had not caught German measles this would never have happened to my child." "I feel so guilty that I did not know she was deaf until she was almost 3 years old—how could I not have known?"

I also spoke of the effects these feelings often have on hearing-impaired individuals, causing them to arange their lives or the lives of the hearing-impaired child so as to avoid threatening contacts. Sullivan (1956, p. 145) states:

The awareness of inferiority means that one is unable to keep out of consciousness the formulation of some chronic feeling of the worse sort of insecurity, and this means that one suffers anxiety and per haps even something worse, if jealousy is really worse than anxiety. The fear that others can disrespect a person because of something he shows means that he is always insecure in his contact with other people, and this insecurity arises, not from mysterious and somewhat disguised sources as a great deal of our anxiety does, but from something which he knows he cannot fix. Now that represents an almost fatal deficiency of the self system, since the self is unable to disguise or exclude a definite formulation that reads, 'I am inferior. Therefore people will dislike me and I cannot be secure with them'.*

Such feelings are usually present to some extent in all hearing-impaired persons and in the parents of hearing-impaired children. Most can handle them with only minimal help, others will need a prolonged helping relationship, and still others will have problems of a severity necessitating professional psychological guidance. Usually, this latter group of people have personality problems that the hearing difficulty aggravates.

The problem, then, is to create a climate in which a change in the clients' perceptions of their difficulties can occur and in which these clients can explore new ways of solving them. If behavior is to change, the self-concept must change. "The most important single factor affecting behavior is the self-concept. . . . the beliefs that people have about themselves are always present factors in determining their behavior" (Combs et al. 1971, p. 37).

You must seek, therefore, to establish a climate to facilitate change. The requirements of such a climate have been described by Combs et al. (1971, Chapter 11). They include:

1. Establishing conditions for the confrontation of the problems by the client. This will be best achieved by offering guidance and understanding and by proceeding in a mutual exploration of the problem with the client's help.
2. Bring the client into dialogue with some new experience, a stage the authors describe as the informational phase. I discussed this earlier, as it concerns problems created by a hearing deficit and by amplification. I would include, in this section, the help that may be afforded the client by group sessions with other hearing-impaired persons.
3. The person must discover the personal meaning of the new information.

To achieve this climate, the client must be convinced that you and they are, as Combs et al. (1971, p. 215) say, "partners in the helping encounter." This, they state, determines the direction of that encounter by serving a model, by pointing the way to the most fruitful paths of exploration, and by suppressing or extinguishing less profitable routes. They then list (Combs et al. 1971, p. 220) four criteria in an atmosphere that permits growth, they explain that the client must feel: "(a) that it is safe to try, (b) reassured that he can, (c) encouraged to make the attempt, and (d) satisfied to do so."

Finally, Combs et al. state:

Freeing atmospheres provide the stage on which exploration of self and the world takes place. For effective practice, a large portion of the helper's atten-

---

*Reproduced from Sullivan HS: Paranoid dynamism, in Perry HS, Gawel ML, Gebbon M (eds): Clinical studies in Psychiatry. New York, Norton, 1956, p 145. With Permission.

tion and efforts will need to be devoted to the creation of atmospheres which make exploring possible and encourage students and clients to make maximum use of relationships. When this is done well, the need of the individual for adequacy can be counted on to supply the impetus for movement.*

*Reproduced from Combs A, Avila D, Purkey W: Helping Relationships: Basic Concepts for the Helping Professions. Boston, Allyn and Bacon, 1971, p 230. With permission.

REFERENCES

Atherley GRC, Noble WG: Clinical picture of occupational hearing loss obtained with the hearing measurement scale, *in* Robinson DW (ed): Occupational Hearing Loss. London, Academic Press, 1971

Brammer L: The Helping Relationship: Process and Skills (ed 2). Englewood Cliffs, NJ, Prentice Hall, 1979

Combs A, Avila D, Purkey W: Helping Relationships: Basic Concepts for the Helping Professions. Boston, Allyn and Bacon, 1971

Downs MP: The establishment of hearing aid use—A program for parents. Maico Audiol Libr Serv 4:5, 1966

Downs MP: Maintaining children's hearing aids—the role of parents. Maico Audiol Libr Serv 10:1, 1971

Freedman J, Doob A: Deviancy. New York, Academic Press, 1968

Gargiulo R: Working with Parents of Exceptional Children. Boston, Houghton Mifflin, 1985

Giolas TG: The measurement of hearing handicap. Maico Audiol Libr Serv 8:6, 1970

Goffman E: Stigma. Englewood Cliffs, NJ, Prentice Hall, 1963

Hansen J, Stevic R, Warner R: Counseling: Theory and Process (ed 3). Boston, Allyn and Bacon, 1982

High W, Fairbanks G, Glorig A: Scale for self-assessment of hearing handicap. J Speech Hear Disord 29:215–230, 1964

Horton KB, McConnell F: Early intervention for the young deaf child through parent training. Proc Internatl Congress Education Deaf (Stockholm) 1:291–296, 1970

Kodman F: Techniques for counseling the hearing aid client. Maico Audiol Libr Serv 4:8, 1966

Luterman D: A parent-oriented nursery program for pre-school deaf children—A follow-up study. Volta Rev 73:106–112, 1971

Luterman D: Counseling the Communicatively Disordered and Their Families. Boston, Little Brown, 1984

McConnell F: Proceedings of the conference on current practices in the management of deaf infants (0–3 years). Nashville, Tennessee, Vanderbilt University, The Bill Wilkerson Center, 1968

Newby H: Audiology (ed 2). New York, Appleton-Century-Crofts, 1964

Niemeyer W: Psychological aspects of hearing-aid fitting. J Audiol Tech 12:3, 1973. Reprinted in Maico Audiol Libr Serv 12:3, 4, 1974

Noble WG: The measurement of hearing handicap: A further viewpoint. Maico Audiol Libr Serv 10:5, 1972

Noble, WG, Atherley GRC: The hearing measurement scale: A questionnaire for the assessment of auditory disability. J Aud Res 10:193–214, 1970

Paulos TH: Short-term rehabilitation program for hard-of-hearing children. Hear News 29:4–7, 1961

Ramsdell DA: The psychology of the hard-of-hearing and deafened adult, in Davis H, Silverman SR (eds): Hearing and Deafness (ed 3). New York, Holt Rinehart and Winston, 1970

Rogers C: Client-Centered Therapy. Boston, Houghton Mifflin, 1951

Ross M, Tomassetti C: Hearing Aid Selection for Preverbal Hearing Impaired Children, in Pollack MC (ed): Amplification for the Hearing Impaired (ed 2). Orlando, FL, Grune & Stratton, 1980

Rousey CL: Psychological reactions to hearing loss. J Speech Hear Disord 36:382–389, 1971

Sanders D: Aural Rehabilitation (ed 2). Englewood Cliffs, NJ, Prentice Hall, 1982

Sandlin RE: The psychology of the hearing impaired. Hearing Instruments 25:22–23, 1974

Shore I: Hearing aid consultation, in Katz J (ed): Handbook of Clinical Audiology. Baltimore, Williams & Wilkins, 1972, p 656

Stark RE: Sensory Capabilities of Hearing Impaired Children. Baltimore, University Park Press, 1974

Sullivan HS: Paranoid dynamism, in Perry HS, Gawel ML, Gebbon M (eds): Clinical Studies in Psychiatry. New York, Norton, 1956, p 145

Tyler L: The Work of the Counselor (ed 3), Englewood Cliffs, NJ, Prentice Hall, 1969

Appendix A

**Profile Questionnaire for Rating
Communicative Performance
in a Home Environment**

1. (a)   In my living room, when I can see the speakers face, I have:

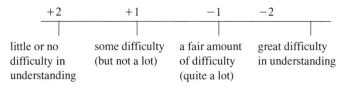

little or no   some difficulty   a fair amount   great difficulty
difficulty in   (but not a lot)   of difficulty   in understanding
understanding   (quite a lot)

    (b)   This happens:

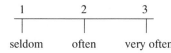

                    seldom   often   very often

2. (a)   If I am talking with a person in my living room or family room while the television,
          radio, or record player is on, I have:

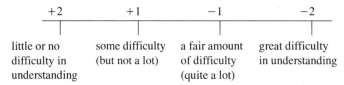

little or no   some difficulty   a fair amount   great difficulty
difficulty in   (but not a lot)   of difficulty   in understanding
understanding   (quite a lot)

    (b)   This happens:

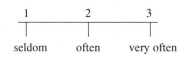

                    seldom   often   very often

3. (a)   In a quiet room in my house, if I cannot see the speakers face I have:

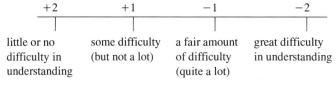

little or no   some difficulty   a fair amount   great difficulty
difficulty in   (but not a lot)   of difficulty   in understanding
understanding   (quite a lot)

    (b)   This happens:

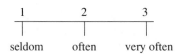

                    seldom   often   very often

4. (a) If some one in my house speaks to me from another room on the same floor, I experience:

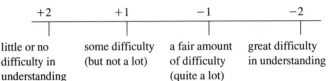

little or no   some difficulty   a fair amount   great difficulty
difficulty in   (but not a lot)   of difficulty   in understanding
understanding   (quite a lot)

(b) This happens:

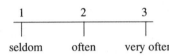

      seldom   often   very often

5. (a) If someone calls me from upstairs when I am downstairs, or from the window when I am in the garden, I will experience:

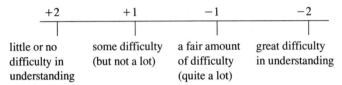

little or no   some difficulty   a fair amount   great difficulty
difficulty in   (but not a lot)   of difficulty   in understanding
understanding   (quite a lot)

(b) This happens:

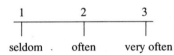

      seldom   .   often   very often

6. (a) Understanding people at the dinner table gives me:

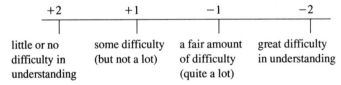

little or no   some difficulty   a fair amount   great difficulty
difficulty in   (but not a lot)   of difficulty   in understanding
understanding   (quite a lot)

(b) This happens:

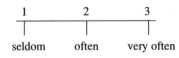

      seldom   often   very often

7. (a) When I sit talking with friends in a quiet room, I have:

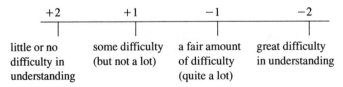

little or no   some difficulty   a fair amount   great difficulty
difficulty in   (but not a lot)   of difficulty   in understanding
understanding   (quite a lot)

(b)   This happens:

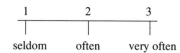

```
        1              2              3
```
        seldom   often   very often

8.   (a)   Listening to the radio or record player or watching TV gives me:

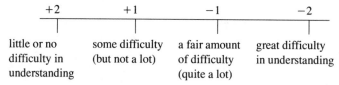

```
    +2              +1              -1              -2
```

little or no   some difficulty   a fair amount   great difficulty
difficulty in   (but not a lot)   of difficulty   in understanding
understanding   (quite a lot)

(b)   This happens:

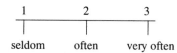

```
        1              2              3
```
        seldom   often   very often

9.   (a)   When I use the phone at home, I have:

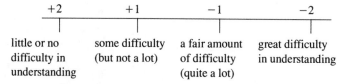

```
    +2              +1              -1              -2
```

little or no   some difficulty   a fair amount   great difficulty
difficulty in   (but not a lot)   of difficulty   in understanding
understanding   (quite a lot)

(b)   This happens:

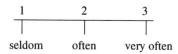

```
        1              2              3
```
        seldom   often   very often

Appendix B

**Profile Questionnaire for Rating
Communicative Performance
in an Occupational Environment**

1. (a) In talking with someone in the room where I work, I have:

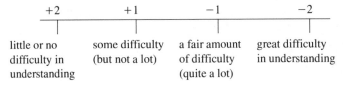

+2	+1	−1	−2

little or no
difficulty in
understanding

some difficulty
(but not a lot)

a fair amount
of difficulty
(quite a lot)

great difficulty
in understanding

   (b) This happens:

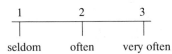

1	2	3

seldom   often   very often

2. (a) When I am in a room at work where there is noise, I have:

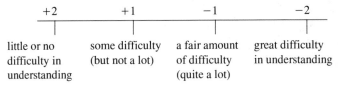

+2	+1	−1	−2

little or no
difficulty in
understanding

some difficulty
(but not a lot)

a fair amount
of difficulty
(quite a lot)

great difficulty
in understanding

   (b) This happens:

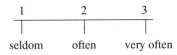

1	2	3

seldom   often   very often

3. (a) When I am at a meeting with a small group of people, around a table in a fairly
quiet room, I have:

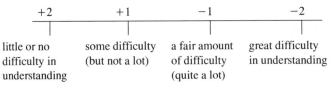

+2	+1	−1	−2

little or no
difficulty in
understanding

some difficulty
(but not a lot)

a fair amount
of difficulty
(quite a lot)

great difficulty
in understanding

   (b) This happens:

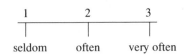

1	2	3

seldom   often   very often

4. (a) If I have to take notes by dictation in a fairly quiet room, I have:

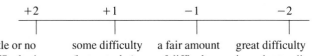

+2	+1	−1	−2

little or no   some difficulty   a fair amount   great difficulty
difficulty in   (but not a lot)   of difficulty   in understanding
understanding   (quite a lot)

(b) This happens:

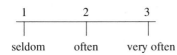

1	2	3

seldom   often   very often

5. (a) If I have to make notes at a meeting, I have:

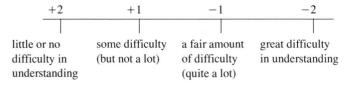

+2	+1	−1	−2

little or no   some difficulty   a fair amount   great difficulty
difficulty in   (but not a lot)   of difficulty   in understanding
understanding   (quite a lot)

(b) This happens:

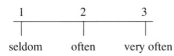

1	2	3

seldom   often   very often

6. (a) If I have to use the phone at work, I have:

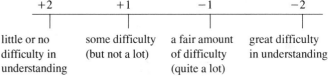

+2	+1	−1	−2

little or no   some difficulty   a fair amount   great difficulty
difficulty in   (but not a lot)   of difficulty   in understanding
understanding   (quite a lot)

(b) This happens:

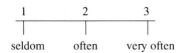

1	2	3

seldom   often   very often

Appendix C

Profile Questionnaire for Rating
Communicative Performance
in a Social Environment

1. (a) If we are entertaining a group of friends, understanding someone against the background of others talking gives me:

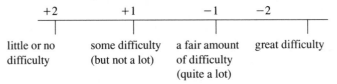

little or no   some difficulty   a fair amount   great difficulty
difficulty   (but not a lot)   of difficulty
                                         (quite a lot)

    (b) This happens:

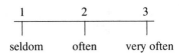

seldom   often   very often

2. (a) If we are playing cards, understanding my partner gives me:

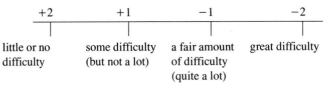

little or no   some difficulty   a fair amount   great difficulty
difficulty   (but not a lot)   of difficulty
                                         (quite a lot)

    (b) This happens:

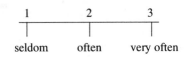

seldom   often   very often

3. (a) When I am at the theatre or the movies, I have:

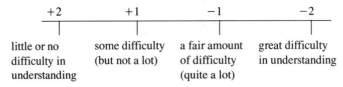

little or no   some difficulty   a fair amount   great difficulty
difficulty in   (but not a lot)   of difficulty   in understanding
understanding   (quite a lot)

    (b) This happens:

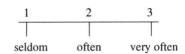

seldom   often   very often

4. (a) In church, when the minister gives the sermon, I have:

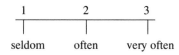

little or no   some difficulty   a fair amount   great difficulty
difficulty in   (but not a lot)   of difficulty   in understanding
understanding   (quite a lot)

(b) This happens:

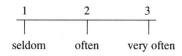

            seldom   often   very often

5. (a) In following the conversation when we eat out, I have:

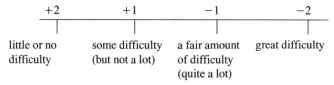

little or no   some difficulty   a fair amount   great difficulty
difficulty   (but not a lot)   of difficulty
                                                (quite a lot)

(b) This happens:

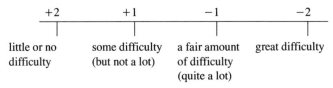

            seldom   often   very often

6. (a) In the car, I find that understanding what people are saying gives me:

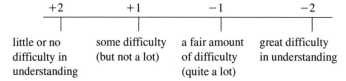

little or no   some difficulty   a fair amount   great difficulty
difficulty   (but not a lot)   of difficulty
                                                (quite a lot)

(b) This happens:

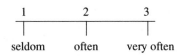

            seldom   often   very often

7. (a) When I am outside talking with someone, I have:

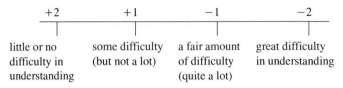

+2	+1	−1	−2
little or no difficulty in understanding	some difficulty (but not a lot)	a fair amount of difficulty (quite a lot)	great difficulty in understanding

(b) This happens:

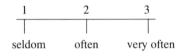

1	2	3
seldom	often	very often

Appendix D

**Profile Questionnaire for Rating
Communicative Performance
in a School Environment**

1. (a) When I am working with Mary, individually, at my desk, she is able to understand what I say with:

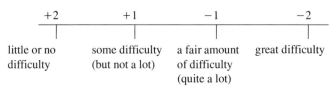

little or no   some difficulty   a fair amount   great difficulty
difficulty   (but not a lot)   of difficulty
                                          (quite a lot)

(b) This happens:

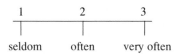

seldom   often   very often

2. (a) When she is one of a small group of children in a learning situation, she understands what I say with:

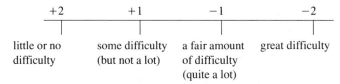

little or no   some difficulty   a fair amount   great difficulty
difficulty   (but not a lot)   of difficulty
                                          (quite a lot)

(b) This happens:

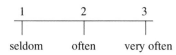

seldom   often   very often

3. (a) In a small group she understands what the other children say with:

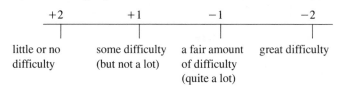

little or no   some difficulty   a fair amount   great difficulty
difficulty   (but not a lot)   of difficulty
                                          (quite a lot)

(b) This happens:

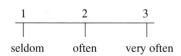

seldom   often   very often

4. (a) When I speak to the class as a whole, Mary is able to understand with:

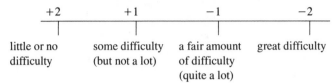

little or no   some difficulty   a fair amount   great difficulty
difficulty   (but not a lot)   of difficulty
                                        (quite a lot)

(b) This happens:

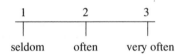

seldom   often   very often

5. (a) When we watch a movie film, television program, or filmstrip, she seems to
         understand with:

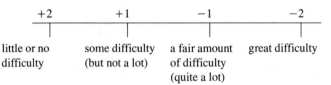

little or no   some difficulty   a fair amount   great difficulty
difficulty   (but not a lot)   of difficulty
                                        (quite a lot)

(b) This happens:

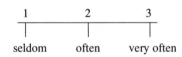

seldom   often   very often

6. (a) In playground or gymnasium games or in activities, she is able to follow verbal
         directions with:

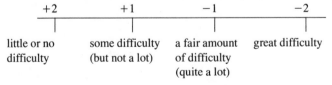

little or no   some difficulty   a fair amount   great difficulty
difficulty   (but not a lot)   of difficulty
                                        (quite a lot)

(b) This happens:

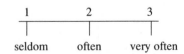

seldom   often   very often

7. (a) In her contact with the other children in class, and in social activities during break
        periods, she seems to understand with:

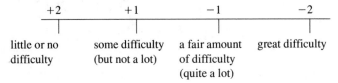

+2	+1	−1	−2

little or no   some difficulty   a fair amount   great difficulty
difficulty   (but not a lot)   of difficulty
                                          (quite a lot)

    (b) This happens:

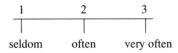

1	2	3

seldom   often   very often

Robert G. Glaser
Michael C. Pollack

11
Private Practice and Hearing Aid Dispensing

As more and more audiologists enter private practice and begin selling hearing aids, two dramatic shortcomings in our graduate training become apparent. Very few of us received any formal training in business management, how to start a business, how to choose the optimal avenue of entry into private practice, how to effectively market our services and products, and how to utilize a computer in our practices. All of these deficiencies in our training make it much more difficult to succeed.

Bob Glaser and I prepared this chapter as a primer for the entrpreneurial audiologist. It presents an overview of this much-needed information. The chapter is by no means all encompassing, but, rather, is a starting point. If the material contained herein assists you to avoid making some of the mistakes that many of us have made, our purpose has been achieved.

MCD

Success in the private practice arena depends on three factors. The first centers around *excellence in clinical acumen and academic training.* Few can argue that audiologists are uniquely prepared in both academic and practicum parameters to provide diagnostic and rehabilitative evaluations and planning necessary to optimize improved communicative performance. By virtue of having an evaluation and a treatment modality, the audiologist is able to function as an independent practitioner in the health care delivery industry.

The second success factor is a *systematic business approach to the practice of audiology.* Common sense and data-based decision making, as well as intelligent

AMPLIFICATION FOR THE HEARING-IMPAIRED, THIRD EDITION
Copyright © 1988 by Grune & Stratton, Inc.

397

use of advisers, are keystones. Of course, a business degree would be helpful, but few graduate-trained disciplines require a course in business issues, let alone a formal degree.

The third factor may be considered a hybrid of the first two. It requires superlative *patient-centered attention to details*, from office furnishings to follow-up care strategies, to issues in maintaining long-term, continuous relationships with patients and referral sources.

DECISION TO ENTER A DISPENSING PRACTICE

Without question, the most difficult professional decision to be made by potential private practitioners will be whether or not to enter the business arena. McCormack (1984) provides a pointed statement to examine decision motives: "If you want to be in your own business because you are 'sick and tired of being told what to do,' because you want more 'freedom,' or because you are unappreciated or undervalued, forget it. These are not reasons for starting a business; these are reasons for running away from your present job."

Job dissatisfaction may be one reason to consider entering private practice. It should not be the sole reason. Private practice can provide a great deal of personal and professional satisfaction. It can offer better control over your own fate—both financial and professional. It can enable you to reap the rewards of your diligence. Understandably, there are drawbacks. Hours are usually long, and time not spent with patients must be used efficiently in planning, promoting, and evaluating the business as a financial entity. Paid sick days become a luxury. Vacations in the formative years of the practice are few, always brief and frequently nonexistent. Collecting monies owed to you for your valued services provides a lesson in professional humility. Aggressive competition for an ever-shrinking health care dollar, professional jealousy, and occasional unethical practices can quickly jade the new practitioner or dissuade those considering the venture.

Critical evaluation requires brutal honesty. Consideration must be given to your personal and emotional needs and whether they can be met in the private practice arena. *Can you emotionally afford the stresses of running a business? Can your spouse or family handle the long hours and the financial burdens associated with starting a practice? Do you have the perseverance and ingenuity to try different approaches to problems that you have not encountered before? Can you listen to criticism and turn it into rational business plans for restructured success?*

Others factors must be considered. A warm, personable manner with people is essential. Excellent oral and written communication skills are necessities. The successful practitioner must be able to establish rapport quickly and impart information on a variety of academic levels. This ability is an asset when dealing with patients and professional referral sources alike. You must possess an ability to complete tasks and follow through on plans or promises. Both patients and referral sources will respect the practitioner who will follow up and offer closure to a situation or topic.

Accurate assessment of your financial capabilities is another key to evaluating your readiness to enter private practice. The first step is to estimate your *net worth*. Net worth evaluation offers information about what you have versus what you own; net worth equals assets minus liabilities. An accurate net worth assessment should guide the method and style of entry into the market. It will be of value to your banker or other potential partners in your venture. It may also serve to prudently delay start-up until enough money to adequately capitalize the practice has been accumulated (see Table 11-4, later in this chapter).

METHODS OF ENTRY

There are a number of ways to enter private practice. Each has its advantages and disadvantages, as well as relevance to financial circumstances:

Degree to Shingle

Starting a practice immediately after completion of professional education and certification/licensure requirements has been done in other disciplines for many years. Despite the discipline, it requires patience. You will be required to build your patient load, reputation, and referrals and pay bills as well as salaries. This takes time and meticulous planning. Be prepared to starve for awhile. This method is difficult to do with little or no experience in a private practice setting.

There is always a home-town advantage in starting a practice. People might recognize your family name and contacts may be easier to make. Your knowledge of the market and its physical and socioeconomic boundaries could help in location selection and marketing plans. Of course, if your plans do not include establishing the practice in your home-town, this information will have to be gleaned from other sources. Chambers of Commerce, Jaycees, County or City Councils, or Offices of Development are good places to start searching for information.

If you are considering a private practice while still in graduate school, capitalize on your position. Take business management courses, including bookkeeping and marketing. Other courses might include computer applications and business software evaluation. Software packages for word processing, data filing, accounts receivable and billing, marketing plans, and financial spreadsheets should be studied carefully. Anytime you go to school, you have to pay tuition. It is less expensive to take courses in the college classroom than to purchase the services in the business world. If nothing else, business courses will orient your decision making and provide an understanding of when to contact an expert for consultation.

Easing In

A less strenuous way to enter private practice is to "ease in" while remaining employed elsewhere. It will require Saturday and evening work. I (R. G. Glaser) was able to purchase hearing testing equipment and place it in an otolaryngologist's office. The office staff scheduled appointments and billed the patients for audiologic services. A portion of the collected revenue was exchanged for rent and other overhead, with a profit margin for the physician that offered an incentive to refer patients for evaluation.

From that beginning, I (R. G. Glaser) was able to start a business and use tax exemptions to my advantage. I was able to accrue adequate capital to open an independent practice on a full time basis. There were long hours; 40 hours at a regular "job" and 20–25 hours at the private office. Eventually, the private practice enabled a better financial opportunity than the "job" and I went into full-time private practice.

Joining an Existing Practice

Many of the most visible professionals—attorneys, physicians, and dentists—are really employees of an established practice. Frequently these individuals will work as employees and later buy into the practice as partners. When you join a private practice, you may be joining as an employee. The option to become a partner may not be a consideration of the owner. However, you can learn the workings of private practice and develop your own business style. As time goes by and your experience and professional development grow, you might approach the owner about partnership. We know of one case where the individual worked in a private practice and proposed that a branch office be opened. He became the manager of the branch office and part owner. As the branch grew and the potential became evident, the manager bought the concern from the original owner and maintained a good relationship with his "competition."

Buying an Existing Practice

Buying a revenue generating practice is probably the easiest, and possibly the most expensive, way to enter private practice. The purchase may include established patient files, repeat business, and referral sources. Depending on the terms of the sale, a completely outfitted office and all necessary professional equipment may be included. In short, you may be ready to assume the practice the day your purchase agreement is completed. You will have to do as much work getting your patients acquainted with the new management as if it were a new practice. Visits to referral sources will have to build confidence that those patients sent will have as good or better care under your management.

If the previous owner had problems with patients, referral sources, or financial woes, you will inherit them all. Prior headaches can be disastrous. Take care to evaluate the practice from as many angles as you and your advisers can imagine. The more you evaluate the practice and identify areas in need of change, the better your chances of success. Careful evaluation of the last three year-end financial reports along with both corporate and owner income tax returns would enable you and your advisors to better evaluate your purchasing positioning. Talk to a few of the referral sources before you buy the practice. They can provide insight into any service delivery problems that may have created difficulty for them in the past.

If you carefully analyze the business and evaluate your position, buying a viable practice may be a good professional and financial opportunity. *It goes without saying that your accountant and attorney should be consulted.* The accountant can help you determine the financial fairness of the offered price and verify the business reports relative to the tax filings. The attorney will offer advice about the legality of the purchase agreement and its terms and conditions, provide you with a clear picture of potential liability, and aid in the negotiations concerning the purchase agreement and its attendant stipulations.

Franchise Opportunity

Entering private practice by purchasing a franchise package places you in a system of selective distribution and guidance, reducing some of the risks of initiating a new practice.

A franchise enables you to market a specific brand of hearing aid in a prescribed, systematized way. The franchise is traded for a fee, usually a percentage of the profits and the franchisee's agreement to maintain standards of delivery dictated by the franchiser. There are several advantages. Start-up costs can be lower than if you would start your own practice. Management expertise is readily available to assist in the daily running of the business. A good franchise system will include a professionally managed promotion program that should generate leads and patient flow shortly after the opening.

The disadvantages of entering private practice by purchasing a franchise require frank consideration. A franchise operation may be your primary investment but not your singular creation. The franchiser may control many practice parameters such as hours of operation, location selection, hiring of personnel and even decor of the office. The franchiser becomes your partner and shares in the profits that you have generated. The franchiser may define patient boundaries in your area, which could have a significant effect on your earning potential.

Before you consider purchasing a franchise, have your lawyer and accountant review the franchise agreement, its limitations, buy-out clause, and dispute settlement policy as well as the method by which the territory will be determined.

CHOOSING KEY ADVISORS: LAWYER AND ACCOUNTANT

One of the worst mistakes beginning entrepreneurs make is to consider their attorney or accountant as problem solvers. They erroneously rely on them in an after-the-fact situation as defense in court or during an Internal Revenue Service audit. You can seriously impair your advisor's effectiveness by relying on their expertise after you have made bad decisions that have resulted in problems.

Use their services in the planning stages so that they may offer guidance, suggestions, and business structure to avoid difficulties. Their advice should be considered optimal when it is preventive rather than curative.

Choosing Your Attorney

Lawyers are helpful in many ways. When you decide to start a private practice, join or purchase an ongoing concern, or consider entering a franchise system, *you should seek legal counsel.* This legal counsel will provide information about contractual obligations and personal or financial liabilities. The attorney is charged with protecting your interests and the interests of the business and will also provide the legal expertise to offer advice as to which type of business form would be best for your circumstance—sole proprietorship, partnership, standard, or "S" corporation. If you are arranging loans from lending institutions or from private-equity lending sources, the attorney can evaluate the loan agreements for accuracy and your protection. Your legal counsel will make sure that you are aware of federal, state, and local laws and how you can best comply with them. This attorney will represent you in the event of litigation (lawsuit), or, if your attorney is not a trial lawyer, will refer you to competent trial co-counsel.

Finding the right attorney can be difficult. Start the search by asking questions. Friends or professional colleagues and other business owners can offer opinions based on their information and experience. Your accountant, if you already have one, can recommend several competent attorneys. Your search should be geared to finding an attorney who can offer expertise on small business operations. This individual should be reasonable in their approach. A good attorney should be able to evaluate both sides of an issue in a logical, concise manner and offer clear alternatives and consequences of the action. Your approach to business should be compatible with all of your advisors. *Do not hesitate to make appointments to "interview" prospective lawyers (as well as accountants) on a "no fee" basis, so that both of you can determine whether your approaches are compatible and you can work together.* If any prospective lawyer (or accountant) is unwilling to meet with you on this basis, look elsewhere.

FEES

Attorneys are paid by retainer or hourly fee. Retainers are periodic, fixed payments covering an agreed-on length of time. Retainers may be good for your business in the early, start-up stages when you will need freer access to the attorney's time. Hourly payment, however, is probably the most common and equitable method of payment. You pay for the time used. Document preparation or incorporation procedures may be charged at a flat rate—one price for the service or documents rendered.

You and the attorney should discuss fees and payment arrangements during the initial interview so that both parties understand the financial arrangements necessary to obtain competent, reliable, and accessible legal counsel.

Choosing Your Accountant

The accountant will provide the framework for your business and will help in setting up the core of your business venture. The accountant should be responsible for establishing the type of accounting system used (cash or accrual) and the method of bookkeeping (from a pegboard system to a computerized spreadsheet), providing periodic financial reports on profitability (financial and profit and loss statements) and advising you of your tax status. The accountant will complete appropriate tax reporting forms and optimize deductions that will decrease your tax liabilities. Your accountant should explain IRS points and offer a balanced view on deductions relative to your tax status. *Tax evasion and tax avoidance differ substantially.* The former is illegal: the latter is not. Failure to report income is considered fraud, while overclaiming expenses may or may not be. Thus, in preparing a tax return or considering a tax position, your accountant should identify those transactions with options and explain all possible outcomes (Churchill and Werbaneth 1979).

Your accountant and attorney should be able and willing to work closely together, when necessary, to serve your best interests. For day-to-day operations, your accountant is the most valuable, and often most accessible advisor. *Listen carefully to your accountant's advice. Choose your advisors wisely and understand that money spent on their expertise may be the best investment you will make in your business.*

PRIVATE PRACTICE FORMS

There is a growing sense of confusion in our profession about what constitutes working in private practice versus actually functioning as private practitioner. There are several forms that private practice can take, depending on market requirements and personal and financial ability to enter the business of private practice.

Independent practitioners are in a solo practice situation. They are not tethered to an agency or other practitioner in any fiscal manner. They may depend on agency or other referral sources but are not financially obligated or otherwise encumbered. If the business is a success, independent practitioners reap the financial rewards directly. They pay no dividends to shareholders or royalties to franchisers. The success of the business rises and falls with their efforts or the efforts of those they managed. Independent practitioners may provide services on a contractual basis to agencies such as health maintenance organizations (HMOs), preferred provider organizations (PPOs), or hospitals. Although working in a setting outside the business office, they will submit a bill for services rendered to the agency and be reimbursed according to the contract negotiated. From that revenue, independent practitioners pay their own health care costs, retirement, taxes, and other business-related expenses. Subcontracting in our field and other health care disciplines is becoming more attractive to administrators facing the rising cost of employee benefits packages. It is sometimes more cost-efficient for the administrator to pay a subcontractor for services at a higher hourly wage than to pay the benefits costs of a full-time staff person.

Practitioners engaged in an *affiliated* or *associated practice* differ from the independent practitioners in that they are fiscally linked to another person or entity. The practice may be shared by one or more practitioners with like interests or with similar, complementing interests. An example is three practitioners working in a group practice arrangement wherein one is an audiologist, one a speech-language pathologist, and the other a psychologist specializing in learning disabilities. Each practitioner offers different yet complementary services. The group could foster in-house referrals and provide an attractive "package" for those in need of comprehensive evaluation or therapy for children with hearing dysfunction and learning and language disabilities.

Many audiologists are employed in private practice settings working for physicians, other audiologists, or hearing aid dispensers. They receive a salary and usually a benefits package. In the strictest sense, some argue, they are not private practitioners because they are not involved in the entrepreneurial aspects of the practice. They share in no revenue generated as dividends. They are paid by the hour, are salaried, work on a commission basis, or a combination of salary and commission. Their position depends on their productivity and participation. As employees, they are not strapped with the responsibility of managing the business unless it is included in the job description. Work schedule, vacations, sick days, wages and benefits, retirement funding, and attendance at professional meetings are at the discretion of the employer.

BUSINESS FORMS

Sole Proprietorship

A sole proprietor is an individual engaged in an unincorporated business for profit. It is probably the easiest way to enter business and requires no special filings or legal documentation. The proprietorship has no legal identity apart from its owner, as do corporations. As such, the owner is liable for all claims against the business. If there are losses, and debtors obtain judgments against the business, the owner must pay the debts with either business or personal assets or both. In other words, business and personal assets and liabilities are one and the same.

Income taxes are reported on Schedule C, Profit (or Loss) from a Business or Profession. Receipts, depreciation, rent, repairs, salaries and wages, insurance commissions, legal and professional fees amortization, pension and profit-sharing plans, employee benefit plans, interest on business indebtedness, and other business expenses are calculated to determine net profit or loss. These figures are entered on the owner's Form 1040, Individual Income Tax Return. Receipts entered into the ledger not paid out for services or consultants become taxable income to the owner. Except for Keough plans, there are few deductions available to the sole proprietor.

Partnership

A partnership is a relationship between two or more persons joining together to carry on a trade or business, with each contributing money, property, labor, or skill, and all expecting to share in the profits or losses of the enterprise. Partnership profits are not taxed. Profit and loss information is filed with the IRS on an informational return. It contains each partner's share of profits, gains, losses, and deductions. The partners file their personal tax forms, reflecting the data supplied on the informational return filed on behalf of the partnership. Each partner is responsible for self-employment Social Security payments.

An attorney should create a partnership agreement, that covers several important aspects of the business. The amount of capital investment should be delineated in the agreement. A buy/sell section should outline an equitable course of action in the event of the death of one of the partners, since death of a partner causes automatic dissolution of the partnership. A buy/sell agreement must provide a method of purchasing the deceased's interest. The agreement should provide a fair means of calculating the accumulated worth of each partner's equity. A partnership is likewise dissolved when one (i.e., a principal) sells one's interest, is ejected from the partnership, or declares bankruptcy.

Partnerships are not without problems. Personal liability is no less in jeopardy than in the sole proprietorship. Indeed, liability is shared across the partners; each individual is liable for the actions or omissions of any partner. There are more tax advantages in the partnership than in the sole proprietorship. It enables a greater latitude in retirement plans and health care packages, depending on the agreement of the partners.

Partnerships can be rewarding when the right mix of personalities and talent are assembled with common goals. Conversely, if you fail to choose the right partners, your daily business life can be miserable to unbearable. McCormack (1984) suggests

There are situations in which the strengths and weaknesses of each partner are well balanced and the business benefits from them. But the odds are a lot greater that the partnership itself will become the business's worst enemy. It is probably not an accident that some of the greatest entrepreneurial successes have been solo acts. *

---

* Reproduced from McCormack M: What They Don't Teach You at Harvard Business School. New York, Bantam Books, 1984, p. 32.

Standard (C) Corporation

Corporations pay taxes and therefore stand as legal entities that can own property, execute contracts, incur indebtedness, and perform business as an individual. The officers and stockholders of the corporation are liable for the debts of the corporation to the limit of the assets held by the corporation. This limiting of liability protects the personal assets of an individual (Sullivan 1986). A drawback to the standard corporation is double taxation; corporate income is taxed, as are the dividends dispersed to the shareholders. Unlike partnerships, corporations have an unlimited lifespan unless otherwise specified. Buy/sell agreements are still needed, but only to establish how the deceased's equity will be disbursed to that person's estate; the corporation does not dissolve. Likewise, buy-out agreements should also be established. An attorney will need to create documents that establish the corporation and describe the nature and intent of its business. Each state has different rules for incorporation. The attorney will file the articles of incorporation with the state. The combined legal fees may exceed the benefits of incorporating. These factors should be discussed with an accountant, as well as an attorney, before incorporating.

"S" Corporation

The "S" corporation is a legal entity that does not pay taxes, yet can enter into contracts, create indebtedness, own property similar to a standard corporation. As in a standard corporation, "S" corporations offer the limited liability aspects of incorporation without the double taxation dilemma. Profits or losses of an "S" corporation are reported on the tax returns of the shareholders, as in a Partnership. "S" corporations may be a good alternative for a beginning practice with high start-up costs of equipment, office outfitting, and so on. These costs flow through to the shareholder's tax returns as deductions relative to that person's share of the corporation's net operating loss.

EXPENSE EVALUATION AND REVENUE PROJECTION: THE PRACTICE PLAN

A practice plan is a structural compilation of real and projected data that will enable you to view your venture with perspective. It provides direction and a means to establish and accomplish goals. It serves to educate your supporters—bankers, lawyers, accountants, and prospective partners—about your professional activity and how you propose to implement your practice plan. It offers comprehensive descriptions of fiscal, personnel, equipment, and workspace needs. It lends justification to marketing plans and attempts to realistically project revenue parameters for 3–5 years. Four important headings should be included in a practice plan: *purpose*, *service market*, *financial*, and *workspace/equipment*.

Purpose

Clearly written statements of the business goals and objectives should open this section. All services to be offered must be described in terms easily understood by nonaudiologists. Hearing examinations, hearing aid evaluations and fittings, aural rehabilitation and counseling, vestibular testing, and evoked potential studies are service topics that should be concisely described so that the reader understands the steps a patient will need to take in the clinical journey. Potential referral sources should be identified in terms of their need for and probability of using your services. References should be made to the equipment necessary to provide the services, with complete descriptions to follow in the more technically oriented equipment section.

Service Market

Prospective patients, referral sources, and area demographics or market analyses are presented in this section. Defining your targeted market delineates patients and potential referral sources alike. Both the quantity and quality of existing service providers found in the intended market segment should be analyzed and pragmatic market share projections reported. Promotional planning relative to the market structure should be evaluated. Demographic information is readily available from a variety of commercial sources. Precisely defined lists of residents are available with information on family income, house ownership, car ownership, and the like. The local newspaper(s) can provide information about the composition of its readership by religion, age, political party, or just about any parameter that might be important to you in defining your targeted market area.

Financial

The financial section is the most critical segment of the practice plan. Clearly delineated operating expenses will enable you to appraise the direction and style of your practice in the crucial start-up phase. Careful, exacting cash flow projections tied to realistic time schedules can provide incentive deadlines as your enterprise grows.

Projecting income is always a difficult task. It requires accurate, objective estimates of the revenue to be generated and the timeframe within which it will be recorded as receipts in your ledger. Parish (1986) states:

Most new business owners tend to underestimate their expenses and overestimate their income. Try to be as reasonable and realistic as possible in your projections. When determining expenses project at least for the first two years.

It is always a good idea to project expenses and income on the assumption that you will not see a single patient for at least the first six months of the practice, and that you will not break even for at least a year.*

Although the thought of not seeing a patient for the first 6 months seems severe, it signals a need to consider the lean times encountered by the beginning practitioner. It instructs us to be careful in projecting income parameters. Optimism and inexperience can be efficient masking devices. It is advisable to have someone else evaluate your projections. If you are unsure of your income prospects, you are really not going into business—you are gambling.

Evaluate your potential referral sources as well as the immediate competition. Scout the market and design your promotional activity accordingly. The longer it takes for you and your services to be recognized by the population to be served, the greater the probability the business will fail. Quick recognition takes planning and work that can be done during the times when patient flow may be at a minimum. Contacts with referral sources must be made and follow-up correspondence should be prompt.

Projecting expenses is less difficult than forecasting income. It is no less important. You must thoroughly itemize all expenses to be encountered in the practice and be able to meet three kinds of expenses: *capital, fixed, and variable.*

Capital expenses are those costs occurring during the start-up phase of the business. They are one-time-only expenses. Testing equipment and office furnishings are examples of capital expenses. *Fixed expenses* are those that require payment on a regular basis. Debt service on a business loan, as well as rent and equipment lease payments, are examples of fixed expenses. *Variable expenses* are those that fluctuate or are unpredictable. Telephone bills, utilities, and the cost of items for resale (hearing aids, earmolds, batteries) are examples of variable expenses. Variable expenses are difficult to prepare for and require contingency funds in the form of cash reserves. Table 11-1 provides expanded listings of capital, fixed, and variable expenses.

Workspace and Equipment

This section must include items and policies that will ensure smooth office operations. Descriptions of furnishings and room sizes, lighting and restroom facilities, coat racks and magazine holders, to filing systems and day-to-day supplies are only a few of the important operating items to be considered. Equipment necessary for office operations and clinical services should be specified in great detail, with attendant cost factors. Alternatives should be described in the event that less expensive items are needed, based on other projections and cost variables.

---

* Reproduced from Parish R: Constraints and commitments: An introduction to the financial aspects of private practice, in Butler K (ed): Prospering in Private Practice. Rockville, MD, Aspen Publications, 1986, p. 90.

Table 11-1
Capital, Fixed, and Variable Expense Item

Capital Expenses	
Audiometer(s)	Typewriter or word processor
Testing booth(s)	Computer and initial software
Tympanometer(s)	Billing system
ENG equipment	Calculator(s)
Evoked potential equipment	Safe
Sound-level meter	Water cooler
Hearing aid adjustment tools	Legal and accounting fees associated with start-up
Hearing aid electroacoustic test system	Promotion/advertising associated with grand
Hearing aid accessories	opening
Initial battery supply	Lease deposit
Initial hearing aid inventory	Leasehold improvements and decorating
Desks	Telephone deposit
Chairs	
Charts or models	

Fixed Expenses	
Rent	Taxes
Building maintenance/cleaning	Repetitive advertising such as Yellow Pages
Lease payments	Answering service
Debt service on loans	Petty cash
Insurance	Wages and withholding
Professional dues or memberships	Retirement contributions
Journal or magazine subscriptions	Retained accounting or legal services
Licenses	Equipment repair contracts

Variable Expenses

Telephone bills
Utilities
Customer service—complaint resolution
Overtime
Additional temporary wages
Commissions
Unscheduled equipment repair and maintenance
Travel and entertainment
Seminar expenses
Auto expenses
Inventory for resale, ordered as needed

A budget must be developed that covers at least the first 18 months of operation. Fixed and variable expenses, as well as payroll, must be included. As mentioned previously, contingency funding should be included in the budget to cover the variable (unforeseen) expenses.

Beside describing office outfitting, physical plant, and equipment, this section must contain a comprehensive office procedural manual. The manual should have five sections: *personnel, fees, collection policy, patient records, and calendar of operation.*

The first section contains all staff responsibilities. These job descriptions need to be encompassing. They should delineate duties and responsibilities, yet not serve to limit staff participation beyond the job description. A sample job description outline is seen in Figure 11-1. It is a comprehensive outline for an office coordinator in charge of the management and coordination of a multifaceted audiology and speech pathology practice. The personnel section should also include dress codes, method of performance evaluation, causes for dismissal, licensing and malpractice insurance requirements, wage and benefits information and mileage, travel, and seminar and educational reimbursement policies.

The fee section should define all services and offer appropriate procedural codes [such as the current procedural terminology (CPT) codes] with associated charges. This section will be reviewed and updated from time to time to reflect the changing costs of service delivery and instrument charges. Many offices post a summary of the fee schedule in the waiting room.

The collection policy of the office can have a profound effect on the accounts receivable side of the ledger. It can make or break a business. It dictates the policy to the office staff as to how and when debts are to be collected. A well-written and strictly enforced collection policy can take the heat off the office staff. They should not deviate from the collection policy unless the executive officer grants permission for the variance. If a patient is not satisfied with the collection policy, the office staff should explain the policy and refer that patient to the executive officer.

Payment should be expected the same day services are provided. The patient should be informed of the costs prior to the visit. If unable to pay in full, a partial payment is expected. Patients often claim that their insurance company will pay for the service provided. Merit to that statement depends on each patient's individual policy and carrier. Provide an option to pay for the service—at least partially, but preferably in full—and submit the charges to the patient's insurance company.

In other words, *do not accept insurance assignment*, if you can avoid it, except in those cases where doing so is a prerequisite to being a provider (union hearing aid benefit plans, etc.). Each patient should be informed of the office policy on outstanding accounts; thus, all accounts are turned over to a collection agency after 90 days. Once an account is turned over to collection, it is not removed and the collection agent has the opportunity (with your permission) to file suit in a small claims court to recover the money or place liens against property, after all usual collection attempts have been made. Only a small percentage of accounts end up with the collection agent. Obviously, the fewer that go to collection, the more money is retained in the practice, because collection agents retain a judgmental percentage for their services. You can assist your collection agent by having a patient intake or information sheet that requires listing places of employment, nearest relative other than spouse and their phone number, and other cross-identifying references that can assist in finding the "skippers." The intake sheet should also have a clearly written agreement to pay for the services rendered,

Description of office coordinator responsibilities

Name _____ Effective Date _____

1. Accounts Receivable
   a. Billing and collections
   b. Day sheet posting and checkbook
   c. Window receipts and collections
   d. Third party payments and collections
   e. Coordination with collection agent
   f. Monthly reporting of accounts receivable

2. Accounts Payable
   a. Patient overpayments and refunds
   b. Taxes: corporate, payroll, FICA, etc.
   c. Supplier payments
   d. Legal and accounting retainers
   e. Other fixed-expense payments
   f. Monthly reporting of accounts payable
   g. Payroll: compilation of hours and deductions

3. Patient Records Management
   a. Report coordination and transmittal
   b. Report filing
   c. Coordination of all facility schedules
   d. Coordination of patient scheduling
   e. Coordination of hearing aid repairs, rechecks, fitting, and follow-up visits
   f. Mail in and out

4. Office Management and Maintenance
   a. Office equipment and supplies
   b. Professional equipment and supply orders
   c. Forms management and supply
   d. Rooms and office orderliness
   e. Petty cash management
   f. Fiscal reports as needed and directed

Fig. 11-1. Example of job description headings for office coordinator.

whether covered by third party payment or not. The form should be signed and witnessed by one of the office staff, thus binding them to a contractual obligation to pay their bill. An example is seen in Figure 11-2.

Patient records are the heart of the practice. Records of active clients (those who return periodically for service or retesting) should, of course, be kept indefinitely, but inactive records can usually be "retired" after 3 years of inactivity (Rowland 1986). Procedures for transmitting information, timeliness of reporting results, report formats, and procedures for protecting the confidentiality of the records should be precisely delineated in the operations manual. Examples of all forms to be used in the practice should also be found in this section.

Today's date _____

Patient's name _____ Date of birth _____ Age _____
Address _____ City _____
State _____ Zip _____ Home phone _____
Responsible party _____ Spouse _____
Social Security number _____
Employer _____ Work phone _____
Employer (spouse) _____ Work phone _____
Nearest relative or friend _____ Phone _____
Referred to us by _____
Family doctor _____
Insurance company _____ Policy or group No. _____
Medicare No. _____ Medicaid (Welfare) ID No. _____

Please read these next sections very carefully and ask office staff questions if you do not understand the information.

Insurance policies and extent of coverage vary. Some plans pay all charges. Others pay a percentage, and a few pay nothing at all for the services you are to receive. The amount your insurance company will pay is between you and your insurance carrier. You are responsible for the determination of coverage.

You are responsible for paying all charges. Payment is expected the same day services are rendered unless you are in the hospital or prior arrangements have been approved by the office manager. Accounts not paid within 90 days will go to a collection agent and your credit status may be in jeopardy. Please feel free to discuss our payment policy with us.

I have read and understand the above and agree to pay all charges. I authorize payment for the services rendered. Release is hereby granted to send results as considered necessary by this office.
Signature _____
Witness _____

Fig. 11-2. Example of patient information sheet and contractual obligtion to pay for services.

The last section includes the calendar of operation and establishes the hours and days of operation, scheduled vacation days, and holidays.

ESTABLISHING FEES

Determining prices for various services and products is not a haphazard undertaking. Many factors need to be considered.

Usual and customary fees in your geographic area are quite important. Be careful not to price yourself out of the market. A survey of fees in the area will provide a low to high range. Fees should, in general, be at neither extreme.

Overhead and profit are vital considerations. Whatever fees you establish must be enough to pay your expenses (including salaries and taxes) and allow some profit. Too many audiologists have approached the setting of fees in a disorganized manner, only to discover (often too late) that they were losing money. One of the reasons that hearing aids and hearing test cost as much as they do is because they are a low-volume item. If each of us performed 500 or more audiologic evaluations and sold 100 or more aids per month, prices *could* be significantly less. If wholesale sales exceeded 2,000,000 units per year, the price from the manufacturers *could* be less. However, this is not the case.

Analysis to determine pricing must be twofold: *estimation of the number of services and products to be sold each month and careful determination of overhead factors that need to be included in pricing them.* If this analysis reveals that you must charge more than the "going rate" in order to break even, it will be necessary to reduce enough expenses so that your fees will be appropriate.

Table 11-2 is an example of a service and product sales estimation. You may have more or fewer items on your list. In estimating monthly occurrence of each, be conservative. It is better to do more business than you expected, and make a greater profit, then to do less, and risk losing money. Remember that these should be averaged monthly figures, taking into account those months when business may be slow. Also, keep in mind that it will take time to build business volume to these levels. That is why it is wise to have enough capitalization to cover your expenses for *at least* 6 months.

Overhead factors are critical. They are not estimates, but actual costs. Table 11-3 presents an example of overhead determination for an independent practice with two audiologists (you are one) and one secretary-receptionist, with a 1000-square-foot office. It is assumed that there is the usual complement of instrumentation and supplies (described above). It is also assumed that products for resale (hearing aids, assistive devices, batteries, etc.) are acquired for the best available prices. Furthermore, we are assuming that this practice advertises itself and its products regularly. This hypothetical practice has estimated income figures based on the sources delineated in Table 11-2, below. It is a business that, at least initially,

Table 11-2

Example of Estimation of Monthly Service and Product Sales

Service or Product	Estimate of Monthly Occurrence
Hearing tests, including impedance	100
ENG	5
BSER	5
Site of lesion evaluations	10
Hearing aid evaluations	20
Batteries (no. of packs)	200
Hearing aids	20
Repairs (no. charged)	12
Assistive devices	5

Table 11-3
Sample Determination of Monthly Overhead

Fixed Expenses	
Rent (1000 sq. ft.)	$ 1,200.00
Phone (2 lines)	135.00
Yellow Pages ad (line/display)	200.00
Utilities	100.00
Insurance (product/professional liability, fire, theft, major medical/dental, flood, etc.)	750.00
Secretary-receptionist salary	1,100.00
One Audiologist (salary plus commission)	2,500.00
Payment on bank loans	500.00
License fees	20.00
Dues for professional organizations	20.00
Additional books and journals	15.00
Magazine subscriptions for waiting room	5.00
Subtotal	$ 6,585.00
Variable expenses	
Your salary	$ 3,000.00
Acquisition cost of aids (20 @ $180.00)	3,600.00
Acquisition cost of assistive devices	300.00
Advertising	800.00
Office supplies	150.00
Hearing aid and earmold supplies	75.00
Batteries (including 1 pack given with each aid sold)	400.00
Earmolds	250.00
Hearing aid repairs (12 @ $35.00)	420.00
No charge repair costs (postage, insurance, etc.)	30.00
Equipment maintenance and calibration	50.00
Accounting and legal fees	500.00
Postage	50.00
Bad debts, including third-party reimbursement less than charges	300.00
Auto and travel	100.00
Printing	50.00
Taxes (personal property, FICA, unemployment, workers compensation, business income, etc.)	1,000.00
Cost of no charge follow-up visits (2 hours/day @ $30.00)	1,320.00
Bank charges	20.00
Payroll charges	30.00
Miscellaneous	400.00
Subtotal	$ 12,945.00
Total monthly	$ 19,530.00
Total annually	$234,360.00

does a moderate amount of business in both testing and product sales, perhaps with an emphasis leaning toward hearing aid dispensing.

In addition to the items listed in Table 11-3, there may be other expense factors that you will need or want to consider and to plan for unforseen financial emergencies.

According to this example,the revenues generated must be $19,530.00 per month ($234,360.00 per year) *just to break even.* Assuming an average of 21 working days a month, you must generate collectible revenues of over $900.00 *every* day. This daily figure rises when you consider vacation time for professional, sick days, and so on.

To determine pricing, we will make some additional assumptions: (1) over a period of time, battery sales (gross) pay for the rent ($1,200.00); (2) all testing fees pay fixed expenses and your salary ($9,585.00); and (3) other sources of income, excluding hearing aid sales, will be minimal.

The balance of expenses (approximately $10,000.00) will be covered by the sale of the 20 hearing aids a month. Therefore, each aid must sell for $500.00 *to break even.* It is appropriate to add some figure to this for business profit and building reserves for expansion, new equipment, and other expenses. In this example, we will add $75.00. Thus each aid should retail for $575.00.

However, since some hearing aid sales will be through third-party payers (insurance companies, medicaid, etc.) who will reimburse less than $575.00 (reducing the profit), a factor should be included to compensate. For this example, we will add $50.00, bringing the retail cost of each aid to $625.00.

FINANCIAL MANAGEMENT

Capitalizing the Venture

One of the leading causes of small business failures in this country is under capitalization. Whether starting a new practice, buying into an ongoing practice, or purchasing a revenue-generating concern, adequate capital is required.

In order to open the doors, or in some cases, keep the doors from shutting, bills must be paid. Start-up and operating expenses as well as salaries and suppliers' bills must be planned for and paid in a timely fashion. Credit ratings must be considered, and employees deserve to be paid on time. Contingency funds should be accumulated to defray any unexpected operating expenses or to cover costs during seasonal business slumps. Your salary should be realistic in terms of both your personal fiscal needs and the neonatal position of the business venture. Judicious conservatism should be used in establishing this salary figure.

Unfortunately, most of us are unable to personally finance the costs associated with entering private practice. Since there are attendant risks involved in any fledgling enterprise, it is unadvisable to put all your money in the venture. Contingency funds should be retained if possible. An often repeated, yet rarely written guideline is "if you are going to fail, do it with someone else's money. . . ."

Financial assistance may take one of several forms. Lending institutions, for example, are willing to bankroll a good risk and can be helpful in objectively estimating start-up costs relative to your particular financial needs. Careful planning and accurate expense and revenue projections will enable you to determine a break-even point. *Breaking even is that point in your business' life where collected revenue equals expenses.* The most difficult part of the start-up assessment is accurate calculation of the amount of money needed to carry the practice through the period of negative cash flow, when expenses exceed collections. Allow for a margin of error in the projections. The long-term goal is to create positive cash flow in which collected revenues surpass operating expenses. Collection time must be kept in perspective. If 10 hearing aids are dispensed and 20 hearing evaluations are done the first week in business, it may be 2–3 months before all the money is collected, depending on the office payment policy and the speed with which third-party payers remit payment for services or instruments provided.

SOURCES OF CAPITAL

The first source of capital to be considered includes personal finances. To determine your fiscal position, a detailed assessment of your finances is needed. It requires brutal honesty, and few of us are satisfied with the analysis. Net worth calculation identifies your assets and financial liabilities. Figure 11-3 provides a simple worksheet for calculating net worth. Not all the items on the worksheet can be as easily determined as cash on hand. Fixed assets such as real estate do not provide readily available funding. The value of fixed assets may, however, provide equity or collateral useful in securing business loans. Every possible asset and liability must be considered to accurately reflect your current fiscal position. The more realistic the estimate, the greater the chances for accuracy when projecting capital needs. Precise net worth assessment provides you, your partners, or your bankers with a clear picture of what you are able to bring to the venture.

Assets		Liabilities	
Cash on hand and in bank	$ _____	Notes payable to bank	$ _____
Government securities	_____	Notes payable to others	_____
Stocks and bonds	_____	Accounts and bills due	_____
Accounts/notes receivable	_____	Alimony or child support	_____
Real estate owned/equity	_____	Real estate mortgage	_____
Automobile	_____	Student loans	_____
Cash surrender value on life insurance	_____	Credit card liabilities	_____
Personal (jewelry, trusts, coins, etc.)	_____	Other debts	_____
Other assets	_____		
Total assets	$ _____	Total liabilities	$ _____

Calculation

Net worth = (total assets) − (total liabilities)

Fig. 11-3. Net worth worksheet.

Equity financing may be obtained from relatives, friends, or others in the business community who may view your venture as an investment opportunity. Potential investors must be convinced that your ideas and capabilities will prove successful. They will need information on your net worth and should carefully review your practice plan (discussed above). Equity investors rarely are interested in a rapid return on their investments. They want assurances that their financial contribution is relatively safe and will appreciate over a reasonable period of time. Equity financing results in having "concerned individuals" who will deserve to know what is going on with their money and how the business is faring from time to time. Unfortunately, if you do not choose these minority partners well, you will not only be sharing some of the profits but also, to some extent, some of the control of the business. If you have to engage equity financing, make every effort to retain a majority interest in the practice. Consult your accountant and attorney for fiscal and legal advice and documentation when the autonomy of your business is at the slightest risk.

Equity financing may be most valuable in times of "tight money," when the cost of a bank loan is excessive, or if loans are difficult to secure. Lending institutions have streamlined the procedure for securing business capital. The bank or savings and loan makes its money by lending capital to individuals or groups meeting their requirements. The lender will consider you as a partner. Fiscal officers will not lend money unless they are convinced that you have a high probability for success and at least a reasonable capability to repay the note. Generally, they are conservative lenders. They will rarely loan the entire amount of start-up costs for new ventures. An accurate net worth assessment demonstrates that you have sufficient capital of your own to warrant a lending institution's taking a reasonable risk by advancing part of your financial needs.

The lender will want to know more about you than is available on a net worth assessment form. Your resume, practice plan, assessment of the market potential for your practice, any prior business or management experience and how you plan to use the loan will serve to clarify questions about your academic, professional, and business background. You may need to orient the lender to contemporary audiology and provide statistics on practice trends. There is no substitute for personal contact with the lending institution's officers and staff. Your goal should be to win their confidence, so that you can return when it is time to expand your business. Make your banker a part of your team.

EQUIPPING THE OFFICE

Office Waiting Room

Since the reception area or waiting room is considered nonrevenue generating space, it is usually the smallest and often most neglected area when planning a private practice. That is a mistake. After the initial phone contact, the next most important patient impression generator is the waiting room. It strongly influences the patients' attitudes about the practice and the practitioners. The style of decor should be professional, yet not stuffy or cold. It should convey the idea that sensitive care and professional services are available. Patients should feel at home and be able to spend time in a comfortable environment. A television mounted in a corner, toys and books for children, a variety of reading material for adults, and, perhaps, a display of assistive listening devices, should keep your waiting patients occupied and less conscious of the wait. Promotional and informational brochures about the practice and available services should be available. Additionally, the receptionist should be available and able to answer questions.

Waiting areas should be cheerful and well illuminated. Fluorescent lighting can be harsh and unflattering. A mix of incandescent and "soft" fluorescent lighting, coupled with warm wall colors or washable wallpaper, can establish a relaxed mood. Comfortable armchairs should be available so that elderly patients can move easily. A closet or coat rack should be provided, and toilet facilities should be readily accessible. Depending on your approach, a fee schedule and payment policy can be posted next to the receptionist's window. Wall hangings should be tasteful and provide interesting opportunities for children and parents to interact. Interesting posters are available from several hearing aid manufacturers that incorporate pictures and drawings that are not solely relegated to mundane anatomic diagrams of the human ear. A chalkboard mounted to accommodate children will be used frequently.

Business Office

Patients are the most important component to your practice. Your office staff runs a close second. They are responsible for collections and appointments. They work hard at what they do, and they, like the patients, deserve to feel comfortable and at home in a warm, relaxed atmosphere. Adequate space should be allocated for files, business machines, and computer equipment. Good lighting increases work efficiency. The receptionist must have full view of the waiting room and be able to discuss billing or collection topics in a semiprivate area, out of range of the other patients in the waiting room. Patient movement from waiting area to examination or consulting room should be made as easy as possible. An intercom facilitates communication and enables the receptionist to better manage office traffic and telephone calls.

Personal Office

Your private office can be used to counsel patients and meet with others regarding business matters. It can also provide an interruption-free refuge where you can complete necessary work. Knowing that a private office is a luxury in a beginning practice, you must remember that there will be times when you will need to hold private meetings about the business or with staff, or take private calls out of earshot of patients and office personnel.

The need for other rooms will depend on the extent of your practice. For a hearing aid dispensing practice, there should be at least one hearing evaluation area with appropriate sound room and equipment; a room for taking earmold impressions and fitting hearing aids; a space for a workshop; and space for inventory, records, and patient file storage. Other rooms for special testing procedures such as electronystagmography or evoked potential studies may be needed, depending on the scope of the practice. Of course, if you have speech-language pathologists working with you, additional space will be needed for therapy areas and office space.

Office space is expensive, and it is always a good policy to obtain enough space to conduct your business in a professional, efficient manner. It is difficult to predict space needs when you are getting started. Give yourself plenty of room for additional staff or adding new procedures or services. Decide on the amount of space you need to get started, as well as what you conservatively project you will need over the term of your lease. It may be wise to limit the duration of the lease to your projected expansion timetable, so that you can move or renegotiate the lease to include greater space. If that is not possible, then obtain the space you need for expansion at the first writing of the lease, even though it will mean increased overhead at a time when you can least withstand the financial burden.

EQUIPPING A HEARING AID/EARMOLD LABORATORY

In addition to the office and professional equipment, your office will require a fully equipped hearing aid/earmold workshop. Table 11-4 presents a listing of various supplies, equipment, and tools needed. In addition, it is important that you have a hearing aid test box in order to determine whether new, used, and repaired aids meet manufacturers' specifications. Ideally, you will also have a real-ear probe microphone test system, as described in Chapters 2 and 5.

ACQUIRING AIDS FOR RESALE

Unless you are buying enough instruments from a manufacturer to qualify for their maximum discounts, it is likely that you can purchase aids at a lower cost from one of two sources. Additionally, when you receive referrals for fittings of brands you do not typically use, you can save money by purchasing from one of these sources.

Wholesalers

There are a variety of hearing aid wholesalers today. All offer discounts ranging from about 7 percent to about 15 percent off single-unit pricing for most

Table 11-4
Hearing Aid Office Supplies, Equipment, and Tools

Hearing Aid Supplies	Earmold Supplies	Tools and Equipment
Batteries	Stock molds	Battery testers
Loaner aids	Prebent tubing in various sizes	Tubing scissors
Tone hooks	Impression material	Tubing expander
Dehumidifier kits	Otoblocks	Hot-air blower
Hand mirror	Mixing cup	Sonic cleaner
Repair order forms	Spatula	Cleaner liquid
Battery mailing envelopes	Syringe	Tubing inserter
Manufacturer catalogs	Pipe cleaners	Buffer/grinder
	Tubing cement	Otoscope
	Build-up liquid	Stethoscope
	Order forms	Earmold reamer
	Shipping boxes/labels	Otolights
	Earmold lab catalogs	Small files
		Small screwdriver
		Needlenose pliers
		Bench drill bits
		Tweezers
		Contact cleaner

manufacturers. Generally, the discounts from different wholesalers do not vary considerably on any particular brand, so determine the terms and perquisites when selecting a supplier.

Buying Cooperatives (Co-ops)

A number of cooperatives (co-ops) have been formed in recent years. They differ from wholesalers in that you must be a member to take advantage of the special discount structures. By combining the buying power of a number of dispensers, co-ops have the ability to negotiate substantial discounts from a variety of manufacturers. These usually equal or exceed maximum published discounts. Regardless of how many or few aids an individual member purchases, the larger negotiated discount applies. This can be especially helpful for someone who does not dispense a large volume of instruments each month and for obtaining aids for brand-specific referrals.

LOANER STOCK

It is vital for you to have a selection of used aids to loan to patients during repairs. Initially, you may need to purchase some reconditioned instruments from manufacturers. Later, your stock will grow with trade-ins and donated aids. Having a sizable stock of loaners provides an important service to your patients. It is one of the factors that keep them returning to you.

MARKETING FOR A SUCCESSFUL DISPENSING PRACTICE

A Fairy Tale — or Is It?

Once upon a time, long, long ago in the Land of Beeps and Tones there was a nicely ordered society. At the top were those who cared for the people's medical ills (we will call them the "treaters"). At the bottom were those who sold things to people who could not be helped by the others (we will call them the "sellers").

In the middle of these two segments of society was a very austere group of people. No one really knew from whence they arose or even if they truly owned their name, much less what their name really meant. They lived in ivory towers, usually covered with ivy. They studied, taught, and did research. They even joined together to form a ruling body that promulgated rules of behavior, telling everyone what was right and what was wrong.

In the hierarchy of the land of Beeps and Tones, these people (we will call them the "professionals" for the sake anonymity) defined people's problems, tested them for these problems, sent them either to the treaters or the sellers and sometimes tried to teach them rather esoteric things for their own good.

For many years the professionals believed that it would be very wrong for them to be sellers. That would be "unprofessional" and would surely taint the purity of what they did. After all, how could a professional make objective, unbiased recommendations to people if that person was also a seller? They would not dirty their hands with money (they also did not earn much money).

The professionals continually told the other two groups how things should be. Unfortunately, very few people ever listened to them. They were so concerned with trying to tell the other groups what to do that they forgot to communicate with the common folk.

One day, some of the professionals began to think that this situation was not right. They thought, "If we really know as much as we think we do and know how to take care of people's problems, then why do we not do it ourselves?" They became sellers (we will call them "dispensing professionals" to avoid confusion with the "regular" sellers and "regular" professionals). Naturally, the rest of the professionals were very upset with these radicals. Their ruling body even exiled some of them.

Curiously, in the early days of this revolution, neither the treaters nor the sellers were very concerned. As time went by, however, more and more professionals became dispensing professionals. Some even went to work for sellers! Everyone became upset and started calling each other names.

And so, as many professionals joined the revolution, the ruling body saw that it could not stop this flood of defections and changed its rules, making it acceptable for professionals to become dispensing professionals. The ruling body even went so far as to declare that it was okay to advertise what they were doing.

As more and more professionals left their ivory towers, many of them realized that they needed to communicate not only with the treaters but with the common folk as well. After all, if the common folk did not know about the wonderful things they sold and services they offered, how would the common folk ever be able to take advantage of these wonders? Strangely enough, the sellers had known this for years. Some of the professionals, and even some of the dispensing professionals, did not think this was right and stayed in their Ivory Towers, looking down their noses.

This brings our story to a close. Unfortunately, it cannot be said they lived happily ever after as in other fairy tales. Perhaps they never will.

Reality

"Changing patterns in the delivery of health care has resulted in a shift in focus from the provider to the buyer. As a result, it has been necessary for providers . . . to recognize that the health care field is not exempt from the cardinal rule of marketing—the customer is king" (Skafte 1986). Gone forever are the days when audiologists could hang a shingle and expect the public to beat a path to their doors.

As more and more audiologists enter some form of hearing aid dispensing, competition increases. This situation makes it incumbent on us to increase our efforts to attract patients and customers. Those (audiologists or hearing aid dealers) who do the most effective and consistent job of promoting their products and services will be the most successful. Marketing is necessary to create a demand and let the potential customer know how that demand can be fulfilled. It is a process that moves products or services to market effectively and, therefore, profitably.

Some believe that we must market only to referral sources and advertise only generic, public information material. For example, Loavenbruck (1986), when discussing "hard-sell marketing techniques by audiologists" (advertising special price promotions, open houses, free hearing tests), states that "it is a style that reduces us to 'giveaways' of our professional services as the item of value." Also, Hampton (1986), when discussing audiologists adopting a retail hearing aid model, states, "we now see audiologists involved with telemarketing, free hearing tests, battery promotions, and other product-oriented marketing tactics that are only somewhat different from the door-to-door tactics that audiologists have criticized in the past."

Audiologists have been critical of commercial marketing practices in the hearing aid industry. Some of those criticisms were accurate and justified. From the isolated perspective of audiology in the 1950s, 1960s, and 1970s, *all* the criticisms appeared appropriate. However, the marketplace and the consuming public have been changing dramatically. Attitudes about marketing in audiology appear to be changing at a slower pace than those found in the real world of the marketplace. Many audiologists, however, have come to realize that some of these previously criticized advertising approaches are necessary components of a total marketing plan for a successful practice.

As a profession, we have done a poor job of informing the public about who we are and what we can offer. On the other hand, the hearing aid industry and dealer organizations have done a much better job, especially in recent years. The average person has never heard the terms *audiologist* or *audiology* and has no idea we exist or what we do. Millions of hearing-impaired individuals do not use hearing aids. The reality is that the number of nonusers would probably be much higher had it not been for the "hard-sell marketing techniques" of the hearing aid industry.

The distinctions among the professions that make one group more or less aggressive in marketing than the others are rapidly breaking down as the competition for clients becomes more acute. In order to survive in this highly competitive marketplace, audiologists must inform the public who and what we are and induce them to seek our specialized services, especially since formerly reliable referral sources are dwindling as more audiologists and Otologists enter the dispensing area. Realistically, after emphasizing quality of service and benefits of amplification, people, especially those on a fixed income, need an additional reason to act. In many cases, the reason to act is generated by offering a new product or a reduced cost promotion. Advertising gets the message across. It is necessary for our professional survival.

HIA Survey

The Hearing Industries Association (1985) recently completed a survey of the hearing-impaired population of the United States. Some of the data thus obtained are significant in terms of deciding whether to comprehensively market a dispensing practice and in planning a marketing strategy. The study indicates that there are approximately 10 million hearing-impaired people in this country who do not yet use hearing aids, 78 percent of whom report communication difficulty some or most of the time, and 44 percent of whom report a hearing loss in both ears.

Of the nonowners of hearing aids, 45 percent believe that their loss of hearing is not severe enough to justify use of an aid. This suggests that a major thrust of our marketing should be geared to demonstrate to consumers that use of hearing aids will make a noticeable difference in their lives.

The results of the study also contradict some of the beliefs of many on the hearing health care team:

1. The anticipated cost of amplification is *not* an important factor in explaining why nonowners have not yet purchased an aid.
2. Cosmetic factors are *not* a significant influence in an individual's decision to buy a hearing aid, although they may be once the decision is made.
3. Hearing-impaired persons who believe that family members, friends, co-workers, and their physician think that they should use a hearing aid tend to have a substantially more favorable attitude about hearing aid use than those who do not so believe.

Based on these and other results of the study, it is apparent that we need to plan our marketing strategies to accomplish certain specific goals. Among them are:

1. Promoting the attitude that use of a hearing aid will make a significant positive difference in the lives of the hearing-impaired.
2. Supporting the family, friends, and co-workers of the hearing-impaired to encourage them regarding hearing aid use and to convince the hearing-impaired that these people want them to use amplification.
3. The most effective way to influence nonowners is through family physicians, otologists, and the Yellow Pages.
4. Since about 27 percent of nonowners are between 30 and 50 years of age, marketing strategies and materials must be made attractive to a younger population.
5. With over 64 percent of non-owners over age 50, other approaches must be designed to appeal to this group.
6. Educate physicians and other health care providers about the benefits of amplification in general, and its benefits to the mildly and unilaterally impaired.
7. Promote binaural fittings for

Marketing In A Dispensing Practice

There is a distinct difference between marketing and selling. *Marketing* is what you do to attract new or repeat patients or customers to the practice. *Selling* is what you do after they arrive. This chapter will not concentrate on selling. The reader is referred to an excellent series of articles on selling hearing aids by Caruso (1985a,b,c; 1986).

Marketing is both a process and a way of thinking. It is defined by the American Marketing Association as *"The process of planning and executing the conception, pricing, promotion, and distribution of ideas, goods and services to create exchanges that satisfy individual and organizational objectives"* (Pfeil et al., 1985). In a sense, marketing is an exchange process wherein all parties benefit—the seller obtains more sales and the consumer obtains a product or service he needs or wants.

Marketing is a critical tool in the business world. It offers an opportunity to instruct the hearing-impaired public about our professional acumen and expertise. It enables us to overcome our low professional visibility and offer accountability the average consumer knows little about. Consumer attitudes and increased competition for the same health care dollar dictates the need for a solid marketing plan. Consumers are sophisticated and interested in quality service for their health care dollars. They are willing to shop around until satisfied and if dissatisfied, will seek care elsewhere.

As the service or product delivery systems change and as competition and consumer awareness increase, we are faced with a situation in which our "professional" view of marketing is no longer sufficient. To meet these changes, it is necessary for us to expand our view of how we can "get our message to the people."

HISTORICAL PERSPECTIVE

When most audiologists worked in universities or various agencies, there was little concern about or need for marketing. Referral sources were developed and generally remained constant. Audiologists were not dispensing hearing aids. When an instrument was recommended, the patient was referred to one or more of the local hearing aid dealers.

There were problems inherent in that system. Often, the greatest of these were the audiologist's dissatisfaction with some or all of the local dealers and the feeling that the audiologist should and could provide all the services. In the early 1970s a few audiologists began dispensing hearing aids. Later in that decade, the number of dispensing audiologists grew. Today, there are 2500–3000 audiologists involved in some form of hearing aid dispensing (Cranmer 1986). Many of these individuals are involved in private practice.

Audiologists choose to dispense hearing aids because it is a natural outgrowth of their training in aural rehabilitation. Dispensing enables the audiologist to manage all aspects of the patient's rehabilitative progress. The financial advantages are obvious; it enables the audiologist to increase practice revenue.

Marketing as an Ongoing Process

Marketing is not something you do once or once in awhile. To be successful, it *must* be a continuing program. The sale of your services and products begins months or years before an actual purchase is made. When dispensing hearing aids, it must be remembered that *the instrument is something few people want to buy and only a limited segment of the populace actually needs.* The marketing process, therefore, begins by building an awareness in the consumer's mind that *hearing aids can have a positive effect on the quality of that person's life.* Attitudinal changes such as these do not happen overnight.

Marcus (1986) states: "Today in the competitive marketplace, the process that ends in closing the sale is increasingly elaborate and requires strategy and skill" and that it "begins with the conscious decision to grow and compete, departing substantially from serendipity," "moves to developing a marketing plan and strategy strategy and then executing that plan," and "includes learning and practicing new skills performed by others."

Time and money spent on marketing and promotion is an investment in the practice. When a successful marketing plan is followed, new patients, a broadened market base, and increased visibility will be the results.

Types of Marketing

There are two basic types of marketing as they apply to a dispensing practice; *public relations and advertising*. Both have the same goal—*to increase the number of patients coming to the practice.*

PUBLIC RELATIONS

Public relations covers three areas; *generating referral sources, increasing public awareness of audiology, and hearing health care and keeping in touch with the existing patient/customer base.*

Generating referral sources involves both maintaining close contact with existing referral sources and promoting new ones. In the past, the primary referral base for dispensing audiologists consisted of Otolaryngologists, Otologists, and other nondispensing audiologists. Since each group is increasingly entering dispensing, the numbers of available referrals are dwindling. Efforts must now concentrate on nondispensing Otolaryngologists (or the audiologists working for them) and non-ENT physicians.

In addition to well-prepared and expeditious patient reports, there are other proven marketing approaches to increase referrals from the medical community. They include:

1. Arranging to speak at hospital general or specialty staff meetings
2. Offering a series of lectures to family practice or other specialty resident training programs
3. Including area specialty physicians (especially ENT, internal medicine, family and general practice, pediatrics, psychiatry, emergency medicine, gerontology, physiatry, neurology and neurosurgery) on the mailing list for a practice newsletter
4. Preparing brief, periodic (every 6–8 weeks) informational letters to area specialists, each covering a different aspect of audiology such as overview of audiology, diagnostic benefits of impedance measurements, diagnostic import of vestibular testing and evoked potentials, audiogram and tympanogram interpretation, orientation to hearing aids, psychology of hearing impairment, new developments in the field, and new equipment or services in the practice.
5. Preparing an informational packet welcoming new physicians to the area.
6. Personal phone calls to referring physicians to discuss interesting cases or to periodically inquire about their level of satisfaction with your services.
7. Submission of formal service and/or product contract proposals to the administrators and medical directors of area HMOs, PPOs, hospitals without existing audiologic services, and large practice medical clinics.
8. Informational brochures and proposals to area geriatric and mental retardation/developmental disability (MR/DD) extended-care facilities.

The more that can be done to keep a practice name or logo in front of a potential or existing referral source, the greater the likelihood referrals will be sent.

PUBLIC AWARENESS

Today's consumers are interested in information about health care. Most of them are uninformed about or refuse to acknowledge that they have hearing problems. You can provide a meaningful public service and increase awareness about the profession and practice by undertaking a campaign of public awareness marketing. Some aspects of such a program cost little, if anything. A few examples include soliciting invitations to radio and TV talk shows, press releases, and public service announcements (PSAs) to daily and weekly newspapers, speaking at area services clubs and other community organizations, and offering hearing screening programs at health fairs and senior citizens residential complexes and recreational centers. These opportunities may be exhausted quickly and cannot be relied on as a sole means of promotion. Regular "informational" ads may be placed in local newspapers and can follow on the first wave of some of the aforementioned opportunities.

The results of these efforts will not materialize quickly, as it takes time to increase awareness of hearing problems and the benefits of amplification. *Be patient.* The time and money you invest in this type of program will, over time, be rewarded with increased numbers of patients and profits.

EXISTING PATIENT/CUSTOMER BASE

An often neglected segment of a dispensing audiology practice is that group of patients previously fitted with amplification or those evaluated but not following the recommendation for hearing aid fitting. Generally, after the first postfitting year, patients should be contacted to return at least annually. The annual visit provides a time to repeat hearing examinations, evaluate the electroacoustic status of the instruments, and provide adjustments and new earmolds. It also provides an opportunity to dispense new hearing aids when needed. Those patients not responding to annual recheck announcements should be contacted by phone. From a marketing standpoint, *if 30–50 percent of hearing aids dispensed are not resales to prior patients (after 3–5 years of practice), the "in-house" marketing plan needs reevaluation.*

Proven techniques for marketing within an established patient/customer base include:

1. A thank you note after the trial period indicating appreciation for the patient's confidence in you and encouraging follow-up visits.
2. A birthday card.
3. A Christmas card or annual calendar with logo or practice name, location, and phone number.
4. A thank you note and complimentary pack of batteries on referral of a new patient.
5. Recall notices for annual hearing and hearing aid rechecks.
6. Notices of new product developments.
7. Notice of trade-in promotions for aids at least 3 years old.
8. Battery club promotion

PRIVATE LABEL BATTERIES

When you dispense a hearing aid, the user generally receives very little material containing your name, office address, and office phone number; the sales contract; an instructional booklet; and a business card. None of these are typically kept out for periodic reference. One item that must be used is the battery pack. If your identification information was imprinted on it, the pack would serve as a constant reminder of you. Then, when more batteries are needed, the user is most likely to return to you rather than buying them at a drug store. If there is no brand name on the package, many people will assume that they can obtain the batteries only from your office. There are a number of programs currently available that inexpensively provide major brand batteries in private label packaging.

BATTERY CLUB

Many dispensers have found that a Battery Club serves two important functions: it helps cash flow by requiring patients to pay in advance for a supply of batteries and it increases the chances that patients will remain with you since they have prepaid for a large supply of batteries.

The basic format is one in which a customer prepays for a specified number of packs of battery (e.g., five), has them mailed as needed, and receives one free pack when the prepaid supply is exhausted. When the free pack is sent, a renewal notice is included. There are a number of variations of this format that can be utilized.

PRACTICE NEWSLETTER

The last marketing program related to referral sources and existing patient base to be considered is the practice newsletter. It is an excellent vehicle that can effectively inform and orient patients and referral sources. You can subscribe to a commercially produced newsletter that allows you to personalize a portion of the content, or you may write your own. Newsletters offer a convenient format for patient education and lend favorably to professional credibility among the referral sources. They can be an effective and acceptable method of keeping new developments and important events about the practice in front of patients and referral sources. Articles for the newsletter could include topics such as causes of feedback, the importance of annual hearing rechecks and hearing aid service, various styles of hearing aids, tinnitus, advantages of binaural amplification, professional meetings attended by staff, and biographies and personal items about staff members. Some dispensers allow patients to "subscribe" to the newsletter for a nominal fee. The newsletter can assist in updating patient records. Each issue can include a coupon with which the recipient can send notification of an address change. Additionally, each issue should have "Address Correction Requested" imprinted on the address label portion. It is well worth the postal service fee to acquire and utilize this information.

The writing style should be simple, concise, and personal. Type faces, paper stock, and format should be easily read. Design should be attractive, and photographs and drawings should be used. A quarterly publication schedule which does not interfere with holidays is optimal: January, April, July, and October appear to be the best months (Mahon 1984).

A Total Marketing Plan

Quite a few audiologists take a negative position regarding marketing, especially the advertising aspect of it, saying "I have tried lots of advertising—newspaper, radio, mailings—at various times. I tried things that other people said worked. But nothing has worked well for me; I don't think advertising really sells hearing aids." Such statements suggest a haphazard approach and a violation of the cardinal rule of marketing: *a successful marketing approach is one that is carefully researched, planned, and carried out.* It must involve the strategic development of a *total marketing plan.* Solitary advertisements or occasional direct mailings do not yield successful results.

A successful marketing campaign should include, in addition to those elements noted above, *consumer education, display advertising, direct mail, and special promotions.* The objective is to systematically increase visibility and become recognized as "THE" source of services for the hearing-impaired.

Brown (1984) described six steps to be considered in the strategic planning of a marketing program:

1. Identify *personal goals.* How much income do you want for the year? How many hours a week will you work?
2. Identify *practice goals.* By how much do you want the practice revenues and profits to increase this year? How many hearing aids do you project selling per month? What additional referral sources do you want to acquire this year? What new contracts for services do you project acquiring this year? What percentage of hearing aid sales will be to previous users?
3. Identify *target markets.* This usually requires some market research, either on your part or by hiring a marketing consultant. It could be money well spent, especially if you do not have sufficient time or capability to do it. As part of the analysis, you first need to *segment* the market to identify to whom you will direct your efforts. *Each segment you identify is a separate target market.* Segmentation involved determining various characteristics of the population demographics, including number of people in various age groups, socioeconomic makeup, any unusual incidence of hearing loss, potential referral sources, attitudes about hearing aids, and current users and nonusers.
4. Analyze *target market needs.* How much do the people in your target markets know about hearing loss and hearing aids? What are nonusers' values about better hearing? To what types of marketing are they most likely to respond? What is the consumer's orientation about spending their money for what they may consider "luxury" items, such as hearing aids? Much of the data regarding segmentation and market needs are readily available from such sources as recent census figures, state and county Department of Health records, the recent Hearing Industries Association national survey concerning hearing aids and the public's attitudes, and local university Marketing Department surveys (you might even convince the Marketing Department to conduct a specific survey for

you as a class or thesis project). Another aspect of determining market needs is to analyze the competition. Who are they? What kinds of marketing do they use? How successful are they? What services and promotions can you provide that they do not?

5. Formulate *marketing plan*. Brown (1984) states that "many health care professionals misunderstand the true meaning of professional marketing . . . most either view the activity far too narrowly and/or have a negative attitude toward the term/activity." *There is nothing inherently unprofessional about marketing, including advertising. At the heart of establishing a profitable business is reaching the consumer.*

6. Evaluate *effectiveness of plan*. The marketing plan you develop should have a specified life (e.g., 1 year). It is vital to periodically evaluate the results of its implementation, perhaps monthly or quarterly, and to adjust the plan on the basis of its results. If these results do not appear to be headed toward your stated goals, carefully reevaluate each step. Are your goals realistic? Are the marketing tools being used reaching the desired segments? It may prove beneficial to shift the emphasis of some parts of the plan, that is, better designed ads and direct mail pieces, more direct mailing, less radio advertising, and more or less frequent newspaper display ads. Such reorientation will increase the likelihood of reaching your overall goals.

Kofski et al. (1986) state: "Long-term success in the hearing health care field is not dependent on the success of a single element or action. Effective marketing, superior service or product alone will not serve to optimize a business' share of the market. Instead, all of these factors must be developed equally to assure success in modern retailing." This statement reinforces a belief that marketing is an ongoing process that requires a mix of many media to effectively reach all targeted segments of the population.

We have described the parts of a plan aimed at three market segments: referral sources, existing patients, and public relations. The balance of this discussion will focus on that aspect of marketing generating the most controversy: *advertising*.

ADVERTISING

"How can you expect to sell a service or a product to the public when you fail to tell the public what you are selling, and why it should be bought from you?" (Gluck 1986)

Advertising is *the process of disseminating information about who is selling what, for what purpose and at what price*. Its primary purpose is to generate interest and attract new and old customers. Although image building, consumer education and new product announcement advertising can be important, *the most effective advertisements are those designed to trigger a specific response*, such as "call today for an appointment," "come in and let us check your aid this week," and "this special price is good only until Friday."

Reasons for advertising. Gluck (1986) describes 10 reasons for advertising.

1. *New prospects*—to attract both nonusers and users who are new to you. Ours is a mobile society. Nearly 20 percent of all families, including senior citizens, will move this year.

2. *Continuous advertising*—to be effective, an advertising campaign needs to be a continuing, long-term program, even if it is limited at times to small weekly or monthly image-building advertisements. Many dispensers do not market during "slow" periods such as January–March or July–August. These are the times to direct your major emphasis. Do not write off the "slow" periods just because revenues have been down in the past. You can convert those valleys into peaks through effective advertising.

3. *The competition is not quitting*—advertise to secure your share of the market and, perhaps, reduce that of your competitors.

4. Advertising in a troubled economy gives a business a distinct *advantage over competitors who cut back*. Hearing aid sales figures, published annually in trade journals, show that they are not significantly effected by inflation, recessions, or unemployment. It is a matter of being able to tap new sources of referrals and third-party payments.

5. *Advertising sets the record straight* by correcting gossip, and misinformation, advertisements project a positive image. Studies indicate that most Americans have a favorable attitude about advertising and agree that it is necessary (Gluck 1986).

6. *Strengthen your image* for today and tomorrow through continuous advertising. Remember Chrysler? Hearing aids have a negative image at worst, or a neutral image at best. That is likely the reason that most people are reluctant to use amplification. They do not become converted overnight. Their loss did not occur rapidly and their enthusiasm for your product will not do the same.

7. *Advertising works.* In my practice (M. C. Pollack), hearing aid sales spike during those months in which specific promotions are featured that are geared to elicit action.

8. *Advertising generates office traffic.* Getting people into your office for evaluation is the first step in making the initial sales and selling additional products and services in the future.

9. *To maintain internal morale.* The office staff may become demoralized when they think you are cutting back and/or when patient flow is down.

10. *Expenses already exist.* Your doors are open, so why not advertise to generate a steady flow of customers?

Advertising focus. An effective marketing mix is one that includes a variety of messages. It is necessary to understand buyer incentives that successfully sell products to the greatest number of people. Some will respond better to ads that feature hearing aid size (ITE and ITC) and price reductions. Others will respond better to approaches that stress the benefits to be gained through the use of amplification. Still others will take action in response to descriptions of "new and better" products (better understanding in noise).

Because people respond differently, it is necessary to create a variety of messages in your advertising. A single advertisement can convey multiple messages, such as benefits, size, price, and new products in order to appeal to a greater number of people. At other times, a continuing campaign can consist of a variety of ads, each appealing to a different segment. Such a mix can be very effective. Whatever approach you use in any individual advertisement, *always* give the consumer a reason to act now; provide incentives such as limited-time offer, free hearing tests, new product introduction at a reduced price, or out-of-town "expert" visiting to consult with consumers.

CHOOSING THE MEDIA

There are a number of advertising media available: television, radio, newspapers, senior citizen and other specific market publications, direct mail, and the Yellow Pages.

Electronic media. The production and air time costs for radio and television can be cost prohibitive for the intended market and therefore may not provide cost-efficient, high-return benefits. On the other hand, electronic media are excellent sources for "nonadvertising" marketing—especially PSAs and talk shows.

Newspaper. Display advertisements in newspapers can be expensive, depending on the rates and readership characteristics. If properly designed and placed, however, newspaper advertising can be quite effective, especially if used consistently and in conjunction with direct-mail campaigns. Advertisement location in the newspaper is critical. If the focus is on senior citizens, usually the Society section and Obituaries will be read most frequently. Day of the week is also important. Sunday issues typically have a higher readership. Consult the advertising manager of your newspaper(s) for readership and other important demographic data. Smaller, weekly papers usually have lower advertising rates (and lower readership), and can be effective for targeted ads.

Direct mail. One of the most popular and successful forms of advertising among hearing aid dispensers is direct mail. With proper design, careful mailing list selection, and judicious choice of mailing date, this method of advertising has proved to be highly cost-effective. As with any form of marketing, the direct-mail message can be *general* (benefits of amplification, information about your practice) or *specific* (special promotion, new product introduction, or special offers).

The five key elements in a direct mail program are: *mailing list, message, package* (mailing piece), *offer,* and *fulfillment.*

Mailing lists are available from a number of sources. They are typically updated once or twice a year, although none are ever perfect. These companies obtain their information from various sources. You can select carefully segmented lists by age, head of household, zip code, income level, or any mix thereof. This allows you to target your mailing to a specific group.

The most economic method of mailing is *bulk mail*. You purchase a permit from the post office and enjoy lower postal rates. Bulk mail goes third class, is not returned and has a slower delivery time.

Direct mail has a relatively low response rate. A 1 percent response is considered extremely good. The response tends to increase if a newspaper advertisement is run a few days following the mailing. The ad reminds many people of the mailing they received and triggers action.

The *message* or content is critical to the success of a direct-mail promotion. A well-balanced message mix, including benefits of amplification, hearing aid size, and price parameters in a focused, simple and to-the-point format, optimize chances for a response.

Packaging of the mailer piece should be simple and readable. Most of the mailings will be to senior citizens, whose eyesight may be impaired. Select type faces and paper stock and ink colors that optimize readability.

The *offer* is the stimulus to take action now. It should be specific and time-dated, such as the introduction of a new product at a reduced price before a certain date, an open house with a manufacturer's representative or out-of-town expert, or a trade-in allowance on an old aid when buying a new one.

Fulfillment pertains to the results of the mailing. How successful was it? Did you reach the goal you set? If not, why not? What can you do differently next time to improve the results.

Yellow pages. For a new practitioner, the Yellow Pages can be the most effective means of gaining visibility and making the phones ring for appointments. For an established practitioner, it can be the most potent reminder of an ongoing practice's services and reputation. Best of all, the results in terms of new patients can outweigh the cost (Walker 1985). Approximately 80 percent of adults referring to the Yellow Pages are seeking information about professional services—lawyer, accountant, dentist, physician and so on; 85 percent of these follow the reference with action—a phone call, visit, or letter to the professional selected (Swerdlow 1981).

There are many kinds and sizes of advertisements to be used. Evaluate the competition and decide what you need to compete or gain a marketplace advantage. A display advertisement listing multiple locations or a map to the office with a readable listing of services offered are only a few of many options available. Space, size, and special features, such as multiple colors or boldfacing, can escalate the price of the placement dramatically, yet may be critical to heighten consumer appeal. The Yellow Pages offer complete art work and design, usually at no charge. They are willing to help and can be a great source of assistance in deciding what approach is best within the limits of an advertising budget.

MARKETING BUDGET

It is necessary to allocate funds to accomplish most of your marketing goals. This must be done within the context of your overall overhead expenses and has to be done judiciously. A typical advertising budget should be at least 6–10 percent of total practice revenues (Cranmer 1986). How you allocate this budget will be determined by your marketing plan.

CONCLUSION

Brown (1984) discussed the importance of *word-of-mouth* advertising. This can be your best or worst form of advertising. It is a reflection of the care people receive in your office, as well as their satisfaction with the hearing aids you have sold them. Patients who are satisfied will tell four or five others about their positive experience. However, consumers tell more than twice as many others about a negative experience. Related to this are *reasons why customers cease to be your customers*.

- 1 percent—death of customer
- 4 percent—customer moves away
- 11 percent—competitive inroads
- 16 percent—product dissatisfaction
- 68 percent—reaction to an attitude of *indifference* by someone(s) in your organization

Think about it! The following quotation is from Gluck (1986):

WHY IS IT?
A man wakes up in the morning to an
advertised alarm clock, and
pulls off *advertised* pajamas,
takes a bath in an *advertised* tub,
washes with an *advertised* soap,
uses an *advertised* toothpaste,
puts on *advertised* clothes,
sits down to breakfast with an *advertised* coffee,
puts on an *advertised* hat,
rides to work in an *advertised* car,
writes with an *advertised* pen. . .
Then refuses to *advertise*, saying he
can't afford to *advertise*.
Then, if business is not good enough to *advertise*,
He *advertises* it for sale.*

---

* Reproduced with permission from Gluck LD: Advertising builds business. Hearing Instruments 37:13, 1986.

THE COMPUTER IN A DISPENSING OFFICE

Introduction

Profit in any business can result only from an increase in revenue (sales) or a decrease in expenses, or both. Many hearing aid dispensers have discovered that one way to increase revenue is by using an office computer system. Technological advances have made computers and software packages more available and affordable. Dispensers are facing a decision as to whether to introduce computers into their professional practices. This chapter section is not intended as a computer short course, but, rather, as an overview of the many uses to which a system can be put in your practice.

One basic premise in this chapter is that, with the exception of formal not-for-profit settings, *any hearing aid dispensing practices operating to make enough profit to support all business expenses and salaries (including the owner), and, hopefully, have some bottom line profit left over.* When operating any business, an astute owner/manager has set certain specific short-term and long-term goals, along with methods of achieving these goals. Naturally, all goals have the intent of improving the fiscal and operational situation of the company. Computers may be viewed as tools for reaching certain of these goals, thereby improving the operation and profits of the business.

For most of us who began our practices more than a few years ago, computers were not something we considered. In fact, there are probably many "old timers" who know so little about computers that they are very resistant to using them, just as many of us were resistant to using ITE aids when they were first introduced some 20 years ago. Old habits are hard to change. However, as today's new practices begin, computers are frequently included as a start-up expense, along with audiometers, typewriters, and calculators. A recent report (Cranmer 1986) estimates that nearly 37 percent of hearing aid dispensers and dispensing audiologists use computers in their practices, and that another 20 percent are planning to purchase a computer in the near future.

Why should you spend up to $15,000 dollars for a computer system? No wise business person should be enthusiastic about spending such a sum for a capital expenditure unless there is a realistic assurance of a return on the investment. In other words, will the computer pay for itself and increase my profits?

At the outset of this discussion we pointed out that increased profits must result from either more sales or less expenses. It is unlikely that computer usage will result in significantly reduced expenses. However, through more effective marketing of products and services, it is likely that revenues will increase.

Classification of Computer Usage

The uses to which any business can put a computer can broadly be classified into two categories: *revenue generating uses and operational efficiency uses.* If done properly, the former will almost certainly increase profits and the latter will likely reduce expenses and may result in some increased revenue.

REVENUE GENERATING USES

While operational uses, which will be described below, are very nice and can lessen the workload, they do not directly produce revenue for the practice. Therefore, the primary purposes for which any hearing aid dispensing practice should acquire a computer system are those that will directly increase revenues and profits. This can be done in a number of ways.

Marketing your existing customer base. By increasing contact with your patients or customers it is likely that you will see an increase in revenues. With appropriate data entry, you may recall patients for annual hearing tests, annual hearing aid servicing, hearing aid check-up just prior to warranty expiration, hearing aid replacement, date-specific insurance eligibility for a new hearing aid, consideration of a second hearing aid for a monaural user, update information on new products or assistive devices for certain patients, and special promotions such as a trade-in special or an open house. Battery club notices, special occasions announcements, and birthday or holiday greetings can be filed in the computer for retrieval by date, name, or service to be provided. Anything that will favorably impress your patients and keep them thinking of you will also keep them returning to you.

New customers and referral sources. A computer can be used to generate labels to mail notices regarding special promotions, open houses, new products, and so on, intended to generate new business for you. Sending thank you letters to referral sources along with a report of the outcome of the consultation is a very effective tool to keep your name in the consciousness of those referral sources. Such communication is only one of many ways to market your referral network. It is also important to generate new referral sources by disseminating professional information about services and products to the professional community. Lists of members of local medical societies, organized by specialty, can provide the names of potential referrers. This information can be entered for use in producing labels and personalized letters. These endeavors will likely result in increased referrals, therefore increasing your customer base and your revenues.

OPERATIONAL USES

Patient records. Patient identification parameters; address, phone number(s), insurance policy number(s), dates of first and most recent visits, hearing test data, hearing aid fitting, follow-up and repairs, instrument type and serial number, and history of battery usage may be included in programs to facilitate retrieval. Detailed information enables   recall for marketing, practice growth pattern analysis, or billing purposes.

Receivables. Accounts receivable and billing may be computerized. It can keep your receivables current and permits analysis of accounts by 30-, 45-, 60-, or 90-day periods. By aging the accounts, those exceeding tolerable limits may be "flagged" for immediate attention by the office staff or collection agent. Tracking accounts gives you a clear picture of your collection program's efficiency. Additionally, the computer can be programmed to produce monthly statements for private paying customers and complete billing forms for insurance companies and other third party payers.

Accounts payable. Just as a computer can assist in keeping track of receivables, it can also assist in keeping track of accounts payable (the bills you owe). Payment dates can help to establish necessary payment times. By paying bills on time, not before not later than needed, cash flow becomes less of a problem. Deadline dates to qualify for early payment discounts can be used to maximum efficiency when date sensitive payment information is reviewed. Rent, payroll taxes and other important fixed or variable expenses may be placed in the computer for timely response and attention.

Insurance or medicaid billing. The clerical burden of third-party payments can be reduced considerably by computerization. Several programs are available that print the form at the same time it fills in required data. Other programs can be easily adjusted to accommodate a variety of billing formats.

Business records. In addition to customer accounts, accounts receivable, and accounts payable, many other general business record-keeping functions can be handled very efficiently with a computer. These include posting to a general ledger, payroll, tax information, and management of inventory.

Coordination of branch offices. Computer terminals in various locations can be "networked" together to improve communication between satellite offices and also improve business record keeping between branch offices. In lieu of networking, data on disks can be carried with ease from office to office.

Trends analysis. An important consideration in the successful management of any business is to be able to identify, analyze, and react to trends that have been developing in the business over a given period of time. Such an undertaking allows retrospective analysis of the methods that you have used to achieve your various goals. What has worked? What hasn't worked? What procedures and marketing approaches should be changed to increase their effectiveness? Having trend data readily available makes such analyses much simpler and more effective and can be used as the basis for future decisions in terms of the growth of your practice.

Hearing aid selection and fitting. In Chapter 7, Berger very thoroughly describes the various formula fitting approaches that are currently being used today in selecting hearing aids for a given patient. Most of these prescriptive approaches are available as computer programs. These methods provide a means of matching hearing aid specifications with audiologic data. Thus the computer can sort through the many hearing aids available to you and identify those that, according to the criteria of the prescriptive program you are using, appear most appropriate for the patient. Please refer to Dr. Berger's chapter for an in-depth discussion of this material.

Word processing. Preparation of professional reports to referral sources can be greatly simplified by using a word processing program. Routine reports, letters, and specific phrases can be stored in memory and recalled as needed. Some programs permit report building where phrases may be selected to yield a composite report.

Storage of test results for research data. Although this is not a use that most private-practicing hearing aid dispensers will be interested in, the capacity does exist to store detailed audiologic data for later recall for statistical analysis as part of a research project. However, potentially profitable use of such data would be in the analysis of specific trends in terms of answering specific questions. Have you been less successful in fitting hearing aids to individuals with certain kinds of hearing loss? If so, perhaps identifying such a trend will give you a clue to improve case management.

All of these operational uses are intended to increase the efficiency of your practice, improve your time management, and save money on taxes and professional expenses. Therefore, these operational uses can reduce your expenses, thereby increasing your profits.

Choosing the Computer

With the many computer systems and software packages on the market today, there is no specific computer recommendation that can be made for the specific needs of every practice. However, there are some general guidelines that must be considered in selecting computer hardware and software.

1. *Evaluate your needs* and be clear about the intended purpose of the system.
2. *Investigate the availability of software and plan ahead for usage.* Buy equipment that is expandable. The ability to add on storage capacity is a must. The more you use a computer, the more familiar and comfortable you will become with it and the more demands you will place on its use. The cost of adding more storage, such as a hard disk, is minimal compared to the cost of replacing an entire system.
3. *Investigate the compatibility of the various systems with your other office equipment, both business and clinical.* Some electronic typewriters are compatible with certain computers for use as word processing systems, although most electronic typewriters are not as efficient and durable as standard computer

printers. Some audiometers are computer-compatible, allowing for rapid and efficient storage of audiologic data.

4. *Evaluate the ease of use of both the hardware and software components you are considering.* Any system you purchase must be "user-friendly." Such a system does not require a degree in computer programming but, rather, allows even the most inexperienced operator to easily use the system effectively.

5. *Investigate the availability of local support.* This includes back-up support for your service warranty and training. These services are a must. If you purchase a system from outside your immediate area, or purchase a system that is not available nationwide, such as one of the many IBM clone systems on the market today, first determine that there are local personnel available for the servicing of such a system and to provide you with a service maintenance contract.

6. *Use proven software.* Software should be selected first and hardware second. The cost of developing a software program can run into thousands of dollars. Therefore, it is imperative that you look for programs that have been tested in hearing aid offices. Two examples of such systems that are on the market at the time of this writing are the "Hearing Aid Office System" from RJS Acoustics, Inc., in Portland, Oregon and the "EARS2 YOU: Software For the Dispensing Office" available from Hearing Associates, Inc. in Kansas City, Missouri. A practical software program should be versatile, allowing you to input varied data, perform some of your bookkeeping and billing chores, and scan for particular patients exhibiting certain characteristics for follow-up and marketing. Specifically, the program should include the following: patient general identification information; hearing aid information, audiogram data, daily financial activity, billing and statement generation, and scanning for select data. Figures 11-4 through 11-6 present three computer screens with data of a hypothetical patient. Note that some of the fields use a coding system for the data. You will be able to devise codes to meet your specific needs.

Figure 11-7 presents scanning options for this software program. You can choose one or any combination of these items to select patients for a mailing. For example,

```
PATIENT RECORDS

------------------------------------------------------------------
|  Account Number:    715                                        |
|  1) Title:   Mr.              16) Referral:        Dr. Otol    |
|  2) First:   John             17) Loss Type [R]:   S2G         |
|  3) MI:      Q.               18) Loss Type [L]:   S2G         |
|  4) Last:    Public           19) Insurance:       BXBS        |
|  5) Street:  3272 Malleus La. 20) Ins Group Id:    123-45-6789 |
|  6) City:    Anytown          21) Status:                      |
|  7) State:   US               22) Special Codes:               |
|  8) Zip:     00000-           23) Misc Codes:                  |
|  9) Phone:   (   )555-4321    24) Associate:       MP          |
| 10) SSAN:                     25) Fitting:         2B          |
| 11) Sex:            M         26) Comment: POOR DISCRIMINATION |
| 12) Birth Date:       07/21/21                                 |
| 13) Last Visit Date:  05/24/87                                 |
| 14) Last Test Date:   02/22/87                                 |
| 15) Mail Class:                                                |
------------------------------------------------------------------
```

Fig. 11-4. Sample patient identification computer screen with data for a hypothetical person.

```
    Account Number: 715
    Name:   Mr.  John          Q.  Public


            1)        2)        3)     4)     5)     6)
           -----------------------------------------------------------
 1) Ear     :R        :L        :      :      :      :      :
 2) Manufac :XYZ      :XYZ      :      :      :      :      :
 3) Model   :GUDEAR   :GUDEAR   :      :      :      :      :
 4) Serial # :12345   :12346    :      :      :      :      :
 5) Pur Date :03/05/87 :03/05/87 :     :      :      :      :
 6) Warr Exp :03/05/89 :03/05/89 :     :      :      :      :
 7) Price   : $623.00  : $623.00 :     :      :      :      :
 8) Fit Date :03/05/87 :03/05/87 :     :      :      :      :
 9) Battery :13Z      :13Z      :      :      :      :      :
10) Specs   :         :         :      :      :      :      :
           -----------------------------------------------------------
```

Fig. 11-5. Sample computer screen with hearing aid data for a hypothetical user.

TEST RESULT (AUDIOGRAM) RECORDS
                          ALL TEST RESULTS
    Account Number: 715
    Name: Mr. John Q. Public

		AIR			BONE				SPEECH		
			MASKED			MASKED					
		L	R	L	R	L	R	L	R		L	R
250 Hz	|	10	10			NT	NT			| AVG PT	33	33	|
500 Hz	|	20	20			20	20			| SRT	30	30	|
1000 Hz	|	35	35			35	35			| MCL	70	75	|
1500 Hz	|	NT	NT			NT	NT			| UCL	90	90	|
2000 Hz	|	45	45			45	45			| DISC %	60	64	|
3000 Hz	|	NT	NT			NT	NT			| PRES LVL	70	75	|
4000 Hz	|	60	60			60	60			|			|
6000 Hz	|	65	65			NT	NT			|			|
8000 Hz	|	75	75			NT	NT			|			|

```
    Air Unmasked Test Date: 02/22/87     Bone Unmasked Test Date: 02/22/87
    Air Masked Test Date:                Bone Masked Test Date:
                                         Speech Test Date: 02/22/87
```

Fig. 11-6. Sample computer screen with audiogram data for a hypothetical patient.

PATIENT INFO SCAN ITEMS   HEARING AID SCAN ITEMS

 1) Scan for ZIP CODE   15) Scan for MANUFACTURER
 2) Scan for BIRTH DATE   16) Scan for MODEL
 3) Scan for AGE   17) Scan for SERIAL NUMBER
 4) Scan for last VISIT date   18) Scan for PURCHASE date
 5) Scan for last TEST date   19) Scan for WARRANTY expiration date
 6) Scan for MAIL CLASS   20) Scan for FIT/DELIVERY date
 7) Scan for REFERRAL   21) Scan for BATTERY number
 8) Scan for loss type LEFT EAR   22) Scan for SPECIFICATIONS
 9) Scan for loss type RIGHT EAR
10) Scan for INSURANCE
11) Scan for SPECIAL CODES   23) Scan for All patients regardless
12) Scan for MISC CODES   of characteristics for merge list
13) Scan for ASSOCIATE
14) Scan for FITTING

Fig. 11-7. Scanning/sorting options.

you might opt for last test date (scan item 5) and warranty expiration date (scan item 9) for recall purposes. You may choose one or more codes for loss type (scan items 8, 9) to notify certain patients of a new hearing aid model appropriate for them. Another useful scan item is purchase date (scan item 18). Utilizing this data, you can notify patients when their aids are 3 or 4 years old, suggesting they consider upgrading. Refer to the discussion on marketing for more ideas of how to utilize your customer data base.

7. Consider hiring a consultant. It is worth spending a few hundred dollars to get advice about software and hardware from someone who has been through computerization and knows what your objectives are. Many larger accounting firms have computer consultants on their staffs. All cities have computer consulting services available. Ask any colleagues in your area who are using computers whether they are familiar with any of the computer consulting services. The advice of the consultant may result in you selecting a less expensive and/or more efficient system, thus saving money in the long run.

8. When considering various hardware systems, simple considerations such as repair or service availability, place of purchase, or simply knowing someone who has a computer can help you decide. Some of the factors that you should consider in choosing your hardware are speed of operations, storage capacity, terminal capacity, and the ability to add further storage and function to the computer (expandability).

9. Perhaps one of the most important caveats that can be given to the computer user is to always be sure that you make back-up copies of computer records. At least weekly, make an extra set of diskettes with all the records stored in the computer. Then, if something happens that results in a loss of the data, you have an additional copy to use.

CONCLUSION

This chapter has, by no means, been exhaustively comprehensive in its scope. Its intent is as a primer for audiologists considering entering private practice and for dispensers who are interested in upgrading their businesses. The most important statement that we can make is *always consult your accountant and attorney before making any major business decisions.* The advice they give you could save you from making a major mistake. Good Luck!

REFERENCES

Brown SW: Marketing strategies in a changing environment. Paper presented at the 1984 Spring Conference of the Academy of Dispensing audiologists, Tucson, AZ
Caruso B: How to sell the benefits of wearing hearing aids—Part I: The concept. Hearing Instruments 36:8–11, 1985a

Caruso B: How to sell the benefits of wearing hearing aids—Part II: The benefits. Hearing Instruments 36:8–11, 1985b

Caruso B: How to sell the benefits of wearing hearing aids—Part III: The sales strategy. Hearing Instruments 36:14–15,1985c

Caruso B: How to promote the benefits of wearing hearing aids—Part I: Discovering your style. Hearing Instruments 37:28–30, 50, 1986

Churchill N, Werbaneth L: Choosing and evaluating your accountant. Harvard Business Rev May–June, 79–83, 1979

Cranmer KS: Hearing aid dispensing—1986. Hearing Instruments 37:6–12, 141, 1986

Gluck LD: Advertising builds business. Hearing Instruments 37:13–16, 1986

Hampton D: Establishing and equipping an audiology private practice, in Butler K (ed): Prospering in Private Practice. Rockville, MD, Aspen Publications, 1986, pp 135–148

Hearing Industries Association: Executive Summary—HIA Survey of the Hearing Impaired Population, 1985

Kofski MA, McMillon L, Blemaster NL: First impressions—the sell before the sale. Hearing instruments 37:11–12, 40, 1986

Loavenbruck A: Marketing strategies from an audiological perspective, in Butler K (ed): Prospering in Private Practice. Rockville, MD, Aspen Publications, pp 223–236, 1986

Mahon WJ: Practice newsletters: Why and how. Hearing, 37:19–22, 1984

McCormack M: What They Don't Teach You at Harvard Business School. New York, Bantam Books, 1984

Parish R: Constraints and commitments: An introduction to the financial aspects of private practice, in Butler K (ed): Prospering in Private Practice. Rockville, MD, Aspen Publications, pp 88–100, 1986

Pfeil MP, Lampris T, Whitcomb OA: A total marketing approach for greater hearing aid sales. Hearing Instruments 36:26–29, 1985

Rowland R: Legal implications of a professional dispensing practice, in Curran J (ed): Patterns in Private Practice: Hearing Aid Dispensing. New York, Thieme Inc., Semin Hearing 7:193–198, 1986

Skafte M: Don't just sit there. Hearing Instruments 37:4, 1986

Sullivan C: Business and management aspects of private practice in speech-language pathology and audiology, in Butler K (ed): Prospering in Private Practice. Rockville, MD, Aspen Publications, pp 149–166, 1986

Swerdlow RA: Consumer Attitudes toward Professionals who Advertise. Dayton, OH, L. M. Berry & Company, 1981

Walker M: A practical guide to physician's yellow pages advertising. Physician's Marketing pp 1–2, 1985

Kenneth E. Smith

12

Professional Relationships

Over the years there have been various groups of professionals and parapro-fessionals who have been directly involved in the diagnosis and rehabilitation of the hearing-impaired: audiologists; Otologists; teachers of the deaf and hard-of-hearing; and hearing aid dispensers. It is rather ironic that there has been such a great lack of communication between these individuals, all of whom work with communicaton disorders. Starting with the premise that the audiologist should be the case manager, Ken Smith presents rationales and suggestions for improving the rlationships between the audiologist and other team members. While some of his proposals will meet with disagreement from various quarters, Ken's suggestions will undoubtedly lead to much discussion and, hopefully, facilitate improvements in these professional relationships.

MCP

When the first edition of this book was written, I was a university professor with primary teaching responsibilities and a limited clinical load. I evaluated five or six patients each week, but as the semester developed the actual responsibility for patient care was shifted to students. My work with hearing aids was limited to specification of electroacoustic characteristics to fit the hearing loss and postfitting evaluation. Postfitting testing was designed to tell the dealer whether the sale was

AMPLIFICATION FOR THE HEARING-IMPAIRED, THIRD EDITION ISBN 0-8089-1886-9

443

correct according to my recommendation. Day-to-day problems of the hearing aid user were simply not my concern.

During those days, professional relationships were relatively easy to establish but the extent of interaction with other professionals was minimal. I was not dependent on any professional for referrals, since there was an abundance of teaching cases who welcomed my free services.

The second edition of this book was written after 3 years of private practice, casually referred to as the "years of struggle." My patient load and direct responsibility for hearing aid fittings had increased dramatically, and professional relationships assumed primary importance. Those relationships affected my ability to stay in business, as well as the quality of patient care. Much of my time was spent in developing new relationships with other professionals, convincing them (and probably myself) that my service was *worthwhile*.

After 10 years of private practice, my attitude toward professional relationships has undergone further change as my self-confidence and the self-confidence of the audiology profession in general has matured. The development and maintenance of good professional relationships maintains primary importance in my practice, but I now view my services as vital to the total evaluation and rehabilitation of the hearing-impaired patient. This maturation of professional attitude can now be seen in a growing number of clinical audiologists and reflects the movement of audiologists toward professional independence.

The emergence of Clinical audiology as an independent profession has had a profound effect on all types of professional relationships. These relationships reflect a dynamic process, affected by official positions held by national organizations and community norms. Professional roles in the hearing aid evaluation and delivery system have also changed. Common forms of interaction may be outdated as these patterns change, and positions presented in this chapter may be viewed as amusing bits of history in the near future.

Without question, the audiologist's relatively new role in hearing aid dispensing has been a major factor in the development of *private practice*, and such independence is clearly the wave of the future. The audiologist's participation in dispensing may have started as a result of concern for the effectiveness of care provided under the indirect model of dispensing (Goldstein B 1981, Goldstein D 1979). This model provided for the referral of hearing-impaired patients to a traditional hearing aid dispenser following medical and audiologic evaluation and is still practiced in some clinical settings.

The financial advantage of hearing aid dispensing by audiologists allows for both financial independence and total responsibility for the rehabilitation of the patient through one professional source. Despite lingering rigidity among audiologists regarding hearing aid candidacy and the marketing of hearing aids to the public (Goldstein D 1979), a growing number of audiologists are seeking employment in free-standing private practices. This relatively new form of business is beginning to have an impact on the hearing aid industry and the quality of hearing health care available to the public.

ASSUMPTIONS UNDERLYING PROFESSIONAL RELATIONSHIPS

Several assumptions form the basis for professional relationships that affect the recommendation for and delivery of the hearing aid: (1) a hearing health team exists whose activities are in the best interests of the patient, (2) there is a *best* source of service for each individual patient, and (3) professionals will tend to interact in a manner that is in the best interests of the patient.

The hearing health team has been strained, modified, and redefined because of direct dispensing by almost everyone traditionally associated with the team and by the development of audiology as an independent profession. Initial protests of organizations such as the National Hearing Aid Society have changed to both solicitation of audiologists and physicians as members, and to the active recruitment of audiologists by retail hearing aid business operations. One has only to look at classified advertisements in the trade journals to realize that a small revolution has taken place. There are frequent and subtle references to the fact that the clinical-dispensing audiologist is the *expert* of choice in non-medical hearing health care.

The team concept has been further weakened by government regulation. While FDA (April 1976) regulations specify medical examination before the purchase of a hearing aid, examination and medical clearance can be completed by *any* physician. The otologist, who is probably best qualified to evaluate and treat the medical aspects of hearing impairment, is suggested but not required as the examining physician. Newer and more restrictive regulations proposed by the FTC were finally rejected as unnecessary (Hearing Instruments 1985) to the dismay of the American Speech-Language and Hearing Association and the AARP. These regulations would have provided for a mandatory trial fitting and other restrictions on the sale of hearing aids. This lack of government regulation means both relative freedom in the dispensing of hearing aids and a continuing responsibility for competence and fairness in hearing aid sales.

Despite the obvious problems associated with any *team* concept, there are several reasons why effective professional relationships are essential to the audiologist. First, good professional relationships can mean a generally higher quality of patient care. For example, a hearing-impaired patient with chronic otitis media, external otitis or external dermatitis will experience needless setbacks to success with a hearing aid unless the dispensing audiologist and the otologist can coordinate their efforts. Such coordination often involves *cross-teaching* and may require a period of many years to develop.

Second, good professional relationships mean referral of new patients to the audiologist for services. Generally, no single member of the professional team can provide all of the services necessary for management of the hearing-impaired patient. Even in those settings where the *physician is dispensing*, an audiologist or technician is the individual who actually fits the aid and provides long-term follow-up care for the patient. Also, most of the education or rehabilitation activity (speechreading training, aural rehabilitation, etc.) takes place separately from the setting in which the aid is sold.

Too often, professional relationships are based solely on territorial considerations, as if the patient's problems and payments were a piece of property to be
handled in one setting. However, when audiologists, physicians, traditional hearing
aid dealers, and rehabilitation specialists cooperate, the patient can receive a high
quality of care, regardless of the setting or the number of professionals involved in
the process. Professionals should remember that the patient's interests relate to
restoration or improvement of hearing and communication skills through medical
treatment or use of a hearing aid. Modern patients demand a high-quality product,
the *latest* technology, and the lowest price possible. These interests *can* be met if
professional roles are well defined, and if the patient's needs assume primary
importance.

PRIMARY RELATIONSHIPS AFFECTING THE AUDIOLOGIST

The Otolaryngologist

The otolaryngologist (ENT) will always be a necessary part of the hearing aid
delivery model, since certain types of hearing impairment can be improved or
corrected through medical treatment. When medical clearance was the only element
required from the physician before sale of the hearing aid (i.e., FDA, 1976 Regulations), roles were fairly well defined except for the continuing controversy over the
audiologist as an *entry point* in the rehabilitation of the hearing-impaired patient.

Since a growing number of ENT specialists are now including hearing aid
dispensing as part of their clinical management program, the roles of hearing health
team members are less than clearly defined. Only time and further regulation will
clarify what must appear to be a very confusing delivery system to the consumer. As
long as audiologists function as technicians, or "dial twister" or hearing aid fitter,
their role as dispenser in the ENT clinic will remain unchanged. If, however,
audiologists contract for services with the medical practice or enter the practice as a
partner or stockholder, their professional relationships to physicians become critical
to the rehabilitation process. Rather than *suggesting*, audiologists can be in a position of selecting, recommending, and selling the course of nonmedical care directly
to the patient. It can work, but this type of relationship is more exception than norm
at this writing.

Recent apparent changes in the position of the American Academy of
Otolaryngology–Head and Neck Surgery (Goldstein J 1985) may change the relationships between audiologists and ENT specialists. For the first time, this draft
position paper alludes to the independent practice of audiology as a "different
situation." The paper infers that the clinical audiologist can provide a "clinical
quality" of evaluation and is the best trained individual to determine deviation of
hearing levels from normal. While this rhetoric appears at first glance to be a
substantial change in an historically adversary position, the continuing role of the
physician as the primary provider of care is clearly stated. The basic concept and

position, restated in the position paper, is that otologic decisions preceed audiologic decisions. While this may be disagreeable to many independent audiologists (Flower 1985), a dispensing audiologist in private practice should understand that medical cooperation, support, and ongoing care are critical to the audiologist's rehabilitation efforts with the patient.

It is unfortunate for everyone involved that the petty bickering over the point of entry and rights to the patient's care have clouded the image projected by the hearing health care team. There is a practical difference between medical and nonmedical care. The Academy of Dispensing Audiologists' (ADA) position paper (1983) takes the position that the audiologist is the best qualified professional practitioner to assume responsibility for the nonmedical habilitation and/or rehabilitation of the hearing-impaired person. This position reflects the reality of patient care, since once the hearing impairment is defined and surgery or medical treatment (if any) is completed, the physician has minimal interest in or expertise with rehabilitation. Again, cooperation between the audiologist and the ENT specialist can mean quality care for the patient.

This type of cooperative relationship will become more and more difficult to achieve as ENT specialists enter into the sale of hearing aids. The motivation for this type of recent development may be based on the need for more income as the number of surgical cases decreases or on the desire to present a total service in one clinical setting. In most cases, the ENT specialist has little or nothing to do with the hearing aid delivery and rehabilitation process: this specialist's employee, the audiologist, or the hearing aid dispenser provides the actual service.

Despite the apparent conflict of roles, cooperation between the independent audiologist and the ENT specialist is possible and necessary. The dispensing audiologist is in the position of identifying new patients and directing them into appropriate treatment channels. Many of these patients are not candidates for hearing aids or other forms of audiologic rehabilitation and require medical care.

Other patients will be identified as needing only medical clearance before the hearing aid is recommended. If the audiologist's only choice for otologic referral is to a dispensing physician, *pirating* may be a legitimate concern. In most cases, the key to this potential problem is the perception of the audiologist as a valuable source of medical-surgical cases for the ENT specialist and as a source of convenient, competent service for the patient. For example, I frequently refer patients to several ENT specialists who dispense hearing aids in their offices. These referrals are made because of the the skill of the surgeon and geographic proximity to the patient. In turn, patients who are difficult to manage or patients who live near one of my offices are referred to me for hearing aid services. [As Pratt (1978) predicted, few physicians will have the time or expertise needed to deal with the long-range problems of fitting hearing aids on children or other *difficult* patients.] Such a relationship can work to everyone's advantage if both professional and economic factors are considered. This type of relationship will develop only as dispensing audiologists see themselves as independent, contributing members of the hearing health care team.

As audiologists begin to see themselves as independent professionals, they quickly realize that the depth of their knowledge in related fields has a major impact on their professional relationships with physicians. In-depth knowledge of medical management techniques is necessary to relate audiologic data to real-life treatment of the patient's problem. For example, the audiologic evaluation and rehabilitation history should be one of the major factors in directing selected patients toward evaluation for a cochlear implant or other types of medical management. Too often, the dispensing audiologist works with patients who have worn hearing aids for years, unsuccessfully, when correction of an obvious medical problem would have meant a real change in the quality of life for the patient. Such *clinical competence* leads to excellent professional relationships with physicians, respect from the medical community, and a major improvement in the quality of patient care.

Considering the number of hearing-impaired individuals who do not wear hearing aids or do not seek professional help, it would seem to be time to eliminate current divisive issues between physicians and audiologists and to proceed with the identification, education, and treatment of the hearing-impaired public. Recent position changes and cooperative efforts between the AAO, ADA, and ASHA (cited earlier in this chapter) may signal better hearing health care for consumers than was ever available in the past. Mutual case-finding efforts by all concerned specialists may be the best way to educate the public.

The Traditional Hearing Aid Dealer

The traditional hearing aid dealer (*nonaudiologist* or *nonphysician*) represents both competition and opportunity for the dispensing audiologist. When a few renegade audiologists first engaged in dispensing, cries of "foul" were heard from the National Hearing Aid Society, in university settings, clinics, the trade media and (in a few cases) the courtroom. However, as audiologists entered the marketplace on a competitive basis, relationships between the national organizations and individuals involved have changed. Trade publications now reflect more mutual tolerance, common educational training opportunities, and the realization by manufacturers and other vendors that dispensing audiology is a viable occupation.

In April 1978 the Supreme Court ruled that a professional society's canon of ethics having the effect of limiting competition among members was illegal (*United States v National Society of Professional Engineers* 1978). Soon after that ruling the American Speech-Language-Hearing Association (ASHA) adopted Resolution 53 (1978). Resolution 53 gave dispensing audiologists (for the first time) ethical license to dispense hearing aids at a profit as long as the product was part of a rehabilitation plan. The resolution further specified disclosure of the dispensing fee, freedom of choice for the source of services and products by the patient, presale disclosure of fees, and a fitting *evaluation* process (a vague attempt to document fitting success and patient satisfaction). To many audiologists who were dispensing at the time, the resolution appeared to be directed at developing a *clean medical-type model* for sale of hearing aids rather than a *tainted* commercial model as used by the hearing aid dealers.

Happily, those days of interorganizational tension over economic and territorial issues are fading memories. Now, hearing manufacturers recruit audiologists for sales and training, and many hearing aid dealers have hired audiologists as staff members. For the newly trained clinician who wishes to follow the path toward independence, working for an experienced hearing aid dealer can be invaluable. Not only can the day-to-day skills of fitting and caring for hearing aids be learned, but business skills necessary to succeed are available. As any successful hearing aid dealer knows, the best clinical skills are useless if one lacks the business skills to keep the doors open. This type of hands-on training is still not available in most training centers.

Modification of training programs for audiologists is a step in the right direction, if audiologists are to compete and cooperate with the hearing dealer. Both ASHA and the Academy of Dispensing Audiologists (ADA) have been active in this training endeavor, and the long-term effects of dispensing training for audiologists can only benefit the hearing-impaired patient. Postgraduate training in hearing aid design, selection, fitting, sales, service and business development are widely available, but in my judgment, the metamorphosis of the audiologist from a self-concept as a technician to one of an independent professional must begin in the university.

The audiologist's self-concept is a major factor affecting the manner in which this specialist relates to the hearing aid dealer. If the audiologist chooses to follow a traditional, indirect, delivery model, then good communication with the dealer is essential. The audiologist should remain directly involved with the rehabilitation process through postfitting evaluation, hearing reevaluation and counseling. In some cases, the audiologist acts as a *comfortable* source of complaints about dealer services: complaints are relayed directly to the dealer. This may be a desirable model for some, but as the role of clinical audiology changes, this type of relationship will probabaly diminish or disappear.

Other Dispensing Audiologists

Clinical audiology is in its infancy regarding the development of professional relationships between dispensing audiologists. It remains to be seen whether we will cooperate or compete, or whether we will see both factors in our interrelationships. Organizations such as the ADA have made a very real attempt to foster intradisciplinary training and ethical conduct standards, but the future of the professional relationships between dispensing audiologists will vary with the community setting and number of audiologists in the local market. From an economic position, considering the fact that much of the hearing-impaired public is underserved or unserved, it is my strong opinion that there are enough patients for everyone. The real issue is not *who will solicit the most referrals*, but *how we will reach and educate the public.*

The development of *cut-throat* competition would be a diastrous image to project to the public at this point in our professional development. Again, the issue of marketing and advertising must be addressed in training programs and by the organizations that define ethical codes of conduct. The following suggestions may be useful in establishing effective professional relationships with other dispensing audiologists.

First, beware of marketing specialists whose primary goal is to undercut the competition by luring patients from other dispensers. Such a strategy usually is designed for short-term gains and can be destructive to professional cooperation. Development of an image as competent, honest, and reasonable will do more to solidify your business than carnival-type advertising that the public has associated with traditional forms of hearing aid sales campaigns. If you are uncertain about the direction or image your advertising projects, consultation with a marketing specialist who specializes in medical promotion (hospitals, clinics, etc.) can give you a feel for community norms and can probably reduce your advertising budget and hostile comments from other dispensing audiologists.

Second, know other dispensing audiologists in town, and foster a relationship that allows for honest feedback regarding patient care matters. In my experience, initial attempts at cooperation between audiologists are viewed with suspicion, but the advantages of cooperation far outweigh the risks. Formation of professional groups can allow for shared experiences, organized continuing education, and a unified approach to education of the public and medical community about the role and services of the dispensing audiologist.

Third, if you cannot provide quality care to a patient because of geography, time constraints, or other factors, refer them to a colleague. The national directory of dispensing audiologists provided by the Academy of Dispensing Audiologists is an invaluable tool for cross-country referral and provides some assurance that the patient will receive fair, competent services.

Fourth, investigate cooperatives of other dispensing audiologists for the purchase of products and services necessary for your business. Such cooperatives have the advantage of substantial discounts on aids and other supplies but they also allow dispensing audiologists to have a more unified impact on manufacturer's services and the ultimate direction of hearing aid technology. For example, the Audiology Co-op, Inc. of Akron, Ohio provides group purchasing for hearing aids and related products from a variety of manufacturers at substantial discounts. A local cooperative has allowed for group purchases of office supplies and printing. In each example, suppliers are more likely to modify products and services based on demands of a *large* customer than they are on the demands of one individual practitioner.

The result of this type of communication between dispensing audiologists can be improvements in technology (through sharing of common problems and ideas), better case finding procedures in local markets, and better services to the hearing-impaired patient. We risk being no better than our dispensing predesessors if our professional relationships with each other are poor.

Teachers

Successful use of a hearing aid in the rehabilitation-habilitation process depends heavily on the communication level between the educator, parent, and audiologist responsible for the care of the hearing aid. Yet, contacts between audiologists and teachers tend to be sporadic (at best). Teachers complain about the lack of detailed information regarding care and adjustment of the aid, while the audiologist may complain about the teacher's narrow interest in the *perfect* volume control setting.

It is expensive and time-consuming for the audiologist to follow children in a school district, but the final level of benefit the child receives may depend on the amount of effort invested by both teacher and audiologist. Proper classroom care of the hearing aid can minimize repair needs and prolong the life of the hearing aid. The teacher may be very helpful in identifying the need for a new aid, repair, or modification of the current aid or changes in hearing that require attention.

There are two opportune times for the audiologist to establish a working relationship with the teacher: at the time of the initial hearing aid fitting and at the time of annual reevaluation. Feedback on the child's classroom performance with the hearing aid or auditory training system must come from the teacher. Audiologic evaluation and parental feedback are generally insufficient as a data base for hearing aid modification.

The audiologist should keep two factors in mind: teachers appreciate personal feedback on their work (or the audiologist's work with their student), and teachers are busy professionals with multiple responsibilities. Therefore, the following suggestions should be considered when developing an effective professional relationship with teachers:

1. Send an annual summary of contacts with your patient to the teacher. Include test data and information on any problems that might affect the teacher's classroom management.
2. Solicit feedback from the teacher on the hearing aid's effectiveness, problems, and so on. Teachers in small classroom settings can provide rate data on the child's response to voice and environmental sounds with the aid, changes in speech reading, visual awareness, or other behaviors with the hearing aid. If the classroom is large, thus limiting the teacher's data collection time, develop and provide a checklist to identify factors that can help the audiologist determine the quality of the fitting.
3. Attend school-sponsored staffings of hearing aid patients. This is another way to provide a better service to the patient, improve audiologist-teacher communication, and develop community involvement and visability.

All of these activities make the teacher a part of the patient's care. My experience is that personal, patient-related contacts are far more effective in developing effective communication than are workshops or other forms of group training.

In summary, professional relationships that are productive and in the best interests of the patient require time, effort, and a thorough understanding of the prejudices affecting each profession. Flexibility when dealing with other professionals is essential when inevitable conflicts occur. While this chapter reflects current conditions affecting the physician, audiologist, dealer, and teacher, these conditions are susceptible to immediate (and drastic) change. Such changes will occur as a result of economic, legal, professional, and consumer issues and, hopefully, as a result of our perception of the "patient's best interests.".

REFERENCES

Academy of Dispensing Audiologists: Position paper, Adopted November 1983

Flower R: Response to AAO-HNS Draft Guidelines. June 6, 1985

Goldstein B: Factors contributing to the changing hearing aid scene. Ear Hearing, 2:260–266, 1981

Goldstein D: Audiological rehabilitation and hearing aid dispensing in a university teaching clinic. ASHA 21:650–653, 1979

Goldstein J: Otologic referral in the independent practice of audiology—Draft. American Academy of Otolaryngology—Head and Neck Surgery, Inc., Committee on Hearing and Equilibrium, February 25, 1985

Hearing Aid Devices. Professional and Patient Labeling and Conditions for Sale, Department of Health, Education and Welfare, Food and Drug Administration, Federal Register 41(78), April 1976

Hearing Instruments: FTC Decision Terminates Hearing Aid Trade Regulation Rule. Vol 36: 32, 1985

Pratt L: Why physicians may regret a decision to dispense hearing aids. Ear Nose Throat J 1978

Resolution 53 of the Legislative Council of the American Speech and Hearing Association, San Francisco, CA, 1978

United States v National Society of Professional Engineers, No. 76-1767. ASHA 20:542–549, 1978

Index